Using Integrated Behavioral Health in Pediatric Practice

Roger W. Apple • Cheryl A. Dickson
Rebecca Rausch
Editors

Using Integrated Behavioral Health in Pediatric Practice

An Essential Guide to Better Outcomes and Equitable Care

Springer

Editors
Roger W. Apple
Pediatric and Adolescent Medicine
Western Michigan University, Homer
Stryker M.D. School of Medicine
Kalamazoo, MI, USA

Cheryl A. Dickson
Pediatrics and Adolescent Medicine
Western Michigan University, Homer
Stryker M.D. School of Medicine
Kalamazoo, MI, USA

Rebecca Rausch
Pediatric and Adolescent Medicine
Western Michigan University, Homer
Stryker M.D. School of Medicine
Kalamazoo, MI, USA

ISBN 978-3-031-85783-6 ISBN 978-3-031-85784-3 (eBook)
https://doi.org/10.1007/978-3-031-85784-3

This Springer imprint is published by the registered company Springer Nature Switzerland AG
The registered company address is: Gewerbestrasse 11, 6330 Cham, Switzerland

Foreword

Over the years, numerous frameworks have been proposed to improve the American healthcare system. Berwick and colleagues introduced the Triple Aim in 2008, with mutually reinforcing goals of improving population health, enhancing patient satisfaction with care, and reducing the cost of care. Recognizing that provider satisfaction and well-being are critical for meeting these aims, Bodenheimer and Sinsky expanded this framework to the Quadruple Aim in 2014, adding the fourth aim of improving provider satisfaction. They recognized that without addressing provider burnout and attrition, efforts to achieve the Triple Aim would be in vain.

There are social determinants of health that, left unaddressed, may yet impede the success of these aims. The United States is plagued by healthcare inequities to a greater degree than many other developed nations. It has recently been argued by Nundy and colleagues that a fifth aim, health equity, should be championed to improve American healthcare, as it also reinforces the other four aims. Health equity is achieved when all have a fair and just opportunity to attain optimal health regardless of race, ethnicity, disability, sexual orientation, gender identity, socioeconomic status, geography, and preferred language. Without striving to reduce disparities and ensure equity for all patients in our healthcare system, any victory in achieving other aims would be tenuous.

The rise of patient-centered medical homes, integrated care, and team-based healthcare represents a crucial means to achieve all five of these aims. Efforts to reduce the siloed nature of healthcare have given rise to integrated primary and specialty care settings. This book focuses on the integration of medical and mental health care. Various models of integration have demonstrated beneficial outcomes over the decades. These models involve collaboration between primary care physicians and mental health providers, resulting in coordinated care that addresses both the physical and psychological aspects of an individual's health. The robust evidence for integrated behavioral health (IBH) presented within this book highlights the contribution of this treatment model to these aims, including the pursuit of health equity.

It is intended that this book may serve as a guide for medical professionals to advocate for integrated healthcare teams and improve health equity among their patients. The authors' collective expertise provides a comprehensive guide to pediatric IBH, not only in primary care but also in subspecialty settings. Readers may be most familiar with IBH as a term applied to primary care. Here, IBH is broadly applied to the integration of mental and physical health in both primary and subspecialty care. Throughout, there is a specific emphasis on the role of IBH in promoting health equity in pediatric populations. There is also a special emphasis on training the next generation of physicians to work on psychologically integrated teams, as highlighted by some of the chapters' content and medical learner co-authors.

Pediatric and Adolescent Medicine
Homer Stryker M.D. School of Medicine
Kalamazoo, MI, USA

Katherine Tennant Beenen

Contents

Part I
General Pediatrics

Chapter 1
Integrated Behavioral Health: Definitions and Contexts

Nicole Garton, Jocelyn DeLeon, Pradnya Joshi, and Dilip R. Patel

Introduction

Most children with behavioral and mental health conditions initially present in a pediatric primary care setting. The World Health Organization defines mental health as "a state of well-being in which every individual realizes his or her own potential, can cope with the normal stresses of life, can work productively and fruitfully, and is able to make a contribution to her or his community" [1]. It is infrequent for children and adolescents with behavioral and mental health conditions to first present in a specialized mental health care practice [2, 3]. An estimated 50% of mental health disorders have their onset by the age of 14 years [2, 3, 4]. Failure to recognize behavioral or mental health concerns early and suboptimal treatment have been associated with significant long-term adverse outcomes including poor academic performance, increased school absenteeism, substance use, and suicidal behavior [3–8]. When compared to the general population, persons with severe mental illness often die 13–30 years early [3]. Early recognition and optimal treatment of mental illness can reduce the morbidity and mortality associated with mental health disorders.

It is difficult for a typical pediatric practice to deliver behavioral and mental health care effectively and efficiently without collaboration with mental health services [3, 6]. This can be due to several different barriers including lack of time during appointments, concerns about reimbursement, and lack of training [6, 7]. There

N. Garton (✉) · J. DeLeon · D. R. Patel
Department of Pediatric and Adolescent Medicine, Western Michigan University Homer Stryker M.D. School of Medicine, Kalamazoo, MI, USA
e-mail: nicole.garton@wmed.edu; jocelyn.deleon@wmed.edu; dilip.patel@wmed.edu

P. Joshi
Western Michigan University Homer Stryker M.D. School of Medicine, Kalamazoo, MI, USA
e-mail: pradnya.joshi@wmed.edu

R. W. Apple et al. (eds.), *Using Integrated Behavioral Health in Pediatric Practice*, https://doi.org/10.1007/978-3-031-85784-3_1

is also a shortage of child and adolescent psychiatrists when compared to the growing prevalence of mental disorders in the youth population [4]. According to Skokauskas et al., [4] the worldwide ratio of child and adolescent psychiatrists to the population is an alarming 1.19 per 100,000 youth in high-income countries, while in low-income countries, the number is even more distressing—less than 0.1 per 100,000 population. Appointment wait times for these scarce resources can be an additional barrier to mental health care for the pediatric population [9]. Combining mental health services with primary care can reduce costs, improve access to care, increase the quality of care, and, ultimately, save lives [3, 6].

Integrated behavioral health is defined as primary care providers and behavioral and mental health care providers working together to provide comprehensive health care in a cost-effective way. Behavioral health, when practiced within the context of a pediatric primary medical care setting, reflects some level of integration between the two. As most children and adolescents with behavioral health concerns are initially seen in a primary care setting, it is useful to have an understanding of what is considered primary medical care, especially in the United States. There has been a relentless discussion of primary care in the United States on a daily basis in both the scientific and lay media and various other venues of discourse. Many experts contend that primary care, or lack thereof, is the most important aspect of the healthcare system that must be addressed to save or rescue the US healthcare system from impending catastrophe.

Primary Care

In 1961, White et al. first used the term "primary medical care" in their work on the ecology of medical care [10]. The World Health Organization, in 1978, following an International conference in Alma-Ata, elaborated on the need and role of primary health care [11]. Primary care, or primary medical care, is considered the most critical component of healthcare delivery in the United States. Kovener et al. [12] have cited several reasons for this: primary care provides the initial point of contact for individuals seeking medical care, primary care practitioners are essential in the coordination of patient care within the healthcare system, primary care practitioners are able to effectively engage the patient and family in promoting their health, and evidence suggests that increased access to primary care improves the quality of care and reduces the cost of care [12]. Starfield et al. [13] in their extensive review have also discussed the rationale and benefits of primary care for health that includes greater access to needed services, better quality of care, a greater focus on prevention, early management of health problems, the cumulative effect of the main primary care delivery characteristics, and the role of primary care in reducing unnecessary and potentially harmful specialist care [13].

A widely cited definition of primary care is that proposed by the Institute of Medicine [14, 15]:

> Primary care is the provision of integrated, accessible health care services by clinicians who are accountable for addressing a large majority of personal health care needs, developing a sustained partnership with patients, and practicing in the context of family and community.

According to Goroll et al. [16], each of the definitions of primary care has evolved within the historical context at the time. Within the context of the current healthcare system in the United States, the most predominant definition of primary care is based on the functional attributes of the primary care system of care [16]. Goroll et al. [16] have provided the following definitions of primary care [16]:

Systems definition:

The systems definition of primary care integrates the attributes of site of first contact for the patient as well as the continuity of care.

Task-oriented definition:

Another way of defining primary care is a definition based on the work of primary care clinicians. The task-oriented definition includes the following key tasks within the context of primary care: integrating medical and psychological diagnosis and treatment; eliciting and responding to patient attributions, requests, and preferences; mastering the use and interpretation of diagnostic tests; interpreting the medical literature and applying it to the care of individual patients; attending to the patient's social network; and planning for end-of-life care.

Function oriented definition:

Includes the first contact, longitudinal, continuous, comprehensive, and coordinated care.

A cross-disciplinary academic definition:

The cross-disciplinary academic definition encompasses the research and educational domains of primary care. This definition evolved from interdisciplinary research, predominantly with social sciences and includes such other areas with impact on health as economics, communication, epidemiology, and biostatistics.

Professional definition:

This definition is similar to those used by some of the government agencies and organized medicine. It recognizes formal medical specialties of family medicine, general internal medicine, pediatrics, obstetrics and gynecology and other self-designated specialties. The essential characteristic of professional definition of primary care is that the practitioners define their own scope of primary care practice.

Characteristics of Integrated Healthcare

The basic characteristics of integrated health care are coordination, continuity, and comprehensive scope. Both major aspects of integrated health care—care coordination and care continuum—are comprehensive in that they span across different providers, different health care delivery settings, and different levels or intensity of medical care delivered [17–19].

Continuity of medical care should occur on a longitudinal basis, and ideally over the life span of the individual. Continuity of care encompasses the care provided by the same health care provider as well as the same interprofessional team of providers over time.

Coordination of medical care includes timely and efficient sharing of relevant information between providers and different services including community-based agencies. Communication between providers and agencies in a timely manner is an essential characteristic of integrated health care. Individuals should be able to access care when needed and any barriers to care should be addressed, including administrative, financial, or socio-cultural.

Definition of Integrated Behavioral Health

The Lexicon for Behavioral Health and Primary Care Integration, published by the Agency for Healthcare Research and Quality, defines integrated behavioral health care as follows [18]:

> The care that results from a practice team of primary care and behavioral health clinicians, working together with patients and families, using a systematic and cost-effective approach to provide patient-centered care for a defined population. This care may address mental health and substance abuse conditions, health behaviors (including their contribution to chronic medical illnesses), life stressors and crises, stress-related physical symptoms, and ineffective patterns of health care utilization.

Behavioral health can be applied broadly as an integral part of any medical care. The practice of behavioral health in an integrated model will address not only behavioral symptoms but also multiple psychological and behavioral factors that are associated with acute or chronic illness [19].

The core principles of IBH models are applicable across all age groups [3, 17, 18]. Ongoing social, psychological, and cognitive development in children and adolescents is an essential differentiating consideration when applying IBH principles to the care of children and adolescents, especially those with complex medical conditions [3]. When compared to adults, the application and delivery of IBH in the pediatric practice setting differs in three key aspects: (1) sensitivity to social, emotional, and psychological development; (2) the essential role of family and other caregivers; and (3) relatively greater importance of coping strategy and adjustment in treatment plan [3, 17, 18]. Intellectual disability and developmental delay should be considered as part of the evaluation of children and adolescents who have behavioral concerns [3]. In a pediatric setting, normal or typical behaviors of children and adolescents as these relate to health-related lifestyles should also be considered. Behavioral health also includes mental health conditions seen in children and adolescents, which may be recognized as primary concerns or in association with acute or chronic medical conditions [19–21].

Integrated behavioral health is patient-centered in that it respects the participation of the patient in making informed choices related to his or her health or medical care. Collaboration between the patient, family, and health care team is an essential characteristic of integrated behavioral health.

Integration of care by its very nature implies a systems-level approach to care delivery. It is not necessary for all the team members to be physically in the same place to deliver integrated care. Different models of integrated behavioral health have been described (see Table 1.1) [3, 18, 21]. These models exist along a spectrum of progressively higher levels of integration between medical and behavioral health care.

Table 1.1 Comparison of key features of different models of integrated behavioral health care

	Model			
Features	Coordinated care	Co-located care	Collaborative/ fully integrated	Primary care behavioral health
Key Element	Communication	Physical proximity	Practice change	Practice change
Where is care provided?	Separate facilities	In same facility not necessarily same offices	In the same space in the same facility (some to all of the space is shared)	In the same space in the same facility (some to all of the space is shared)
Electronic medical record	Separate systems	May have separate systems or may share some systems	Shared system	Shared system
Treatment plan	Separate treatment plans	Separate plans may be informed by shared information; collaborative treatment planning for specific patients	Collaborative treatment planning for all shared patients	Collaborative treatment planning for all patients
Level of communication/ interaction	Low; primarily triggered by referral/consult; communication rarely occurs in person	Partial; curbside consult; meet occasionally to coordinate plans for specific patients; communication may occur in person or via phone or e-mail	Complete; regular in person communication; have regular team meetings to discuss overall patient care and specific patient issues	Complete
Business model (funding, resources, expenses, billing)	All separate	Separate funding (may share grants), may share facility/office expenses, separate billing	Blended funding, sharing of resources, shared expenses, billing is integrated for single billing structure	Shared funding, resources, expenses, and billing
Population being targeted	Patients for which a referral or consult is placed	Patients for which a referral or consult is placed, shared patients	Subgroup of the larger population-either specific patients or specific conditions	Entire clinic population—including those not seen by BH clinician and those without significant behavioral issues

Models of Integrated Behavioral Healthcare

Coordinated

The coordinated IBH model is at the lower end of the spectrum of integration. The key characteristic of this model is effective interdisciplinary communication that includes the sharing of relevant health-related information between the pediatrician and behavioral health consultant [3, 18, 19]. Increasingly, telephone consultations with child psychiatrists and pediatric psychologists by pediatricians are becoming a common practice. Pediatricians are able to consult with a behavioral health specialist over the phone regarding appropriate intervention and treatment. Sometimes this method can involve care coordinators who serve as the intermediary between physicians and mental health providers. This model can be cost-effective compared to hiring full-time behavioral health consultants by the practice. In a coordinated model, different professional disciplines are not necessarily located in the same practice setting.

Co-located

In a co-located IBH model, both pediatric primary care and behavioral health services are located in the same practice setting. However, each practice operates independently, with patients in need being referred from pediatric care to behavioral health services [3, 18, 21]. Co-location refers to the physical proximity of care rather than collaboration between providers on a patient's treatment plan, as each provider maintains separate treatment plans [15]. Being located in the same setting provides an excellent resource to both the pediatrician and behavioral health consultant being able to access each other and consult when necessary [18, 21]. A potential benefit of co-located services is the ability to share the same electronic medical record, which can effectively enhance access to patient information.

Fully Integrated/Collaborative

Fully integrated models regard behavioral health consultants as members of the pediatric primary care practice. In a fully integrated, collaborative IBH model, the behavioral health consultant is available and consulted during all regularly scheduled pediatric office visits [18, 21]. In integrated care, instead of having two separate treatment plans—one with medical elements and one with behavioral elements—there is a unified treatment plan that includes both pediatric care and behavioral management plans [18, 21]. The integrated model does not necessarily function to replace more extensive regular behavioral health care evaluation and management of children and adolescents. Rather, it functions to augment or complement the timely delivery of behavioral healthcare more efficiently and effectively in the pediatric practice setting [18, 21].

Primary Care Behavioral Health (PCBH)

Reiter et al. [17] described PCBH as "a team based primary care approach to managing behavioral health problems and biopsychosocially influenced health conditions" [17]. The main goal of the PCBH model is to work collaboratively with the primary medical care team in increasing the level of effectiveness of overall care delivery in the evaluation and management of behavioral health concerns seen in the primary care setting [17]. As an integral member of the primary medical care team, the behavioral health consultant is available to participate in the care of all patients seen in the practice. The behavioral health consultant participates in the care of all patients as a routine practice and provides brief office assessments and interventions as indicated, in an efficient manner. Follow-up visits are scheduled, if indicated, for more extensive behavioral evaluation and treatment. The behavioral health consultant is embedded within the medical practice in terms of shared location and resources.

While the PCBH and fully integrated behavioral health care models are similar in principle, they differ in what patient population is served [3, 15, 21]. Many fully integrated behavioral health care programs focus on improving individual patient care outcomes as these programs often target either specific patients or specific conditions. On the other hand, the main focus of the PCBH approach is to improve the care of the entire practice population [17]. PCBH aims to improve population health by strengthening primary care through enhanced access to primary care providers (PCP), increased availability of preventive care, improved PCP competence and confidence in addressing biopsychosocial issues, and the provision of brief, low-intensity interventions to a large number of patients [18].

Hybrid Approach

Different IBH models individually may or may not best serve the needs of the practice, in which case a combination or hybrid approach would be a preferred approach. The specific needs of the medical practice and the patient population it serves are the key determinants of the most preferred IBH model for that practice (e.g., collaborative model providing anxiety intervention and coordinated care with psychiatry) [20]. Hybrid models highlight the very diverse set of services provided by IBH and that IBH models should not be viewed as one-size-fits-all [20].

The delivery of medical care by an interprofessional team that includes behavioral health clinicians is different from typical primary care. In an integrated behavioral health model, each team member brings with him or her a unique set of professional competencies. Each team member must acknowledge and respect the expertise of different disciplines. A clear understanding of one's role on the team and effective communication are essential.

The delivery of integrated behavioral health requires a change in practice operational workflows and a cultural adaptation by the administrative as well as professional staff to work together in a coordinated manner. Systemic or practice-level characteristics are as important as professional competencies in the effective implementation of an integrated behavioral health care model.

Conclusion

Integrated behavioral health care represents a cost-effective way for pediatricians to help their patients receive necessary behavioral and mental health care without requiring physicians to devote substantially more time to provide this care in a quality manner. There are multiple approaches primary care practices can take to implement integrated behavioral health care, making it flexible and adaptable to integrate with existing systems with relatively low friction. Since its implementation can be transformative in pediatric treatment, integrated behavioral health care should be considered when looking to improve existing or new pediatric care programs. While there are several different models of integrated behavioral health care, they all share three basic characteristics: coordination of care, continuity of care, and comprehensive care. Integrated behavioral health care should not be viewed as one size fits all; the model of integrated behavioral health care that a practice chooses to adopt should be based on the specific needs of the practice and the patients that the practice serves.

Key Points

- Most children and adolescents with behavioral and mental health concerns first present to their pediatricians; however, pediatricians have often found it difficult to deliver such care effectively within a typical practice setting and accessing specialty care can be even more difficult.
- Integrating mental and behavioral health care with primary care can lower the costs of care, increase access to mental health care, and improve the quality of patient care.
- Integrated behavioral health is defined as primary care providers and behavioral and mental health care providers working together to provide comprehensive health care in a cost-effective way.
- Different models of integrated behavioral health care represent an increasing level of integration between primary care and behavioral health.

Acknowledgments This chapter is adapted from authors' previous work: Fledderman et al. [22].

Disclosure Statement The authors have nothing to disclose.

References

1. World Health Organization and Calouste Gulbenkian Foundation. Social determinants of mental health. Geneva: World Health Organization; 2014.
2. Kessler RC, Chiu WT, Demler O, Merikangas KR, Walters EE. Prevalence, severity, and comorbidity of 12-month DSM-IV disorders in the National Comorbidity Survey Replication [published correction appears in Arch Gen Psychiatry. 2005 Jul;62(7):709. Merikangas, Kathleen R [added]]. Arch Gen Psychiatry. 2005;62(6):617–27. https://doi.org/10.1001/archpsyc.62.6.617.
3. Integrated Care. National Institute of Mental Health. https://www.nimh.nih.gov/health/topics/integrated-care/index.shtml. Published 2017. Accessed 24 May 2020.
4. Skokauskas N, Fung D, Flaherty LT, von Klitzing K, Pūras D, Servili C, Dua T, Falissard B, Vostanis P, Moyano MB, Feldman I, Clark C, Boričević V, Patton G, Leventhal B, Guerrero A. Shaping the future of child and adolescent psychiatry. Child Adolesc Psychiatry Ment Health. 2019;13(19). https://doi.org/10.1186/s13034-019-0279-y.
5. De Hert M, Correll CU, Bobes J, et al. Physical illness in patients with severe mental disorders. I. Prevalence, impact of medications and disparities in health care. World Psychiatry. 2011;10(1):52–77. https://doi.org/10.1002/j.2051-5545.2011.tb00014.x.
6. Burkhart K, Asogwa K, Muzaffar N, Gabriel M. Pediatric integrated care models: a systematic review. Clin Pediatr. 2020;59(2):148–53. https://doi.org/10.1177/0009922819890004.
7. Wang S, Li Q, Lu J, Ran H, Che Y, Fang D, et al. Treatment rates for mental disorders among children and adolescents. JAMA Netw Open. 2023;6(10). https://doi.org/10.1001/jamanetworkopen.2023.38174.
8. How mental health disorders affect youth [Internet]. Youth.gov. Available from: https://youth.gov/youth-topics/youth-mental-health/how-mental-health-disorders-affect-youth.
9. Cama S, Malowney M, Smith AJB, Spottswood M, Cheng E, Ostrowsky L, Rengifo J, Boyd JW. Availability of outpatient mental health care by pediatricians and child psychiatrists in five U.S. cities. Int J Health Serv. 2017;47(4):621–35. https://doi.org/10.1177/0020731417707492.
10. White KL, Williams TF, Greenberg BG. The ecology of medical care. N Engl J Med. 1961;265:885–92.
11. World Health Organization, United Nations Children's Fund. Primary health care: report of the international conference on primary health care. Geneva: World Health Organization; 1978.
12. Kovner A, Knickman J, Jonas S. Jonas & Kovner's health care delivery in the United States. 10th ed. New York: Springer Pub; 2011. p. 318–20.
13. Starfield B, Shi L, Macinko J. Contribution of primary care to health systems and health. Milbank Q. 2005;83(3):457–502. https://doi.org/10.1111/j.1468-0009.2005.00409.x.
14. Committee on Integrating Primary Care and Public Health, Board on Population Health and Public Health Practice, Institute of Medicine. Primary care and public health: exploring integration to improve population health. Washington, DC: National Academies Press (US); 2012.
15. Donaldson M, Lohr K, Vanselow N, Donaldson M, Yordy K. Primary care: America's health in a new era. Washington, DC: National Academies Press; 1996.
16. Goroll A, Mulley A. Primary care medicine. 7th ed. Philadelphia: Wolters Kluwer Health; 2014.
17. Reiter JT, Dobmeyer AC, Hunter CL. The primary care behavioral health (PCBH) model: an overview and operational definition. J Clin Psychol Med Settings. 2018;25(2):109–26. https://doi.org/10.1007/s10880-017-9531-x.
18. Peek CJ, National Integration Academy Council. Lexicon for behavioral health and primary care integration: concepts and definitions developed by expert consensus. AHRQ Publication No.13-IP001-EF. Rockville: Agency for Healthcare Research and Quality; 2013. Available at: http://integrationacademy.ahrq.gov/sites/default/files/Lexicon.pdf.
19. Soares N, Apple RW, Kanungo S. The role of integrated behavioral health in caring for patients with metabolic disorders. Ann Transl Med. 2018;6(24):478. https://doi.org/10.21037/atm.2018.10.62.

20. Blount A. Integrated primary care: organizing the evidence. Fam Syst Health. 2003;21(2):121–33. https://doi.org/10.1037/1091-7527.21.2.121.
21. Njoroge WF, Hostutler CA, Schwartz BS, Mautone JA. Integrated behavioral health in pediatric primary care. Curr Psychiatry Rep. 2016;18(12):106. https://doi.org/10.1007/s11920-016-0745-7.
22. Fledderman N, Deleon J, Patel DR. Integrated behavioral health: definitions and contexts. Pediatr Clin N Am. 2021;68(3):519–31. Philadelphia: Elsevier Inc.

Chapter 2
Building an Integrated Primary Care Service and Core Competencies

Thomas L. Fisher and Lucie M. Romano

The Rationale for IBH in Pediatric Primary Care Settings

Currently, the vast majority of US children access pediatric primary care services annually, with the top five most common presenting concerns falling under the umbrella of behavioral health [1–3]. As of 2016, approximately one in six US children had a diagnosed mental, behavioral, or developmental disorder, with many more likely going undiagnosed or experiencing sub-clinical threshold symptoms [4]. Recent longitudinal data reflects a concerning increase in depression, anxiety, and conduct problems in children and adolescents [5]. However, many pediatricians feel ill-equipped or unable to appropriately address these concerns, citing short visit times, unclear billing processes, and a lack of specialized mental health training [3]. Left unaddressed, the mental and behavioral concerns of childhood and adolescence have the potential to persist into adulthood, with implications for overall functioning and financial strain on the healthcare system [6]. Thus, Integrated Behavioral Health (IBH) in pediatric primary care settings assists in bridging the divide in traditional care models between evidenced-based interventions for mental and behavioral health concerns and the treatment setting most accessed by children and their caregivers. This chapter begins by covering key considerations for establishing an IBH service in pediatric primary care before highlighting a set of core competencies for providers in IBH settings necessary to ensure optimal patient satisfaction and health outcomes.

T. L. Fisher (✉) · L. M. Romano
Western Michigan University, Homer Stryker MD School of Medicine, Kalamazoo, MI, USA
e-mail: thomas.l65.fisher@wmich.edu; lucie.m.romano@wmich.edu

R. W. Apple et al. (eds.), *Using Integrated Behavioral Health in Pediatric Practice*, https://doi.org/10.1007/978-3-031-85784-3_2

Implementation Overview

The process of establishing an IBH service in the pediatric care home is one that requires careful collaborative planning, assessment, review, and flexible adjustment over the course of the implementation process, which typically takes anywhere between several months to several years. For ease of highlighting the key components of this process, we break the establishment of an IBH service down into three key phases: Assessment and Planning, Implementation, and Evaluation and Refinement. Table 2.1 provides an overview of the activities associated with each phase, which will be addressed in greater detail in the sections to follow. These recommendations for implementation are based primarily on guidance provided by the Substance Abuse and Mental Health Services Administration (SAMHSA), the Advancing Integrated Mental Health Solutions Center at the University of Washington (AIMS Center), and the Adolescent Health Initiative associated with the University of Michigan Medicine, all of which are leaders in advancing the implementation of IBH in primary care settings [7–9]. For a more substantial review of each activity described briefly here, we recommend exploring the various resources made freely available by these organizations, a selection of which are included in this chapter's references.

Assessment and Planning

The first step in launching a pediatric IBH service in the primary care setting is the same as the first step associated with the introduction of any new healthcare initiative: careful assessment and planning. While this process should be done with

Table 2.1 Key activities for implementation of pediatric IBH service

Assessment and Planning
1. Determine and understand your community's need for behavioral health services and your clinic's readiness to provide these services.
2. Select a model of integration that is most feasible for your practice setting.
3. Identify and engage key institutional stakeholders that will support efforts to establish IBH in pediatric primary care.
4. Create a shared vision for IBH service and set clear goals for year 1 of implementation.
Implementation
1. Train providers and physicians including educating them about each role and associated duties.
2. Create a clinic workflow that optimizes resources and centers patient care.
3. Roll out IBH services to patients and their families.
Evaluation and Refinement
1. Revisit IBH's mission and goals to evaluate progress and determine areas for improvement.
2. Make indicated improvements to clinic practices with the goal of enhancing quality of care and patient outcomes.

intention, we emphasize function over form in doing so. That is, assessment and planning may take different forms based on the characteristics of your clinical setting. Despite this variability in form, this phase of implementation should always link back to the overall goal of improving access to behavioral health interventions for children and their families. The following sections outline the basic components of the assessment and planning phase that will aid in launching a successful IBH service.

Determining Community Needs and Clinic Readiness

We recommend beginning by considering the current behavioral health needs of your community. This can be achieved through collaboration with local organizations that are presently responsible for managing behavioral health needs, including your local community mental health organization, school districts, outpatient private practices, residential and outpatient substance abuse treatment centers, your state and county health and human services department, and your own clinic director who can provide information about the utilization of services related to behavioral health concerns. If additional behavioral health services are needed in your community, you must then determine the readiness of your clinic to provide these services. Whether your practice chooses to use formalized readiness measures such as the Collaborative Care Readiness Checklist made available through the AIMS Center or instead adapts a more informal, qualitative approach to understanding your clinic's readiness, we recommend a structured assessment process. This assessment should outline your current approach to managing behavioral health concerns and determine the availability of financial and staffing resources to support an IBH service. Additionally, it should consider the physical infrastructure needed for collaborative care, the clinic's capacity for bioinformatics and outcome tracking, and any other potential barriers or strengths that may impact the sustainability of an IBH service.

Selecting Target Level of Integration

An important determinant of how an IBH service will function is the degree to which it is integrated within the existing pediatric primary care service. The SAMHSA-HRSA Center for Integrated Health Solutions provides a framework of the six levels of integration, ranging from minimal to no collaboration and coordination of care to the most integrated model where both pediatric medicine providers and behavioral health providers function as one integrated medical treatment team [7]. Careful review of your clinic's available resources and these SAMHSA-HRSA guidelines will allow you to determine the degree of integration that is most feasible. While the best model is ultimately determined by the needs of your patients and the availability of resources, we recommend full integration whenever possible to increase the likelihood that children and their families access services that incorporate both medical and psychosocial interventions. Whichever model your team selects during the planning process, it is crucial that all clinic team members are made aware of the defining characteristics of that model and commit to implementing it.

Identifying and Engaging Key Stakeholders and Advocates for IBH

Identifying and engaging key clinic stakeholders is a necessary step in successfully establishing an IBH service. These efforts should convey the value of IBH services, including increased access to care, improved patient outcomes, increased care coordination, and potential cost savings to stakeholders including clinic directors and administrators, other pediatricians, nursing staff, social workers, medical assistants, and facility managers [8–10]. Obtaining the support of these stakeholders helps build institutional support and create a unified effort to integrate behavioral health services into pediatric care, increasing the potential for success.

Creating a Shared Vision and Setting Initial Goals

A successful IBH service is the embodiment of many individuals working together toward a shared objective. Thus, it is necessary that time be spent as a group developing a shared vision for your IBH service. This shared vision should capture your overall approach to serving pediatric patients and their families. It is recommended that included in your vision is a description of the clinical presentations you intend to treat, the types of evidenced-based interventions you will utilize, and the populations that you hope to provide services to. This vision statement should also lay the groundwork for establishing a culture of collaboration and identify the ways in which collaboration will be supported throughout the IBH service [8]. After developing this shared vision, the IBH team should establish metric-based goals related to the volume of patients served, the number of visits completed, patient satisfaction and outcomes, and relevant financial metrics [8, 9, 11]. These goals should be documented and reviewed during the evaluation and refinement phase of implementation.

Implementation

After careful assessment and planning, it is time to begin the implementation phase of establishing an IBH service. This phase begins with the training of the providers that will deliver services in the IBH setting and includes clinic workflow optimization. After this is complete, IBH can begin being presented to patients and their families, as your clinic works toward full implementation.

Provider and Staff Education and Training

Adequate training is crucial for the successful implementation of IBH. First and foremost, the shared vision created in the previous phase should be shared with all providers and staff within the clinic. Subsequently, it is necessary to clearly define the roles of all members of the treatment team so it is clear what role each individual has in the identification of behavioral health concerns, subsequent intervention and follow-up, and relapse prevention. It is recommended to implement training sessions in which physicians can provide education about common physical health concerns to behavioral health providers while they learn about mental health topics from their behavioral health colleagues [8, 9]. It is during this phase that training should also emphasize and seek to develop the core competencies described in depth in subsequent sections of this chapter. While training must occur before IBH services are rolled out, it is also necessary that training occurs on an ongoing basis to ensure adherence to best practices that support patient outcomes.

Clinic Workflow Optimization

It is likely that the greatest growing pains related to establishing an IBH service will be felt in relation to disruptions to the typical clinic workflow. This means it is necessary to clearly outline patient flow through the clinic, beginning with the rooming of the patient and ending with scheduling subsequent follow-up visits. This process should be optimized to ensure that patients receive the services they need, without drastically increasing the time spent in the clinic. It is recommended that each clinic block begins with a team huddle, in which the patient list is reviewed for clear behavioral health needs so the behavioral health consultant can meet with these patients. When possible, physicians should strive to include behavioral health providers in primary care visits as soon as a behavioral health need is identified, allowing the physician to move on to the next patient visit while connecting the patient with the appropriate behavioral health resource. The behavioral health consultant can then provide short, solution-focused interventions to address the concerns and schedule follow-up visits if needed. Designated spaces in the clinic for consultation among team members, follow-up behavioral health visits, and clinical documentation should be established ahead of time to support this process.

IBH Service Rollout

Once all team members feel comfortable with their roles and the workflow of the new IBH service, it is time to roll out this service to patients and their caregivers. During this phase, you may wish to provide written materials in all primary care visits that summarize the new service and that identify presenting concerns appropriate for IBH intervention in the primary care setting. The use of standardized mental health screening tools can be used to help identify patients with specific behavioral health concerns. Physicians should introduce behavioral health consultants as members of the patient's care team and as trusted experts in addressing behavioral health concerns. It is important to emphasize the use of warm handoffs between physicians and behavioral health consultants (BHCs) to maximize patient contact while in the clinic. Treatment planning should center the patient's goals for themselves and should include parents and caregivers in treatment whenever possible. As all providers within the service adapt to the new workflow, take note of any challenges that can be addressed during the next implementation phase.

Evaluation and Refinement

Evaluate Progress Toward Your Goals

Once your IBH service has been launched and a sufficient amount of data has been collected, it is important to evaluate your progress toward the goals you set prior to launching IBH in your clinic. During the planning phase, you should have determined the frequency with which you will check your progress and review goals and ensure that these reviews take place with key members of the IBH service. This process is crucial to evaluate whether you are maintaining adherence to your desired level of integration and that patients are flowing through the IBH service as intended and making adequate progress toward their treatment goals. This review process can also help you track metrics that may be used to increase buy-in from additional institutional leaders to further establish support for the IBH service.

Make Necessary Changes

It is unlikely that the way your IBH service operates in years 2 and 3 will look the same as it did in the initial months of providing IBH services to your patients. Flexible implementation of changes based on a review of your goals is necessary to ensure that you are best able to meet the needs of your patients and their families. You may need to make changes to how patients are screened for IBH-appropriate concerns, how BHCs follow up with patients, how team huddles and communication take place, how and what metrics are tracked, or any other aspects of the clinic workflow that impact patient care. Success in this phase of implementation requires a commitment to the culture of collaboration and a willingness to work through the discomfort that can come with changes to operating procedures. Success also requires the creation of repeated opportunities to develop and refine the core competencies described below. By remaining committed to your IBH vision, you can continually improve your IBH service to increase access to necessary behavioral health services in your community.

Part 2: Core Competencies

When establishing an IBH service, it is important to incorporate practical skills and utilize the basic proficiencies of the various fields involved in the IBH service delivery. In 2014, SAMHSA-HRSA tasked their Center for Integrated Health Services to develop a set of core competencies to assist with the building of IBH services within a primary care setting. To achieve this, the project team conducted structured interviews, reviewed the literature on integration, and conducted a review and analysis of relevant competencies [12]. Through this endeavor, they found that many of the competencies required for integrated care overlapped between those relevant to behavioral health and those relevant to primary care. Additionally, key informants indicated that any distinction amongst the competencies would encourage a divide between the professions for which integration and cohesion are imperative within an IBH model. The CIHS project team identified the following nine competency categories that emerged from their methodological investigation (see Table 2.2 for an abbreviated outline). Thus, we recommend including specific training opportunities for all providers within your IBH team that relate to developing these competencies among all of those delivering services.

Table 2.2 Core competencies by category and key factors

1. Interpersonal Communication Establishing rapport, communicating effectively, and adapting communication to patients, their families, and other providers
2. Collaboration & Teamwork Functioning as an effective member of a multidisciplinary team, respecting the roles of each member, resolving differences, seeking and providing consultation, and fostering shared decision-making
3. Screening & Assessment Conducting brief, evidence-based, and developmentally appropriate screeners and assessments, identifying and responding to risks and complicating factors, and arranging for more detailed assessments as needed
4. Care Planning & Care Coordination Creating and implementing integrated care plans, linking to multiple services, exchanging information with the entire team, including patients and their families
5. Intervention Providing a range of brief, focused prevention, treatment, and maintenance strategies, providing or linking to longer-term services, providing patient education and crisis intervention, and promoting whole health and wellness services
6. Cultural Competence & Adaptation Providing services relevant and adapted to the culture and values of the patient, their families, and the broader community, valuing and striving for health equity, and promoting diversity among the IBH team
7. Systems-Oriented Practice Functioning effectively within the organization and local healthcare system, educating and assisting patients and their families about resources, and adjusting to healthcare reforms
8. Practice-Based Learning & Quality Improvement Implementing evidence-based practices, continually assessing and improving upon services, monitoring patient outcomes and satisfaction and adjusting accordingly, and rapidly addressing and working to prevent future errors
9. Informatics Using technology to support and improve IBH service delivery, providing broader access to care and communication through technology, and ensuring privacy and confidentiality

Interpersonal Communication

Interpersonal communication skills are important for any health service provider, but particularly for providers working within an IBH setting. It is imperative for all team members to be able to leverage this skill so that they can establish and maintain rapport with patients, their families, and other providers. Cultural competence also plays a major role in interpersonal communication skills, as providers must be able to work with diverse populations (for more detailed information on cultural competence within IBH and with specific populations, see Chaps. 8, 9, 10, and 11). Providers must also be able to engage in proficient active listening so that they can understand the presenting concerns, preferences, and potential barriers conveyed by patients. One effective, person-centered method to increase active listening and reflection skills is motivational interviewing [13, 14]. Training in this approach can help to strengthen skills in information gathering, affirmation and validation of patient concerns, and reflection and summarization of pertinent information.

In addition to listening skills, effective interpersonal communication involves the ability to clearly convey important information to patients and other providers without the extensive use of technical jargon and without judgment. In relation to other professionals and providers, this means navigating and using the terminology that is common to the care setting so that collaboration within that setting is successful. In relation to patients and their families, it means using the primary language and preferred communication modality of each individual being served. This can include employing qualified language interpreters and modifying communication styles to more closely match those of the patients and their families so that they can fully understand the information being conveyed. When providing written materials, it is important to ensure that they are at an appropriate reading level so that patients and their families can clearly understand them. These materials should also be used to augment verbal information provided during healthcare visits rather than in lieu of such interactions. Regardless of the forms of interpersonal communication, providers must recognize and manage any personal biases related to the patients, their families, specific health conditions, and other providers or professions. Throughout the process, providers should be able to effectively explain the roles and responsibilities of each team member and how they will be collaborating to provide care to the patients and their families.

Collaboration and Teamwork

All providers within the IBH setting must recognize and respect the unique role that each individual within the setting plays. This includes the patients, family members, behavioral health providers, and primary care providers and physicians. To achieve this, team members must also develop a shared understanding of the roles and responsibilities of each member to promote effective collaboration. Team members must also recognize their own limits and seek assistance from other providers when necessary. Effective teamwork involves effective leadership and response to leadership. These skills assist with collaboration and allow for the multidisciplinary team to capitalize on its strengths toward conceptualizing the patients' concerns. Assessments and treatment should be adapted so that they are rapid and brief, yet still efficacious. The professional opinions of all team members should be able to be expressed and heard and any conflicts should be resolved quickly. This also requires actively sharing relevant information with other providers and team members via HIPAA-compliant and patient-authorized channels.

Effective collaboration and teamwork always include the patients and their families. This includes shared decision-making, responding to expressed needs, and practically and flexibly working toward agreed-upon treatment goals. Providers should work to connect the patients and their families to other team members through face-to-face encounters, or "warm handoffs." Behavioral health and general health interventions should be used in conjunction to enhance patient outcomes, and consultation should occur often and as immediately as possible. Through this collaborative approach, providers should also promote whole-health approaches to patient concerns and should encourage both self-management and peer support models where appropriate.

Screening and Assessment

In order to adequately conceptualize patient concerns, providers must be able to effectively conduct brief evidence-based screeners and assessments. These should be developmentally normed and should be based upon strengths-based, resilience, and recovery models when used in IBH settings. As such, team members should be intimately familiar with the signs, symptoms, and treatments of the most common conditions seen within the setting. Appropriate screeners should be routinely used to identify a variety of concerns and underlying factors such as substance use, mental-health concerns, cognitive impairments, behavior concerns, risk of self-harm or harm to others, environmental safety, impairments in functional living skills, and signs of abuse, neglect, domestic violence, or other trauma. If the screeners are positive for any of these factors, the proper team member(s) should then conduct more detailed assessments of the problem and make accurate diagnoses. Assessments should also be conducted in relation to the patient's social determinants of health, and the team should collaborate to determine the feasibility of providing effective treatment to the patient and their family within the context of the IBH setting and team.

Care Planning and Care Coordination

Because IBH services are collaborative in nature, care plans should be created and updated periodically with the whole team, including the patients, their families, and any other individuals identified by the patients as part of their healthcare team. Plans should address whole health and wellness, and the type, intensity, and frequency of services should match the needs of the patient. Care plans should be utilized so that patients can be linked to the various services, providers, and community resources of the multidisciplinary team. Many patients and their families will present with barriers to care that can be addressed by the IBH team. Financial concerns, transportation, home care, childcare and access to social services, peer support, and treatment are all concerns that the IBH team can provide or arrange access to via the care plan. When patients are unable to be adequately treated by the IBH team or within the setting, team members must effectively connect the patients with other appropriate services.

Intervention

Brief, focused, and multidisciplinary interventions to improve health are of utmost importance and should be of value to any IBH team. All members should be proficient in their ability to engage patients and their families and increase their desire and motivation to improve their health and to adhere to their care plan. Interventions should be evidence-based and best practice for integrated settings. Intervention should always include patient education about conditions, prevention, available treatment options, self-management, peer and community support, and recovery. It is also important for interventions to be trauma-informed, problem-oriented, and solution-focused. Providers should also deliver education and supportive interventions addressing the consequences of illness and injury. This can be especially important when working with children and their families, as accidental injuries are unfortunately common and of great concern but can be preventable [15, 16].

Another common patient concern within pediatric IBH settings is substance use. One in eight high school students has a substance use disorder, and 20–70% have experimented with substances [17].As such, team members must have knowledge of screeners, interventions, and appropriate referrals for substance use in pediatric populations. They must also be able to educate patients and families about risks, and licensed team members must be able to prescribe and manage medications as they relate to substance use disorders and other mental health concerns. For any medication, team members must be able to recognize and to educate patients and their families about the effects, side effects, potential long-term health effects, and interactions of pharmacological interventions.

In some cases, brief interventions or pharmacological interventions are not sufficient. Team members must be able to recognize the need and implement longer-term models of treatment and follow up for persistent concerns. Team members should also support patients in considering and accessing complementary and alternative services. Any IBH model should have a protocol for managing behavioral health crises that includes linking patients and their families to treatment facilities, specialty healthcare, social services, and other resources.

Cultural Competence and Adaptation

Providers within an IBH setting should always focus on health equity by identifying and addressing disparities in healthcare access and increasing the quality of services for the diverse individuals and populations served. This involves adapting the services of the multidisciplinary team to fit the language, cultural norms, and preferences of the patients and their families. It also involves fostering collaborative relationships with other providers and educating team members on the patients' characteristics, needs, behaviors, and views toward illness and treatment. To achieve this skill, diversity should be a strong value within the IBH setting. This includes promoting diversity within the multidisciplinary team in all roles.

Systems-Oriented Practice

Every organization has a culture that is shaped by its providers and its consumers. For an IBH service to be sustainable, team members must understand and practice effectively within the organization, the culture of the multidisciplinary team, the practice setting, and the overall local healthcare system. This involves all team members having knowledge of healthcare benefits, coverage and limitations, utilization procedures, billing, and reimbursement such that they are able to convey this information to the patients with an understanding of the impact of team-based care. Decision-making about the organization and delivery of services should be effective both clinically and financially. Any healthcare reforms or changes in structure should be anticipated and should result in adjustment of care. All services should be planned and delivered with awareness of the healthcare needs of the population being served.

Practice-Based Learning and Quality Improvement

All IBH team members must be able to engage in an evidence-based practice approach by being proficient in searching and evaluating the literature for the most effective interventions and delivering evidence-based, integrated approaches to patient concerns. Team members should recognize and apply guidelines to the delivery of care that are relevant to their own practice. The entire IBH team should assess the fidelity of team-based care, rapidly address any errors in care, and implement policies and procedures to reduce future errors. A successful IBH system must also include procedures to monitor individual outcomes and patient and family satisfaction with services. If either of these measures is lacking for an individual or their families, team members must adjust care plans and practice patterns based on the data and feedback. Additionally, the ability to read, interpret, and monitor aggregate outcome data is paramount. Service system design should be consistently monitored, assessed, and improved upon, and individual providers and the IBH team should have consistent improvement and education goals.

Informatics

The use of electronic medical records and computer-based technology makes IBH service delivery optimal. This allows for more effective and efficient communication between the team and the patients. It also allows providers to screen, assess, and provide services in a more accessible manner such as through telehealth platforms. Providers should assist patients and their families in using technology-based tools as part of their healthcare plan. Although these tools can be beneficial, they are subject to cyber risks. As such, all technology used in the IBH setting must be secure and HIPAA-compliant so that the patients' privacy, documentation, and data remain confidential and protected.

Conclusion

The establishment of IBH services in pediatric primary care represents an important step toward addressing the mental health needs of pediatric patients and their families. By implementing the outlined strategies for assessment, planning, implementation, and evaluation, healthcare providers can effectively integrate an IBH service in pediatric care clinics. The emphasis on core competencies equips IBH teams with the necessary skills to provide effective behavioral health interventions in the context of pediatric primary care. Through collaborative efforts, IBH services have the potential to significantly improve access to mental health care, promote early intervention, and positively impact the well-being of children, families, and their communities.

References

1. Brino KA. Pediatric mental health and the power of primary care: practical approaches and validating challenges. J Pediatr Health Care. 2020;34(2):e12–20.
2. Yogman MW, Betjemann S, Sagaser A, Brecher L. Integrated behavioral health care in pediatric primary care: a quality improvement project. Clin Pediatr. 2018;57(4):461–70.
3. Olfson M, Kroenke K, Wang S, Blanco C. Trends in office-based mental health care provided by psychiatrists and primary care physicians. J Clin Psychiatry. 2014;75(3):247–53.
4. Cree RA, Bitsko RH, Robinson LR, Holbrook JR, Danielson ML, Smith DS, Kaminski JW, Kenney MK, Peacock G. Health care, family, and community factors associated with mental, behavioral, and developmental disorders and poverty among children aged 2–8 years — United States, 2016. MMWR. 2018;67(5):1377–83.
5. Lebrun-Harris LA, Ghandour RM, Kogan MD, Warren MD. Five-year trends in US children's health and well-being, 2016–2020. JAMA Pediatr. 2022;176(7):e1–11.
6. American Academy of Child and Adolescent Psychiatry Committee on Health Care Access and Economics Task Force on Mental Health. Improving mental health services in primary care: reducing administrative and financial barriers to access and collaboration. Pediatrics. 2009;123(4):1248–51.
7. Heath B, Wise Romero P, Reynolds K. A standard framework for levels of integrated healthcare. [Internet]. SAMHSA-HRSA Center for Integrated Health Solutions; 2013 [cited 2024 May 20]. Available from: https://www.integration.samhsa.gov/integrated-care-models/A_Standard_Framework_for_Levels_of_Integrated_Healthcare.pdf.
8. AIMS Center. Collaborative care implementation guide [Internet]. University of Washington Department of Psychiatry and Behavioral Sciences, Advancing Integrated Mental Health Solutions (AIMS) Center; 2024 [cited 2024 May 20]. Available from: https://aims.uw.edu/resource/collaborative-care-implementation-guide/
9. Adolescent Health Initiative. SBHC integrated behavioral health starter guide [Internet]. University of Michigan Health Michigan Medicine; 2023 [cited 2024 May 20]. Available from:

https://umhs-adolescenthealth.org/wp-content/uploads/2023/07/sbhc-integrated-behavioral-health-starter-guide-summer-2023-update-3.pdf.
10. Asarnow JR, Rozenman M, Wiblin J, Zeltzer L. Integrated medical-behavioral care compared with usual primary care for child and adolescent behavioral health: a meta-analysis. JAMA Pediatr. 2015;169(10):929–37.
11. Ouyang JX, Pustilnik S, Cotton A, Fallucco EM, Hopkins M. Building integrated mental health services in pediatric primary care: user guide from the academic trenches. Acad Psychiatry. 2024;48(3):273–9.
12. Hoge MA, Morris JA, Laraia M, Pomerantz A, Farley T. Core competencies for integrated behavioral health and primary care. [Internet]. SAMHSA-HRSA Center for Integrated Health Solutions; 2014 [cited 2024 May 05].
13. Miller WR, Rollnick S. Motivational interviewing: preparing people to change addictive behavior. New York: Guilford Press; 1991.
14. Rubak S, Sandbæk A, Lauritzen T, Christensen B. Motivational interviewing: a systematic review and meta-analysis. Br J Gen Pract. 2005;55(513):305–12.
15. WHO Guidelines Approved by the Guidelines Review Committee. [Internet]. World Health Organization; 2008 [cited 2024 May 05]. Available from: https://www.ncbi.nlm.nih.gov/books/NBK132015/.
16. Sleet DA. The global challenge of child injury prevention. Int J Environ Res Public Health. 2018;15(9):1921.
17. Garofoli M. Adolescent substance abuse. Prim Care. 2020;47(2):383–94.

Chapter 3
Common Behavioral and Cognitive Interventions

C. Dukes, S. Prokos, and J. Vosters

Introduction

Common presenting problems appropriate for IBH are attention-deficit hyperactivity disorder (ADHD), anxiety and depression, behavior problems at home or school, habitual behaviors, eating and feeding concerns, sleep concerns, and toileting [1]. Treatment in IBH consists primarily of behavioral and cognitive interventions [1]. The two main branches of therapy discussed are behavior therapy, which includes parent management training, sleep hygiene, and habit reversal training (HRT), and cognitive behavioral therapy (CBT).

C. Dukes (✉) · J. Vosters
Western Michigan University, Homer Stryker M.D., School of Medicine, Kalamazoo, MI, USA

Department of Psychology, Western Michigan University, Kalamazoo, MI, USA
e-mail: Cassandra.dukes@wmich.edu

S. Prokos
Department of Psychology, Western Michigan University, Kalamazoo, MI, USA

R. W. Apple et al. (eds.), *Using Integrated Behavioral Health in Pediatric Practice*, https://doi.org/10.1007/978-3-031-85784-3_3

Common Components of Behavioral and Cognitive Interventions

Screening Tools

Although treatment varies based on the presenting problem, there are core components of behavioral health intervention relevant to most presenting problems. IBH services often begin with information gathering from the patient's chart, the physician, and the patient and their family. This may be informed by screeners provided to the patient, caregiver(s), and teacher(s) by the primary care physician (PCP) or the behavioral health consultant (BHC) [2]. Common screeners in primary care settings include the Pediatric Symptom Checklist-17 (PSC-17), the Patient Health Questionnaire-9 (PHQ-9), the Screen for Child Anxiety Related Emotional Disorders (SCARED), Strengths and Difficulties Questionnaire, the Generalized Anxiety Disorder-7 (GAD-7), the Modified Checklist for Autism in Toddlers-Revised (M-CHAT-R), and the Vanderbilt (AAP) [2]. Following a positive screen or reported concern, it must be determined whether the patient and presenting problem are appropriate for IBH services. If not, the role of the BHC may be providing resources and referring the patient to alternative services for testing, long-term outpatient therapy, inpatient treatment, or more specialized care.

Psychoeducation and Anticipatory Guidance

Another core aspect of IBH is psychoeducation for the patient and their family. This may involve discussing typical development, diagnostic criteria of a mental health disorder, and/or what might be causing, perpetuating, or compounding a presenting problem. Intervention may also involve providing anticipatory guidance related to the growth and development of a patient.

Caregiver Involvement

Finally, caregiver involvement is an important component of most behavioral interventions with children. Consistency between caregivers is also advantageous during IBH treatment, regardless of whether caregivers are in the same household or not. This ideally also includes consistency across settings like home and school.

Behavior Therapy

Feeding Disorders

Pediatric feeding disorders are most common from 1 to 3 years old and occur in 3–10% of children, many of whom have developmental disabilities [3]. Feeding disorders may also occur in children with various medical issues that may cause pain when eating. Common presentations include food selectivity or refusal, disruptive behavior during mealtimes, and inability to eat age-appropriate textures or amounts of food [3].

Typically, feeding disorders require an interdisciplinary team consisting of a dietician to provide education around nutrition, a PCP to address medical concerns and monitor weight and development, an occupational therapist to address motor skills deficits and sensory aspects, and a psychologist or BHC to implement parent training and behavioral intervention.

Behavioral intervention, in the form of behavioral feeding techniques, is the most empirically supported treatment for pediatric feeding disorders [3]. This begins with a functional analysis to determine the function of the behavior and current intake of food. This may involve the use of a food record to track preferred and refused foods, volumes consumed, and current eating schedule. It then involves teaching the caregivers several different behavioral techniques including either differential reinforcement of an alternative behavior, during which a caregiver would provide praise or reward for engaging in feeding behaviors, or noncontingent attention, during which a caregiver provides attention regardless of the child's behavior during mealtimes. For picky eating treatment in IBH, some recommended techniques are gradual repeated exposure to a non-desired food, starting with just having the food in the room or at the table, and gradually working up to using other senses to experience the food, like touching, smelling, or licking, and finally trying a bite of the new food. Simultaneous presentation of the non-desired food with a desired food can also be helpful in introducing new foods. Finally, caregiver modeling of the consumption of non-desired food can be helpful in providing exposure.

Treatment of feeding and eating disorders may involve addressing anxiety around mealtimes for the caregiver and child [4]. Decreasing stress during mealtimes, using relaxation techniques and later discussed strategies for anxiety, can therefore be beneficial for the whole family. Developing structure and routine around mealtime can increase feelings of stability in children, leading to less anxiety and a consistent appetite [4].

When the above techniques are not successful in reducing the problem or there are associated medical, developmental, or nutritional complications, including meeting criteria for eating disorders, patients should be referred for more extensive and specialized treatment.

Tantrum Behavior, Noncompliance, and ADHD

Parent Management Training (PMT) is a structured therapeutic approach designed to help parents develop effective parenting skills to address behavioral and emotional problems in their children. It is typically used with parents of children aged 4–12 years old who exhibit disruptive behavior disorders, such as ADHD, oppositional defiant disorder (ODD), or conduct disorder (CD) [5, 6]. PMT has been shown to effectively address a wide range of child behaviors, including but not limited to oppositional and defiant behaviors in children—refusing to comply with rules or instructions, arguing, and defying authority; aggressive and conduct-related issues—physical fighting, verbal aggression, property destruction, lying, stealing, and rule-breaking; inattention and hyperactivity—techniques to improve focus, impulse control, and self-regulation; and emotional regulation difficulties—managing tantrums, emotional outbursts, and mood swings by teaching strategies for promoting emotional regulation, coping skills, and problem-solving abilities [5, 6].

PMT is composed of five essential components: (1) skill encouragement, which involves promoting pro-social development by breaking behaviors into manageable steps and providing positive reinforcement contingent upon progress, (2) discipline, which entails reducing negative behaviors through the use of appropriate consequences contingent upon behavior, (3) monitoring or supervision of activities, peers, and locations of children, which aids parents in maintaining a safe environment for their children, (4) problem-solving skills, which assist families in reaching agreements and establishing rules through negotiation, and (5) positive involvement, which supports parents in providing affectionate, positive attention to their children [5, 6].

While implementing PMT in an IBH setting is demanding, it is achievable [7]. It is up to the BHC's discretion to determine which components of the intervention to deliver based on their patients' needs. The section below describes the most common components of the intervention that BHCs can implement in as little as two to four sessions with parents and children [7]. At the beginning of treatment, time is dedicated to psychoeducation with parents regarding behavioral principles such as positive and negative reinforcement, prompting, shaping, and reprimands, among others. Parents are taught multiple techniques such as planned ignoring, the use of behavioral charts and reward systems, timeout procedures, and anger management strategies in order to help reduce their child's disruptive behavior [5]. Planned ignoring involves intentionally withholding attention or reaction to specific problem behaviors that are non-harmful and do not pose a safety risk. The goal is to extinguish undesirable behaviors by removing the reinforcement they receive from adult attention or reactions.

Behavioral charts and reward systems are frequently used in PMT [5]. The behavior chart, a visual tool typically including columns or rows for each day of the week and specific behaviors or tasks that the child is expected to perform, is used to track the child's behavior over time. The BHC can help parents establish clear, specific goals for their child's behavior. Parents and children then collaborate to determine appropriate rewards for meeting the goals or demonstrating the target behaviors. Rewards can vary depending on the child's age, interests, and preferences but may include privileges, activities, small toys or treats, or points that can be exchanged for larger rewards. Once the behavior chart is created and rewards are selected, the reward system is put into action, often with several weeks between sessions to implement the chart, with sessions focusing on troubleshooting any difficulties. Parents consistently reinforce positive behaviors by providing immediate praise, acknowledgment, or rewards when the child meets the specified criteria outlined on the behavior chart. Parents monitor the child's progress on the behavior chart and provide ongoing feedback and encouragement. If the child experiences difficulties or setbacks, parents and BHCs may collaborate to modify the goals, adjust the reward system, or provide additional support and guidance as needed. As the child becomes more adept at demonstrating the target behaviors consistently, the frequency or magnitude of rewards may be gradually reduced or faded over time. This helps promote intrinsic motivation and long-term maintenance of positive behavior patterns.

Timeout is another commonly used strategy in PMT. The timeout procedure involves promptly and calmly removing the child from the situation and placing them in a designated timeout area for a predetermined duration, typically corresponding to their age. During the timeout, parents ignore protesting or escape attempts by the child. After the timeout, parents briefly discuss the reason for the timeout and reinforce positive behavior [5]. In IBH, BHCs can provide guidance around the steps of timeout and role play with parents to ensure they are implementing the timeout procedure properly. It's important to use timeout consistently and fairly, focusing on behaviors that pose safety risks or significantly disrupt the family environment, and to pair timeout with positive reinforcement strategies.

Toileting

There are no standard criteria to define when a child is toilet trained, but the American Association of Pediatrics (AAP) emphasizes the child's ability to sense the urge to urinate, comprehend the need to urinate, communicate this with the caregiver, walk to the bathroom, and use the toilet [8]. Training in the United States begins between 2 to 3 years old, with most children trained by 4 years old. The AAP embraces the "child-directed" approach to training, which emphasizes waiting to train until the child is ready, measured by attaining specific developmental, behavioral, and physiologic milestones rather than chronologic age. Training begins slowly, with gentle encouragement to experiment with toileting behavior—allowing children to see how parents use the toilet, letting them sit on the toilet, and generally nurturing their curiosity [9].

Toilet training can be a difficult process for many caregivers, and it is common to experience temporary setbacks, particularly during times of stress. Common difficulties include nocturnal enuresis, refusal to use the toilet, and functional constipation [10]. While these setbacks are common, urinary accidents become pathological once a child is 5 years old or older, as 24-h continence is achievable at this point. The AAP definition of enuresis is when a child urinates in their bed or on their clothes 2 times per week for 3 consecutive months. Although pathological, enuresis is highly prevalent, with 10% of 6 to 7-year-olds experiencing it. As such, primary care providers should start enuresis evaluation soon after the child turns 5 years old.

The first recommended step is for caregivers to keep a voiding journal to provide additional information. One recorded measurement is the daytime Maximum Voided Volume (MVV)—the highest volume the child urinates during a 24-h period (excluding the first morning void). The second key measurement is the amount of urine produced in 7 consecutive nights (done by measuring the weight of the diaper). It is also beneficial to record the child's eating/drinking and defecation habits, as constipation can affect urinary continence.

Based on the information collected in the journal, there are several first-line treatment options that can be implemented in IBH. Generally, it is preferred to start with simple brief behavioral interventions including motivational therapy, voiding just before bed, waking the child during the night to urinate, retention control training (to increase bladder capacity), and fluid restriction. Specifically, it is encouraged that the child drinks 40% of the daily fluid in the morning, 40% in the afternoon, and the remaining 20% in the evening, with nothing to drink the last hour before bed [11]. Motivational therapy for young children is akin to using a reward system, such as a star chart, to praise the child for positive behavioral changes—for example, earning a star for voiding before bed, dry nights, or helping to change soiled sheets. As enuresis has a significant psychosocial impact, this encouragement empowers children to believe they have control over their bodies. To best understand if these behavioral adjustments are effective, it is recommended to keep a calendar of dry/wet nights.

If these changes are ineffective, another first-line treatment is the enuresis alarm or urine alarm. The alarm attaches either to the child's pajamas or bed and is activated when wet. Thus, when the child urinates while asleep, the alarm will sound, waking them up. Often the caregiver must get up with the child to ensure proper training, as the alarm is only effective when the child immediately goes to the toilet to finish urinating. Over time, this generates awareness training for the urge to urinate. While this method has been proven effective, it takes several months to train the child and make noticeable improvements, requiring significant effort and motivation on the part of the caregivers as well [12].

Thumb Sucking, Nail Biting, and Other Habits

Thumb sucking is a common behavior that young children often outgrow with age, usually before the age of 4 [13]. Therefore, pediatrician guidelines recommend planned ignoring as the first response to thumb sucking. This is also recommended for nail biting and other non-harmful habitual behaviors like rocking. However, there are situations in which this habit prompts further treatment, for example, if thumb sucking is affecting a child's palate or their speech or nail biting or other habitual behaviors are causing tissue damage or significant functional impairment. In addition, if a child is still sucking their thumb after the age of 4, this may require further behavioral treatment [13]. Nail biting may be related to anxiety and can often be treated through addressing the underlying anxiety.

Habit reversal training (HRT) is a common behavioral intervention for habits like thumb sucking, nail biting, and hair pulling. With some modifications to address time constraints, it has been adapted for use in the primary care setting and IBH [14]. HRT traditionally involves awareness training, competing response, and response interruption. In a primary care setting, aversive conditioning may also be helpful as a first option or to supplement other behavioral interventions. This involves frequent application of a bad-tasting substance (ex. Thum Liquid, Control-It) to the child's nail [15]. This could serve as a form of awareness training and response interruption. If the function of this behavior is to self-soothe, the competing response may be the use of relaxation techniques like diaphragmatic breathing and progressive muscle relaxation (PMR). These competing responses are most effective when they are techniques that cannot be done concurrently with the behavior, for example, PMR involving the hands so a child is not able to simultaneously suck a thumb or chew nails. Once patients have developed an awareness of the behavior, this habit, along with other habits, can also be treated in IBH with a similar method to disruptive behaviors. More specifically, treatment may involve a rewards chart to encourage decreasing behavior and rewarding not engaging in this behavior or using an alternative coping technique.

Sleep Problems

Sleep is an active process that has a significant impact on the body's overall health and function [16]. It affects growth, development, memory, synaptic efficiency, immune function, behavioral regulation, and learning [16]. Sleep also fluctuates dramatically across the stages of human development based on the physiologic needs of the body [17]. Newborns, who require feeding every few hours, have a very fragmented sleep schedule that totals 16–18 h of sleep/day. Children 2–12 months require 12–16 h of sleep/day. Children aged 1–3 require 10–16 h of sleep, and aged 3–5 require 11–15 h. Usually, between 3 and 5 years of age, children stop requiring a daytime nap. Adolescents (10–18 years) sleep 9–10 h, with increased daytime sleepiness during puberty.

Parasomnia refers to an abnormal or unusual behavior during sleep, of which there is a wide spectrum. Studies report that parasomnias affect up to 50% of children but often decrease with age [17]. Parasomnias that may be addressed in IBH include insomnia, somnambulism, or sleepwalking, sleep terrors, and nightmare disorder.

As childhood parasomnias are frequently witnessed by a caregiver, their description of events is key to understanding the child's condition [17]. Sleep journals are a useful tool to record bedtime, sleep latency, any sleep fragmentation, wake time, and a description of the concerning events. These journals allow for more interpretation of the episodes and track the effectiveness of interventions. Additionally, the Nightmare Disorder Index—a 5-question diagnostic test—may also be useful in establishing a diagnosis of nightmare disorder [18].

Treatment of primary parasomnias—after ruling out triggers such as obstructive sleep apnea, panic attacks, restless leg syndrome, nocturnal seizures, or adverse medication effects—is predominantly behavioral. The first-line strategy in IBH includes reinforcing good sleep hygiene and providing reassurance that these conditions are predominantly self-limited.

Sleep hygiene is defined as a set of behavioral and environmental recommendations intended to promote healthy sleep [19]. Good sleep hygiene includes setting a consistent bedtime/wake time, avoiding caffeine in the afternoon, being physically active during the day, avoiding excessive napping, creating a relaxing bedtime routine, avoiding screen time in the hour before sleep, and sleeping in a dark and quiet environment [20]. Daytime behavior has a substantial influence on sleep quality. Decreasing stimulation and promoting a relaxing environment are simple first steps in the treatment of parasomnias.

Additional brief behavioral interventions for somnambulism, sleep terrors, and nightmare disorder include scheduled awakenings, home safety counseling, and increased total sleep time [17]. Scheduled awakenings can be used when the child has consistent, predictable parasomnias. In such cases, the caregiver preemptively wakes the child 15–30 min before their episode every night. Once the child is aroused briefly, they may go back to sleep. This interrupts the child's sleep cycle before the parasomnia occurs, resetting the cycle for that night [21]. The caregiver must continue waking the child at the same time every night for 2–4 weeks for the parasomnia to subside [22]. Home safety counseling is vital to maintaining the child's well-being during episodes. Parasomnias, particularly the non-REM subtype, involve unregulated movement. Whether the child is sleepwalking or thrashing, it is important to make sure they won't become injured during an episode. Safety precautions include placing the mattress on the floor, removing sharp or dangerous objects from the bedroom, using bed/door alarms to alert the caregiver that the child is out of bed, and locking exterior doors/windows [23]. Increasing total sleep time is another essential component of treatment. It is believed that sleep deprivation can trigger parasomnias and exacerbate the condition. Therefore, ensuring that the child is getting adequate sleep is a fundamental preventative intervention [24]. Furthermore, CBT treatment for nightmares is discussed in the section below.

In the case of sleep terrors and somnambulism, medical treatment or specialized sleep specialists may be needed if the condition is causing functional impairment and refractory to behavioral interventions.

Cognitive Behavioral Therapy (CBT)

Relaxation Techniques

Relaxation techniques are a core component of CBT and can be beneficial for many presenting problems including inattention and hyperactivity, emotion dysregulation, chronic pain, and anxiety. They can also be taught briefly in one IBH session. Diaphragmatic breathing involves focusing on taking slow, deep breaths. Deep breathing can be tailored using child-friendly approaches, where they might imagine blowing up a balloon or smelling a flower. Progressive muscle relaxation (PMR) involves systematically tensing and then relaxing muscle groups throughout the body to induce a state of deep relaxation. PMR can be adapted into playful games or activities, engaging children in a fun and interactive way while teaching them to recognize and release tension in their bodies. Incorporating elements of play, creativity, and storytelling into these techniques helps make them accessible and engaging for pediatric patients. Relaxation techniques have been found to decrease levels of stress and anxiety and decrease the severity and frequency of chronic pain among pediatric patients [25, 26].

Mood and Anxiety-Related Disorders

CBT is recommended for children and adolescents experiencing anxiety or depression and has shown effectiveness in decreasing depressive and anxiety-related symptoms as part of IBH [26–29]. Components of CBT include exposure, behavioral activation, and cognitive intervention. Solution-focused brief therapy may also be helpful in reliving current stressors that are contributing to depression or anxiety [27].

Psychoeducation in CBT involves addressing the relationship between thoughts, feelings, and behaviors and the role of avoidance in the reinforcement of behavior [30]. The BHC can also introduce relaxation strategies, as described in detail previously, to employ when the child experiences emotion dysregulation or anxiety-related thoughts.

Mood tracking is recommended to determine how engaging in different activities influences mood and, in turn, behavior. Following mood tracking, patients should engage in behavioral activation, which involves increasing participation in activities determined to improve mood, based on mood tracking. This can be done through scheduling time for these activities and engaging in the activities regardless of mood at the time. Exposure for anxiety involves controlled and gradual exposure to previously avoided stimuli or situations [29]. This involves creating a hierarchy of fears, from least to most distressing, and supporting and encouraging children to participate in activities just beyond their comfort level, working through their hierarchy. It also involves praising their ability to handle challenges and helping the child acknowledge the decreased distress from exposure to feared stimuli.

Cognitive restructuring is the other component of CBT for mood disorders and involves investigating and challenging automatic thoughts and cognitive distortions [29]. The first step is identifying unhelpful thinking, often using a thought record [31]. The thought record then aids the patient in challenging the unhelpful thought by questioning the evidence for and against the thought. For younger children, this can be done using the creation of "worry monsters" to create cognitive defusion from anxiety-related thoughts.

Separation anxiety disorder (SAD) is the most frequently diagnosed anxiety disorder in children and accounts for many anxiety referrals in pediatric settings [32]. Separation anxiety is a normal experience in young children; however, this behavior reaches diagnostic criteria if it is no longer appropriate given their developmental level or age [33]. This anxiety can also be exacerbated by parenting behaviors. Therefore, intervention often involves parental behavioral training and/or CBT depending on the age of the child. CBT has been shown to be effective in treating SAD or other anxiety disorders in children over the age of 7 [34–36]. However, children younger than 7 years old may benefit from parent-focused intervention, often in the form of parent management training and employing strategies like creating a consistent routine with preparation for separations. This may include discussing with the child what the separation will look like prior to separation, then leaving and returning from the separation on time to reinforce the child's understanding that they will be reliable.

Patients with severe depression or suicide ideation should be referred to long-term or specialized services. The role of the BHC may be to engage in safety planning with patients with safety risks before referring them for additional services. Referrals should be made for those with severe OCD, phobias, or other complex anxiety-related disorders as well.

Nightmares

Commonly, children's nightmares revolve around survival, security, or physical integrity. Reassurance may alleviate the child's source of stress. Additional interventions include image rehearsal therapy (IRT), a subtype of CBT that focuses on nightmares, which can be adapted for use in IBH settings. IRT invites the child to write or draw their dream. They then imagine themselves acting differently, effectively changing the narrative of the nightmare. This process encourages the child to embrace action, rather than flight, in the new narrative. The child draws or writes these alterations and is urged to repeat the process consistently at home [37].

Chronic Pain

CBT can also be used to treat chronic and acute pain in primary care settings [38]. CBT for chronic pain involves tracking of pain and engagement in activities despite pain, to the extent that they are safe given medical guidelines. This often involves activity pacing as indicated by pain and medical restrictions. It also involves teaching the patient coping and relaxation techniques like diaphragmatic breathing and PMR and skills to challenge negative thoughts. CBT has been found to lead to higher quality of life and better coping skills in children and adolescents with Crohn's disease or ulcerative colitis [39]. Research has also shown that CBT was associated with improved functioning in children with fibromyalgia [40]. Reductions in pain have also been found in children with chronic abdominal pain and chronic headaches who participated in CBT [41, 42].

Outcomes and Equity

In addition to treatment outcomes specific to presenting problems, cognitive and behavioral intervention as part of IBH services has been shown to correlate with general health and mental health outcomes as well. Global mental health functioning, measured by the Behavioral Health Measure (BHM), a 20-item self-report measure, was shown to improve in patients who received IBH services, even in those with severe levels or baseline distress [43–45]. These gains were maintained for an average of 2 years following treatment [45]. Therapeutic alliance, as measured by the Therapeutic Bond Scale, was also found to be greater than that of session four or five of outpatient mental health treatment [44].

Behavioral and cognitive interventions are effective front-line approaches to many mental health problems. However, access to mental health services can be limited for many individuals. By introducing and continuing to expand these interventions to the primary care setting through IBH, more children and families can access these services.

References

1. Talen MR, Burke Valeras A, editors. Integrated behavioral health in primary care: evaluating the evidence, identifying the essentials [Internet]. New York: Springer New York; 2013. [cited 2024 Jun 7]. Available from: https://link.springer.com/10.1007/978-1-4614-6889-9.
2. Trafalis S, Giannini C, Joves J, Portera S, Toyama H, Mehta A, et al. A pediatrician-friendly review of three common behavioral health screeners in pediatric practice: findings and recommendations. Pediatr Investig. 2021;5(1):58–64.
3. Morris N, Knight RM, Bruni T, Sayers L, Drayton A. Feeding disorders. Child Adolesc Psychiatr Clin N Am. 2017;26(3):571–86.

4. Rowell K, McGlothlin J. Helping your child with extreme picky eating: a step-by-step guide for overcoming selective eating, food aversion, and feeding disorders. Oakland: New Harbinger Publications; 2015.
5. Kazdin AE. Parent management training: treatment for oppositional, aggressive, and antisocial behavior in children and adolescents. Fam Ther. 2006;33(3):180.
6. Patterson GR, Dishion TJ, Chamberlain P. Outcomes and methodological issues relating to treatment of antisocial children. In: Giles TR, editor. Handbook of effective psychotherapy [Internet]. Boston: Springer US; 1993 [cited 2024 May 1]. p. 43–88. Available from: http://link.springer.com/10.1007/978-1-4615-2914-9_3.
7. Gomez D, Bridges AJ, Andrews AR, Cavell TA, Pastrana FA, Gregus SJ, et al. Delivering parent management training in an integrated primary care setting: description and preliminary outcome data. Cogn Behav Pract [Internet] 2014 [cited 2024 Jun 10];21(3):296–309. Available from: https://linkinghub.elsevier.com/retrieve/pii/S1077722914000455.
8. HealthyChildren.org [Internet]. [cited 2024 Apr 30]. Potty training. Available from: https://www.healthychildren.org/English/ages-stages/toddler/toilet-training/Pages/default.aspx?_gl=1.
9. Stadtler AC, Gorski PA, Brazelton TB. Toilet training methods, clinical interventions, and recommendations. Pediatrics. 1999;103(Supplement_3):1359–61.
10. Turner TL, Matlock MK. Patient education: toilet training (Beyond the Basics) – UpToDate [Internet]. [cited 2024 May 6]. Available from: https://www.uptodate.com/contents/toilet-training-beyond-the-basics/print.
11. Caldwell PH, Nankivell G, Sureshkumar P. Simple behavioural interventions for nocturnal enuresis in children. Cochrane Incontinence Group, editor. Cochrane Database Syst Rev [Internet]. 2013 [cited 2024 Apr 30]. Available from: https://doi.wiley.com/10.1002/14651858.CD003637.pub3.
12. Tu ND, Baskin. Nocturnal enuresis in children: management – UpToDate [Internet]. [cited 2024 May 6]. Available from: https://www.uptodate.com/contents/nocturnal-enuresis-in-children-management?search=nocturnal%20enuresis%20treatment&source=search_result&selectedTitle=1~39&usage_type=default&display_rank=1#H602906787.
13. Friman PC, Schmitt BD. Thumb sucking: pediatricians' guidelines. Clin Pediatr (Phila). 1989;28(10):438–40.
14. Bruni TP, Tennant K, Lancaster BM. Habit reversal training (HRT) in a pediatric primary care setting. Behav Anal Res Pract. 2019;19(1):39–46.
15. Nasir A, Nasir L. Counseling on early childhood concerns: sleep issues, thumb-sucking, picky eating, school readiness, and oral health. Am Fam Physician. 2015;92(4):274–8.
16. Rana M, Riffo Allende C, Mesa Latorre T, Rosso Astorga K, Torres AR. Sueño en los ninos: fisiología y actualizacion de los últimos conocimientos [Sleep in children: physiology and update of a literature review]. Medicina (B Aires). 2019;79(Suppl 3):25–8.
17. Carter KA, Hathaway NE, Lettieri CF. Common sleep disorders in children. Am Fam Physician. 2014;89(5):368–77.
18. Dietch JR, Taylor DJ, Pruiksma K, et al. The Nightmare Disorder Index: development and initial validation in a sample of nurses. Sleep. 2021;44(5):zsaa254. https://doi.org/10.1093/sleep/zsaa254.
19. Irish LA, Kline CE, Gunn HE, Buysse DJ, Hall MH. The role of sleep hygiene in promoting public health: a review of empirical evidence. Sleep Med Rev. 2015;22:23–36. https://doi.org/10.1016/j.smrv.2014.10.001.
20. Hershner S, Shaikh I, editors. Healthy sleep habits AASM: sleep education April 2, 2021. Accessed 29 April 2024. https://sleepeducation.org/healthy-sleep/healthy-sleep-habits/.
21. Frank NC, Spirito A, Stark L, Owens-Stively J. The use of scheduled awakenings to eliminate childhood sleepwalking. J Pediatr Psychol. 1997;22(3):345–53. https://doi.org/10.1093/jpepsy/22.3.345.

22. Meltzer L, Crabtree V. Scheduled awakenings for disorders of arousal (Parasomnias). In: Pediatric sleep problems: a clinician's guide to behavioral interventions. American Psychological Association; 2015.
23. Zergham AS, Chauhan Z. Somnambulism. [Updated 2023 Jan 9]. In: StatPearls [Internet]. Treasure Island: StatPearls Publishing; 2024. Available from: https://www.ncbi.nlm.nih.gov/books/NBK559001/.
24. Leung AKC, Leung AAM, Wong AHC, Hon KL. Sleep terrors: an updated review. Curr Pediatr Rev. 2020;16(3):176–82. https://doi.org/10.2174/1573396315666191014152136.
25. Eccleston C, Morley S, Williams A, Yorke L, Mastroyannopoulou K. Systematic review of randomized controlled trials of psychological therapy for chronic pain in children and adolescents, with a subset meta-analysis of pain relief. Pain. 2002;99(1):157–65.
26. Holden E. Empirically supported treatments in pediatric psychology: recurrent pediatric headache. J Pediatr Psychol. 1999;24(2):91–109.
27. Bogucki OE, Craner JR, Berg SL, Wolsey MK, Miller SJ, Smyth KT, et al. Cognitive behavioral therapy for anxiety disorders: outcomes from a multi-state, multi-site primary care practice. J Anxiety Disord. 2021;78:102345.
28. Bogucki OE, Craner JR, Berg SL, Miller SJ, Wolsey MK, Smyth KT, et al. Cognitive behavioral therapy for depressive disorders: outcomes from a multi-state, multi-site primary care practice. J Affect Disord. 2021;294:745–52.
29. Maragakis A, O'Donohue WT, editors. Principle-based stepped care and brief psychotherapy for integrated care settings [Internet]. Cham: Springer International Publishing; 2018. [cited 2024 May 6]. Available from: http://link.springer.com/10.1007/978-3-319-70539-21.
30. Sawchuk CN, Craner JR, Berg SL, Smyth K, Mack J, Glader M, et al. Initial outcomes of a real-world multi-site primary care psychotherapy program. Gen Hosp Psychiatry. 2018;54:5–11.
31. Cully JA, Dawson DB, Hamer J, Tharp AT. A provider's guide to brief cognitive behavioral therapy. Department of Veterans Affairs South Central MIRECC; 2020.
32. Cartwright-Hatton S, McNicol K, Doubleday E. Anxiety in a neglected population: prevalence of anxiety disorders in pre-adolescent children. Clin Psychol Rev. 2006;26(7):817–33.
33. Ehrenreich JT, Santucci LC, Weiner CL. Separation anxiety disorder in youth: phenomenology, assessment, and treatment. Psicol Conductual. 2008;16(3):389–412.
34. Barrett PM, Dadds MR, Rapee RM. Family treatment of childhood anxiety: a controlled trial. J Consult Clin Psychol. 1996;64(2):333–42.
35. Kendall PC. Treating anxiety disorders in children: results of a randomized clinical trial. J Consult Clin Psychol. 1994;62(1):100–10.
36. Kendall PC, Flannery-Schroeder E, Panichelli-Mindel SM, Southam-Gerow M, Henin A, Warman M. Therapy for youths with anxiety disorders: a second randomized clinical trial. J Consult Clin Psychol. 1997;65(3):366–80.
37. Gill P, Fraser E, Tran TTD, et al. Psychosocial treatments for nightmares in adults and children: a systematic review. BMC Psychiatry. 2023;23(1):283. Published 2023 Apr 21. https://doi.org/10.1186/s12888-023-04703-1.
38. Steele RG, Roberts MC, editors. Handbook of evidence-based therapies for children and adolescents: bridging science and practice [Internet]. Cham: Springer International Publishing; 2020. [cited 2024 May 6]. (Issues in Clinical Child Psychology). Available from: https://link.springer.com/10.1007/978-3-030-44226-2.
39. Levy RL, Van Tilburg MAL, Langer SL, Romano JM, Walker LS, Mancl LA, et al. Effects of a cognitive behavioral therapy intervention trial to improve disease outcomes in children with inflammatory bowel disease. Inflamm Bowel Dis. 2016;22(9):2134–48.
40. Kashikar-Zuck S, Ting TV, Arnold LM, Bean J, Powers SW, Graham TB, et al. Cognitive behavioral therapy for the treatment of juvenile fibromyalgia: a multisite, single-blind, randomized, controlled clinical trial. Arthritis Rheum. 2012;64(1):297–305.
41. Fisher E, Law E, Dudeney J, Palermo TM, Stewart G, Eccleston C. Psychological therapies for the management of chronic and recurrent pain in children and adolescents. Cochrane Pain, Palliative and Supportive Care Group, editor. Cochrane Database Syst Rev [Internet].

2018 [cited 2024 May 6];2020(10). Available from: http://doi.wiley.com/10.1002/14651858.CD003968.pub5.

42. Huang X, Jia N, Zhang Y, Hao Y, Xiao F, Sun C, et al. Effect of cognitive-behavior therapy for children with functional abdominal pain: a meta-analysis. BMC Gastroenterol. 2024;24(1):62.
43. Bryan CJ, Corso ML, Corso KA, Morrow CE, Kanzler KE, Ray-Sannerud B. Severity of mental health impairment and trajectories of improvement in an integrated primary care clinic. J Consult Clin Psychol. 2012;80(3):396–403.
44. Corso KA, Bryan CJ, Corso ML, Kanzler KE, Houghton DC, Ray-Sannerud B, et al. Therapeutic alliance and treatment outcome in the primary care behavioral health model. Fam Syst Health. 2012;30(2):87–100.
45. Ray-Sannerud BN, Dolan DC, Morrow CE, Corso KA, Kanzler KE, Corso ML, et al. Longitudinal outcomes after brief behavioral health intervention in an integrated primary care clinic. Fam Syst Health. 2012;30(1):60–71.

Chapter 4
Intersectionality Between Social, Behavioral, and Physical Health

Roger W. Apple and Summer Chahin

Introduction

Integrated behavioral health (IBH) services have steadily been increasing in pediatric primary care helping to effectively respond to mental health concerns. Social, behavioral, and physical health do not function in isolation; rather function in complex dynamics. Understanding such complexity can be greatly facilitated by utilizing IBH services in pediatric primary care. Additionally, the role of integrated behavioral health services on outcomes (social, behavioral, and physical health) will be explored.

R. W. Apple (✉)
Pediatric and Adolescent Medicine, Western Michigan University, Homer Stryker M.D. School of Medicine, Kalamazoo, MI, USA
e-mail: roger.apple@wmed.edu

S. Chahin
Homer Stryker MD School of Medicine, Western Michigan University, Kalamazoo, MI, USA
e-mail: summer.chahin@wmed.edu

R. W. Apple et al. (eds.), *Using Integrated Behavioral Health in Pediatric Practice*, https://doi.org/10.1007/978-3-031-85784-3_4

Intersectionality (Social, Behavioral, Physical)

Bronfenbrenner's Ecological Systems Theory and the Assessment of Adverse Childhood Experiences (ACEs)

Bronfenbrenner's Ecological Systems Theory

Bronfenbrenner's Ecological Systems Theory offers a comprehensive framework for understanding human development, emphasizing the importance of the various environmental contexts in which individuals grow. According to Bronfenbrenner, development is influenced by a series of nested structures, each interacting with one another [1].

1. Microsystem: The immediate environment where a child has direct interactions, such as family, school, peers, and neighborhood. These are the closest relationships and settings that directly impact the child [2].
2. Meso system: The interconnections between different microsystems, like the relationship between a child's home life and school experiences. A supportive mesosystem can enhance a child's development, while conflicting connections can pose challenges [2].
3. Exosystem: The larger social system in which the child doesn't function directly, but which still impacts their development. Examples include parents' workplaces, extended family, and community services. These systems impact the child indirectly through their influence on the microsystem [2].
4. Macrosystem: The broad cultural values, laws, customs, and resources that influence an individual's development. These elements shape the child's broader environment and influence the functioning of all the other systems [2].
5. Chronosystems: The dimension of time, which considers the life events and transitions over time that impact the child's development. This could include significant life events like parental divorce, economic changes, or technological advancements [2].

Bronfenbrenner's model highlights how a child's environment is complex and multi-layered, with each layer influencing the others. Understanding these interactions is crucial for comprehensively assessing a child's development.

Assessment of Adverse Childhood Experiences (ACESs)

Adverse childhood experiences (ACEs) refer to potentially traumatic events that occur in childhood, such as abuse, neglect, or household dysfunction (e.g., domestic violence, parental substance abuse). These experiences can have profound, long-lasting effects on a child's development, influencing their physical, emotional, and mental health [3].

When assessing ACEs, it's essential to apply Bronfenbrenner's model to fully grasp the context in which these experiences occur:

1. Microsystem: ACEs often occur within the microsystem, directly impacting the child's day-to-day environment. For example, experiences of abuse or neglect within the family directly impact the child's development. Interventions at this level focus on strengthening the immediate environment, such as improving parenting practices or providing direct support to the child [4].
2. Mesosystem: The connections between the child's immediate environments can either mitigate or exacerbate the impact of ACEs. For instance, a strong, supportive school environment may help buffer the negative impacts of a dysfunctional home life. Conversely, negative interactions between home and school, such as lack of communication or understanding, can worsen the impact of ACEs [4].
3. Exosystem: Factors like parental stress due to job loss or lack of social support can indirectly lead to or exacerbate ACEs. Addressing these external pressures, such as through community programs or support services, can reduce the likelihood of ACEs occurring [4].
4. Macrosystem: Cultural attitudes, policies, and societal norms play a significant role in either perpetuating or preventing ACEs. For example, societal stigmas around mental health may prevent families from seeking help, while robust child protection laws and social safety nets can mitigate the prevalence and impacts of ACEs [4].
5. Chronosystem: The timing and duration of ACEs, as well as changes in societal or family structure over time, are critical in understanding their impact, For example, the long-term impact of chronic poverty or the impact of societal changes such as the Covid-19 pandemic can influence the development and well-being of children who have experienced ACEs [4].

By integrating Bronfenbrenner's Ecological Systems Theory with the assessment of ACEs, practitioners can better understand the multi-faceted nature of trauma in childhood and develop more effective informed interventions. This holistic approach emphasizes that addressing the root causes and broader environmental factors is crucial in mitigating the long-term impacts of ACEs on a child's development [5].

The human experience can be intricate and complicated. The intersectionality of behavior, social circumstances, and physical conditions creates a deep multifactorial reality that is often challenging to separate into its individual components. Understanding how these elements interact is imperative for a comprehensive analysis of the individual and collective experience. As providers, we are at times presented with complicated knots of intertwining strings that we must parse out, but to start the process of unraveling this knot we must better understand how these various factors intertwine and lead to such challenging circumstances.

The Interplay of Behavior, Social Dynamics, and Physical Conditions

Behavior, social factors, and physical health are not isolated entities but are deeply interwoven. This intersectionality means that changes or issues in one domain often ripple through the others, creating a dynamic of interplay that influences overall well-being [6]. For example, consider the impact of chronic illness on an individual's behavior. Chronic conditions can limit mobility and daily functioning, which then impacts behavioral patterns such as activity levels, social interactions, and mental health.

In terms of the social experience, the stigma associated with chronic illness can amplify feelings of isolation and impact self-esteem [7]. For example, individuals with visible disabilities might face societal prejudices that influence their self-perception and social opportunities. This stigma can lead to avoidance of social situations, further compounding feelings of loneliness and behavioral withdrawal.

In regard to physical conditions and functioning, some individuals will develop specific behaviors as a result of their physical functioning and circumstances [8]. For example, individuals with physical disabilities, chronic conditions, or invisible disabilities might start engaging in certain behaviors to compensate for the challenges they experience and may adopt new methods for engagement in play and other social situations. Furthermore, these behaviors can certainly influence social interactions, potentially positively or negatively.

Social Drivers of Behavior and Health

Social determinants such as social support, the neighborhood one lives in, access to healthcare, and education all play a role in shaping behavior and physical health. Individuals with poor access to healthcare can often end up with undiagnosed or poorly managed health conditions. The lack of access to healthcare creates a cycle where poor health limits economic opportunities, which further exacerbates social and behavioral challenges. Researchers have found that a family's socioeconomic status (SES) impacts health status and outcomes over time. Specifically, a youth's family SES influences and predicts their health status into early adulthood [9].

Educational attainment also plays a significant role in intersectionality where higher levels of education are often associated with better health literacy, which influences health behaviors and access to resources [10]. On the opposite end of this spectrum, low educational attainment can lead to misunderstandings about health management and limited opportunities for preventative care, creating a snowball effect on physical, behavioral, and social outcomes.

Additionally, Heerde and colleagues [9] have found that financial insecurity, experience of adverse childhood events, LGBTQIA+ identity, and involvement within the justice system were also all associated with poor health outcomes, especially in the long term. Poor health outcomes associated with these experiences include a high risk of developing a chronic illness, perceptions of low health status, increased mental health symptoms, especially anxiety and depression, and increased diagnoses of mental health diagnoses and substance use or abuse [9].

Behavioral Responses to Physical and Social Challenges

Human behavior is an intricate and powerful phenomenon that can be highly suggestible by a person's genetics, environmental factors, and psychosocial factors. In this section, we will highlight various examples to illustrate the complexities of these interactions. One example of this is the increase in childhood obesity over the last several years [11]. A risk factor for increased risk of obesity is having behaviors that do not align with one's circadian rhythm. This can result in poor sleep and therefore may lead to poor health outcomes such as obesity and poor psychological well-being [12]. To mitigate these risks, providers should encourage families to establish consistent routines around school, sleep, and other daily activities. Children who have structured daily routines, healthy meals, regular physical activity, involvement in sports and extracurricular activities, and consistent sleep schedules are less likely to experience negative health outcomes [12]. Beyond reducing the risk of obesity, physical activity has been found to improve self-esteem in children, positively influencing their self-perception and overall health perception [13]. These factors are especially important in children who come from families with lower socioeconomic status [12].

Another example of how behavioral challenges can arise from physical health issues and social difficulties is a family seeking medical care due to concerns about their child's behavior. Children may begin to exhibit undesired behaviors (e.g., hitting, kicking, biting, scratching) as a response to stress. Stress can stem from various sources, including neighborhood violence, unstable living conditions, familial financial strain, and lack of access to healthcare, among other factors. These behaviors may be further exacerbated by parental stress, as children often observe and mimic how their caregivers cope with their own stress. Furthermore, children may develop undesirable behaviors as a response to experiencing trauma.

Role of Integrated Behavioral Health

Equity

Integrated behavioral health services play a crucial role in impacting numerous aspects of pediatric primary care. These services help reduce healthcare disparities for marginalized populations by offering earlier access to behavioral health interventions and treatment. Additionally, integrated behavioral health services in pediatric primary care can also facilitate communication among all providers and work to reduce the stigma of mental health [14].

Providing integrated behavioral health services within Federally Qualified Health Centers (FQHCs) also works to increase equitable behavioral healthcare; however, there are still gaps in integrated behavioral health equity research. A research study found that children who saw a member of the integrated behavioral health team during their first visit were more likely to attend subsequent visits. Interestingly, diagnoses of ADHD increased while psychotropic medication prescriptions decreased [15].

Equitable Care

Stepped care approaches to psychological services can be useful in triaging psychological concerns that can be easily managed by the primary care team to psychological concerns that require highly trained specialized psychologists. Integrated behavioral health (IBH) services are an ideal location to utilize a stepped care approach to psychological services allowing primary care providers to do their work while the psychologists working in IBH can triage the mental health concerns, and when appropriate, refer to a higher level of psychological service when necessary. Research is needed in such a model to study outcomes and ensure these approaches are efficient and that patients do not prematurely drop out [16].

Outcomes

The implementation of a fully integrated IBH service may be key to improving treatment outcomes for common mental health conditions, particularly depression and anxiety. Several studies have noted a significant increase in the prescription of psychotropic medications for these conditions, yet their prevalence has remained largely unchanged. This phenomenon may occur for several reasons. One possibility is that many patients with these concerns are not being properly identified, or the duration of their illness is not improving. A significant barrier to care could be the competing demands faced by treating physicians, who may lack the time, knowledge, or expertise to effectively address mental health conditions while also managing patients' medical needs. This can lead to delays in treatment. By utilizing a fully integrated IBH model, physicians can focus on the medical needs of the patient while the psychologist can focus on the psychological needs, thus improving the efficiency of the primary care clinic. RCT trials have shown that collaborative care (fully integrated) models are more effective than "usual care" models in primary care [17].

A fully integrated pediatric IBH service can help improve outcomes and access as well as reduce barriers to care. Some barriers include inadequate numbers of psychologists providing IBH services. Utilizing a fully integrated model will also help reduce the stigma of mental health treatment by illustrating that medical and mental healthcare are integrally intertwined. As previously mentioned, a stepped-care approach implemented by a fully integrated IBH model can improve access and outcomes for children and adolescents with mental and behavioral health concerns. Reimbursement policies need to be improved to support the success and sustainability of such models [18].

Outcome measurement, or lack thereof, is one of the barriers to the successful implementation of fully integrated pediatric IBH services. However, there is a position paper by the International Consortium of Health Outcomes Measurement (ICHOM), which reviewed outcome measures for children and adolescents, resulting in 70 possible outcomes and 107 measurement instruments. Seven outcome measures were suggested: the Revised Children's Anxiety and Depression Scale, the Obsessive Compulsive Inventory for Children, the Children's Revised Impact of Events Scale, the Columbia Suicide Severity Rating Scale, the KIDSCREEN-10, the Children's Global Assessment Scale, and the Child Anxiety Life Interference Scale [19].

While fully integrated IBH services are becoming increasingly available in hospitals and large medical settings. IBH services are lacking in smaller private practice settings and primary care offices. In one study, anxiety disorders were the most common in IBH followed by ADHD and then mood disorders. The study also noted significant improvement for those with anxiety and mood disorders and ADHD; however, for mood and anxiety disorders, improvement was noted between 6 and 18 weeks while ADHD showed improvement from baseline to the next follow-up. It is suggested that fully integrated care can provide effective and quality service while improving treatment capacity in primary care [20].

In another study [21], a meta-analysis was completed attempting to show that children who received "medical-behavioral" treatment had better outcomes than children receiving traditional care. Results found that children receiving interventions that included both mental health specialists and medical providers had a 73% probability of achieving better outcomes than children receiving traditional care. Additionally, other mental health treatment modalities were found to have empirical support including Triple P, Incredible Years, interpersonal therapy, guideline medication protocols, and CBT for anxiety and somatic concerns.

Access

Access to behavioral health services can be improved by adding Integrated Behavioral Health services into pediatric primary care. In one study a Behavioral Health Integration Program (BHIP) was used and it was found that utilizing an integrated behavioral health service with pediatric primary care increases access to BH services, improves provider confidence, and works to avoid significant cost increases [22]. Utilizing integrated behavioral health services in pediatric primary care allows for earlier access to behavioral health services than if referred to an outside location. This is critical as many referrals to other locations often have high no-show rates. Additionally, offering a version of integrated behavioral health services within our school systems could allow access for children who would otherwise never receive any behavioral resources due to numerous factors such as lack of transportation or caregivers' work schedules, which are unable to accommodate additional commitments outside of the school day.

Partnerships

Forming partnerships beyond the primary care setting can promote health equity for individuals who may not have access to integrated behavioral health in primary care while also improving overall healthcare outcomes. For example, externalizing behaviors can be addressed within the school system through programs similar to fully integrated IBH services in primary care. Collaborating with willing school systems presents an opportunity to expand access to healthcare services, including mental and behavioral health support, ensuring that more children receive the care they need [23].

Implementation

Planning for IBH in pediatric primary care should be strategically considered and thoughtfully planned for best integration. It has been shown that combining physical and mental healthcare in one setting results in improved care and is more cost effective; however, most healthcare sites fail to strategically plan for this integration or establish clear measurement strategies. It is recommended that organizations develop a logic model that includes all relevant components to guide implementation. Results from previous studies indicate a high level of satisfaction among primary care providers and relatively seamless integration into practice after two years. This study serves as a valuable template for others looking to implement similar models [24].

Conclusion

The vision for the future is that IBH in pediatric primary care will continue to expand and become a fully accepted, standard component of patient care. Recognizing the essential role IBH plays in helping the entire medical team understand the complex intersection of social, behavioral, and physical health conditions will be key to its ongoing success. A strong partnership between IBH and pediatric primary care will help reduce the stigma surrounding mental illness, promote equitable care, improve treatment outcomes, enhance access to services, and foster valuable collaborations. Finally, for those in positions to advocate for and transform pediatric primary care settings to fully integrate IBH services, it is critical to make your voices heard. Organizations that are willing to listen and implement these changes will have the most to gain in improving overall healthcare delivery.

Acknowledgments The authors would like to acknowledge medical student Jeff Nosek for his assistance with the literature search for this chapter.

References

1. Bronfenbrenner U. Toward an experimental ecology of human development. Am Psychol. 1977;32(7):513–31.
2. Crawford M. Ecological systems theory: exploring the development of the theoretical framework as conceived by Bronfenbrenner. J Public Health Issues Pract. 2020;4(2)
3. Shonkoff JP, Slopen N, Williams DR. Early childhood adversity, toxic stress, and the impacts of racism on the foundations of health. Annu Rev Public Health. 2021;42(1):115–34.
4. Lopez M, Ruiz MO, Rovnaghi CR, Tam GKY, Hiscox J, Gotlib IH, et al. The social ecology of childhood and early life adversity. Pediatr Res. 2021;89(2):353–67.
5. Meléndez Guevara AM, Cottam S, Wall C, Lindstrom JS. Expanding ACES in child and family service systems: incorporating context and resilience. Child Prot Pract. 2024;3:100065.
6. Lopez N, Gadsden VL. Health inequities, social determinants, and intersectionality. NAM Perspect. 2016;6(12)
7. Iovino P, Vellone E, Cedrone N, Riegel B. A middle-range theory of social isolation in chronic illness. Int J Environ Res Public Health. 2023;20(6):4940.
8. Short SE, Mollborn S. Social determinants and health behaviors: conceptual frames and empirical advances. Curr Opin Psychol. 2015;5:78–84.
9. Heerde JA, Merrin GJ, Le VT, Toumbourou JW, Bailey JA. Health of young adults experiencing social marginalization and vulnerability: a cross-national longitudinal study. Int J Environ Res Public Health. 2023;20(3):1711.
10. Jansen T, Rademakers J, Waverijn G, Verheij R, Osborne R, Heijmans M. The role of health literacy in explaining the association between educational attainment and the use of out-of-hours primary care services in chronically ill people: a survey study. BMC Health Serv Res. 2018;18(1):394.
11. U.S. Centers for Disease Control and Prevention. Childhood Obesity Facts. 2024.
12. Hart CN, Jelalian E, Raynor HA. Behavioral and social routines and biological rhythms in prevention and treatment of pediatric obesity. Am Psychol. 2020;75(2):152–62.
13. Lubans D, Richards J, Hillman C. Physical activity for cognitive and mental health in youth: a systematic review of mechanisms [Internet]. Rev Article Pediatr. 2016;138. Available from: http://publications.aap.org/pediatrics/article-pdf/138/3/e20161642/1094686/peds_20161642.pdf
14. Arrojo MJ, Bromberg J, Walter HJ, Vernacchio L. Pediatric primary-care integrated behavioral health: a framework for reducing inequities in behavioral health care and outcomes for children, vol. 70. Pediatr Clin N Am. W.B. Saunders; 2023. p. 775–89.
15. Sheldrick RC, Bair-Merritt MH, Durham MP, Rosenberg J, Tamene M, Bonacci C, et al. Integrating pediatric universal behavioral health care at federally qualified health centers. Pediatrics. 2022;149(4)
16. Richards DA. Stepped care: a method to deliver increased access to psychological therapies [Internet]. Can J Psychiatry. 2012;57. Available from: www.TheCJP.ca
17. Sunderji N, Kurdyak PA, Sockalingam S, Mulsant BH. Can collaborative care cure the mediocrity of usual care for common mental disorders? Can J Psychiatry. Sage. 2018;63:427–31.

18. Campo JV, Geist R, Kolko DJ. Integration of pediatric behavioral health services in primary care: improving access and outcomes with collaborative care. Can J Psychiatry. Sage. 2018;63:432–8.
19. Krause KR, Chung S, Adewuya AO, Albano AM, Babins-Wagner R, Birkinshaw L, et al. International consensus on a standard set of outcome measures for child and youth anxiety, depression, obsessive-compulsive disorder, and post-traumatic stress disorder [Internet]. 2021;8. Available from: www.thelancet.com/psychiatry
20. Parkhurst JT, Garcia-Goetting C, Peist E, Ballard R, Romba C, Lavigne JV. Pediatric collaborative care outcomes in a regional model. Front Psychiatry [Internet]. 2023;14:1252505. Available from: http://www.ncbi.nlm.nih.gov/pubmed/38076703
21. Asarnow JR, Rozenman M, Wiblin J, Zeltzer L. Integrated medical-behavioral care compared with usual primary care for child and adolescent behavioral health: a metaanalysis. JAMA Pediatr. 2015;169(10):929–37.
22. Walter HJ, Vernacchio L, Trudell EK, Bromberg J, Goodman E, Barton J, et al. Five-year outcomes of behavioral health integration in pediatric primary care. Pediatrics. 2019;144(1)
23. Rungan S, Gardner S, Liu HM, Woolfenden S, Smith-Merry J, Eastwood J. Ngaramadhi space: an integrated, multisector model of care for students experiencing problematic externalising behaviour, Int J Integr Care [Internet]. 2023;23(4):19. Available from: http://www.ncbi.nlm.nih.gov/pubmed/38107833
24. Mautone JA, Wolk CB, Cidav Z, Davis MF, Young JF. Strategic implementation planning for integrated behavioral health services in pediatric primary care. Implement Res Pract. 2021;2:263348952098755.

Chapter 5
Models of Change for Behavioral and Health Disorders

Katherine Tennant Beenen, Samantha L. Hahn, and Ariana L. Ross Schneiderhan

Introduction

Under the Primary Care Behavioral Health Model [1], psychologists or other licensed mental health providers in integrated behavioral health (IBH) settings are referred to as Behavioral Health Consultants (BHCs). BHCs help patients address a myriad of health concerns. These concerns extend beyond mental health; BHCs also play a crucial role in facilitating patients' behavioral changes, including the adoption of new habits to enhance their physical well-being. In a typical day within a pediatric primary care IBH setting, a BHC may provide interventions for presenting concerns as varied as the management of a chronic medical condition, sleep disturbances, parent behavioral management, management of elimination disorders, and brief cognitive-behavioral therapy.

As exemplified above, the primary goal of IBH and the defining role of the BHC is to help patients improve their overall well-being [2]. Well-being, which in this chapter will be broadly inclusive of mental and physical health, is affected by individual- and systems-level factors. BHCs who understand the micro- and macro-level influences on health-related behaviors and outcomes are well positioned to

K. T. Beenen (✉)
Department of Pediatric and Adolescent Medicine, Western Michigan University Homer Stryker MD School of Medicine, Kalamazoo, MI, USA
e-mail: katherine.beenen@wmed.edu

S. L. Hahn
Central Michigan University College of Medicine, Mount Pleasant, MI, USA
e-mail: hahn4sl@cmich.edu

A. L. Ross Schneiderhan
Western Michigan University Homer Stryker MD School of Medicine, Kalamazoo, MI, USA
e-mail: ariana.schneiderhan@wmed.edu

R. W. Apple et al. (eds.), *Using Integrated Behavioral Health in Pediatric Practice*, https://doi.org/10.1007/978-3-031-85784-3_5

help their patients engage in behavior change to enhance their overall health and well-being.

There are several hypotheses about factors that influence health-related behaviors, which are collectively called models of change. Each model considers environmental factors (e.g., cultural and societal norms) and individual factors (e.g., knowledge, attitudes, and beliefs) to varying degrees. One specific model that will be examined in detail and provide an overarching framework for the chapter is the socioecological model. This model emphasizes how addressing modifiable distal and proximal factors can change individual behavior, emphasizing systemic change while maintaining individual agency.

This chapter provides an overview of factors that affect the uptake of health-related behaviors at both the population and individual levels. It will start by placing the behaviors within the framework of the socioecological model, emphasizing the role of population health in creating behavior change, before moving into hypotheses of health-related behavior within individuals. Within all the covered models, the roles of IBH and BHCs will be highlighted. Two case vignettes will demonstrate the application of the models in the clinical setting to change parent and patient behaviors.

Applying a Socioecological Lens to Behavior Change

The socioecological model provides a comprehensive framework for understanding complex health issues. The primary tenet of this model is that an individual's health status is the product of several interacting spheres of influence (Fig. 5.1). These spheres include macro- and micro-level influences on individual behavior and health outcomes [3]. In this framework, health-related behaviors are impacted by (1) public policy, including local, state, and federal laws and policies that regulate or support health behaviors, along with funding allocated toward health promotion and social equity; (2) community factors, including an individual's built environment, resources, social networks, norms, and standards in the broader community; (3) institutional and organizational factors, including rules, regulations, policies, and informal structures within institutions that limit or encourage behaviors; (4) interpersonal factors, including social support systems such as family, peers, and friends that shape social identity and support; and (5) interpersonal or individual factors, including an individual's demographic characteristics as well as their knowledge, attitudes, and skills.

The socioecological model's framework may effectively inform health promotion interventions [3]. Interventions at higher levels of the model generate downstream effects, enhancing the feasibility and sustainability of changes at the individual level. This top-down approach creates an environment that supports and reinforces these changes over time. By addressing the upstream determinants of health, such interventions can overcome barriers that might otherwise impede individual efforts, making it easier for people to adopt and maintain healthier behaviors,

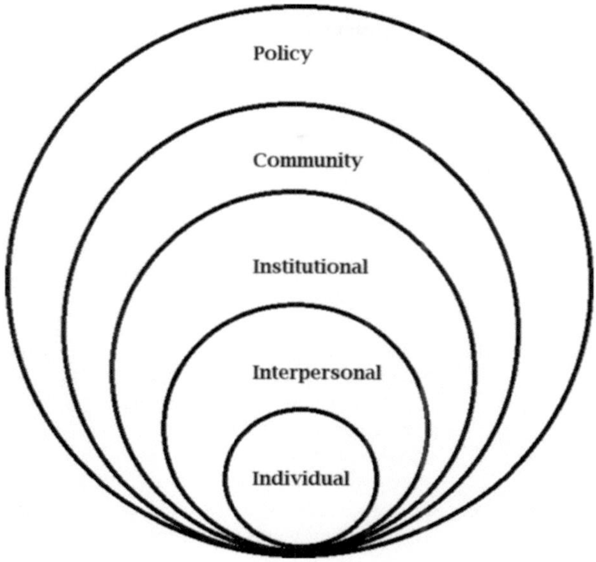

Fig. 5.1 The socioecological model of health promotion. (Adapted from McLeroy et al. [3])

leading to significant and lasting improvements in population health [4, 5]. Enacting higher-level interventions to benefit a greater number of individuals is the goal of public health interventions, which will be touched upon briefly in the next section.

To illustrate a few interventions at the policy level, the Affordable Care Act and the Mental Health Parity and Addiction Equity Act have both expanded coverage of behavioral health conditions through policies requiring parity between behavioral health and medical benefits [6]. In addition, the United States Department of Health and Human Services has outlined several policies to improve access to behavioral health through expansion into primary care settings, including recruitment, training, and support of a diverse behavioral health workforce [7]. The Centers for Medicare & Medicaid Services' update of the Physician Fee Schedule includes payment for behavioral health integration through the inclusion of services provided by clinical psychologists and clinical social workers as part of a primary care team [8, 9].

Through careful application to the socioecological model, it may be demonstrated that the promotion of parity and integration at the higher levels, and the practice of IBH at the lower levels, benefits individual patients (Table 5.1). Interventions at higher levels of influence support the uptake and implementation of IBH, and at lower levels, the work of BHCs impacts institutional and interpersonal outcomes as well as individual health outcomes through tailored interventions.

Patients benefit when BHCs and other healthcare providers consider, and when possible, address, the higher-level influences that affect their health-related behaviors and outcomes. This can also include consideration of the patient's community resources and built environment, for example, their accessibility to safe and convenient spaces to exercise and proximity to grocery stores. Healthcare providers may also have greater success when they consider an individual patient's familial and

Table 5.1 Applying the socioecological model to the promotion and practice of integrated behavioral health

Sphere of influence	Intervention	Example of individual-level impact
Public policy	Payment reforms, parity interventions, and policies to promote integration [6–9].	Patients at Pediatric Office A have greater access to affordable mental health resources like IBH.
Community	Integration potentially reduces the cultural stigma of mental health treatment [10] and improves access and health disparities in underserved and minoritized populations [11, 12].	At Pediatric Office B, patients are more likely to agree to a warm hand-off with a BHC when it is de-stigmatized and viewed as part of their routine care.
Institutional	Integration reduces burnout among physicians [13], reduces the siloed nature of medical care [14], and may improve pediatricians' ability to address their patients' physical and behavioral health problems [15].	Pediatricians at Pediatric Office C refer their patients to the BHC, collaborate on mutual patients, and engage in curbside consults routinely, all resulting in better patient care.
Interpersonal	In pediatric settings, BHCs often work within the family unit to influence change in the patient. IBH also improves the patient–physician relationship and results in more satisfied providers [15, 16].	A BHC at Pediatric Office D provides six sessions in behavioral parent management training to a parent–child dyad involving a 4-year-old presenting with defiance and aggression, improving their interpersonal relationship.
Individual	BHCs meet with individual patients to change knowledge, attitudes, and skills by providing consultation, psychotherapy, and/or referral.	A BHC at Pediatric Office E works with an adolescent patient to change their health-related behaviors, specifically their adherence to type 1 diabetes management.

cultural influences on the manifestation of disordered mental health symptoms and treatment utilization [17–19].

The Role of Public Health Interventions in Health-Related Behavior Change

Public, or population health, is a top-down approach to well-being, focusing on the promotion of health at the population level to create change at the individual level. The overarching goals of IBH, according to the Primary Care Behavioral Health Model, are in many ways shared with the goals of public health. Pediatric IBH may improve public health outcomes by reaching more children, removing barriers to care, and increasing access to evidence-based treatments [14]. The nature of behavioral health treatment in IBH settings is generally short-term and problem-focused. Unlike some traditional mental health treatments, BHCs do not necessarily continue to meet with individual patients through symptom resolution. This practice allows

BHCs to serve a greater number of patients within a healthcare practice. Compared to traditional models of mental health treatment, there is an emphasis on helping many individuals make meaningful small changes to their health behaviors, rather than helping a few individuals make substantial changes [20].

Behavioral health is an integral part of public health, as health behaviors are among the most readily modifiable intervention targets for disease risk and maintenance [21]. Therefore, public health interventions aimed at improving the health of vulnerable populations often target behavioral health, both directly and indirectly, including smoking cessation, seatbelt wearing, breastfeeding, dietary intake, physical activity, increasing screenings and primary care visits, and more. Public health interventions can range from population-level implementations like policies and laws, to community-level outreach efforts aimed at increasing knowledge, to individual impacts such as intervention development and improving intervention utilization.

As an example of the importance of public health interventions aimed at behavioral health, consider smoking cessation. Cigarette smoking is associated with a myriad of negative health effects, including lung cancer and cardiovascular disease [22]. Numerous public health interventions have targeted cigarette smoking and smoking cessation to prevent disease and prolong healthful lives [23]. Public health interventions centered on smoking cessation include FDA regulations (e.g., Surgeon General's warnings on cigarette packaging), laws banning cigarette smoking in public places, banning tobacco sales to minors, and increasing the age of legal purchase from 18 to 21. These policy changes then impact lower levels of the socioecological model; for example, some establishments voluntarily banned smoking, insurance providers began covering smoking cessation interventions, and societal attitudes about smoking shifted, all of which led to shifts in individual attitudes [24]. Ultimately, smoking rates decreased because interventions across all levels focused on discouraging cigarette smoking [25].

Models of Change in Practice

Public health focuses on the prevention of disease to promote long, healthful lives at both the population and individual levels. According to the Centers for Disease Control and Prevention, the five leading causes of death in the United States are cancer, unintentional injury, heart disease, stroke, and chronic lower respiratory disease [26]. Each of these conditions has modifiable behaviors, such as diet, physical activity, smoking, and seatbelt usage, as major risk factors. Among children and adolescents, medical advances in prevention, early detection, and treatment have significantly reduced mortality from infectious diseases or cancer. As a result, injuries have become the leading cause of mortality in the pediatric population. Among the top causes are motor vehicle accidents, firearm-related injuries, suffocation, drowning, and drug overdose.[1] These causes of injury have been labeled as preventable "[socioecological] phenomena" [27].

These examples serve to illustrate not only the importance of addressing modifiable behaviors in healthcare but also how imperative it is to understand how and why people change their behaviors and under what circumstances. BHCs help patients initiate and maintain health-promoting behaviors, and discontinue health-detrimental behaviors. For example, there is evidence that Healthy Steps for Young Children, a program integrating child developmental specialists into pediatric primary care, increases the rate of anticipatory guidance during well-child visits, including topics related to home safety [28].

An understanding of the mechanism by which individuals decide to change certain behaviors can guide the BHC's efforts. At times, patients may be unable to achieve behavior change, particularly as prescribed to them by healthcare providers. There may be barriers to following guidance, including patient and caregiver individual and systems factors. Counseling families on making health-related changes offers no guarantee they will. This sort of paternalistic attitude in medicine is being abandoned in favor of shared decision-making. This provides a means to incorporate patients' and caregivers' preferences into their care. Shared decision-making involves consideration of the patient's or family's own values and expertise rather than treating the provider as the only expert. This builds trust and ultimately leads to a higher likelihood of successful behavior change.

Key Definitions in the Models of Change

At the individual level, behavioral change results from a combination of motivation, information, and support [2]. With the shift toward shared decision-making, there is also greater consideration of individual patients' values, beliefs, resources, and barriers. The different models of change consider the impact of these factors to varying degrees, presenting various entry points for health-related behavior change. This chapter has already described how the models of change can be applied by BHCs in clinical settings and on a population health scale to effect healthful change. This section reviews four of the most common models of change that explain, at a more micro-level, how and why individuals change their health-related behaviors. A brief summary of each of the four models is presented in Table 5.2.

[1] Firearm-related injuries, suffocation, and drug overdose deaths include those that were unintentional and those that were deaths by suicide.

Table 5.2 Key models of change

Model	Description
Transtheoretical model	Behavior change is dependent on a person's readiness to change. Includes a series of stages a person can move between, with interventions for the provider dependent on the stage the client is in.
Health belief model	Behavior change regarding a person's health is based on that person's perceptions of the threat to their health, their susceptibility to the threat, and the benefits of and/or barriers to completing the behavior.
Theories of reasoned action and planned behavior	Behavior change is driven by a person's intention, which is impacted by their beliefs about the behavior, social pressures, and their perceived control over the change.
Social cognitive theory	Behavior change is dependent on the interrelated behaviors of the individual and of the social group, with additional influences from the individual's self-efficacy and expectations of behavior outcomes.

Transtheoretical Model

The transtheoretical model of change posits that behavior change is dependent on an individual's willingness to change, impacted by their self-efficacy and the perceived benefits and drawbacks of the specific behavior change [29]. There are five major stages of behavior change in this model: precontemplation, contemplation, preparation, action, and maintenance. Each stage is characterized by distinct cognitions and behaviors (Table 5.3). Understanding an individual's present stage of change, and their readiness to enact additional change, is important to aid them in moving from one stage to another [30]. This can be determined by a series of open-ended questions that encourage the individual to consider how they feel about the behavior in question and how ready they are to change their behavior. While the goal of healthcare professionals is typically to help the individual move forward to the next stage of behavior change, people may also regress to an earlier stage (e.g., from contemplation to precontemplation). In addition, it is common for patients to spend long periods of time in certain stages, especially precontemplation and contemplation [30]. BHCs are skilled at communicating with patients and eliciting change talk to move them closer to behaviors that align with their health goals, as highlighted in case vignette 2.

Interventions based on the transtheoretical model have been shown to support changes in various health behaviors; specifically in pediatrics, this includes increased fruit and vegetable intake [31–33], increased exercise [34, 35], moderation of weight gain in children with obesity [36], and decreased amount of fat in diets [35]. Important to working with pediatric populations, interventions may also be targeted at parents or the family as a whole, which may result in improved health behaviors [37, 38]. For example, children's food intake is largely dependent on what food is available at school and what food is purchased for them at home. A study on the child-feeding strategies of African American mothers examined their readiness to increase fruit and vegetable intake in their children. The study found that women in

Table 5.3 Stages of behavioral change in the transtheoretical model

Stage	Description	Examples
Precontemplation	The person places minimal to no value or interest in the behavior change in question.	A parent of a child with obesity does not believe there are any concerns with their child's significant amount of daily screen time.
Contemplation	The individual is considering behavior change but is ambivalent and not determined to go through with change. No preparation for behavior change has occurred.	A high schooler thinks there may be some future health consequences of vaping, but she wants to focus on her grades right now.
Preparation	The person is interested in behavior change and has started making plans to best enact change. They have started taking steps in preparation of making change.	A middle-schooler with diabetes has started reviewing his insulin schedule with his parents regularly, with the goal of soon managing his medications more independently.
Action	The person has enacted their plan and has actively changed their behavior. They are working on developing skills for later maintenance.	A teenager has stopped attending parties regularly to avoid binge drinking every weekend—They have been sober for 3 weeks.
Maintenance	The individual has developed the necessary skills, successfully achieved behavior change, and continues to identify and overcome potential barriers to behavior change. This stage is not always mentioned when discussing this model.	A preteen has increased her physical activity regularly from minimal to about 2 h of aerobic exercise weekly. After finding that she is more interested in exercising with others than alone, she joined her track club with a few friends.

later stages reported more actions taken to increase the fruit and vegetable intake of their children, including how food is prepared, having fruits and vegetables available and including them in meals, and replacing junk food with healthier options. In addition, women in the later stages were more likely to model attitudes and behaviors that encouraged children to increase fruit and vegetable intake, such as having children assist in food preparation and eating more fruits and vegetables themselves [39].

There are a few limitations to the transtheoretical model. For example, a multimodal approach may be the most beneficial for behavior change when using this model, as printed materials alone may not be sufficient to help an individual move forward in stage [40]. Additionally, while this model can be used to target families, it is designed to target individuals and does not necessarily take into account the individual's interaction with their greater community, unlike the social learning theory described later in this section. One of the most significant limitations of this model is the minimal consideration of external barriers to behavior change, whether physical, financial, or social, or any other innumerable barriers, perceived or real, to behavior change. Models of change that have these considerations as core pieces include the socioecological model described above, the health belief model, and the theory of planned behavior.

The Health Belief Model

The health belief model (HBM) is a widely applied theoretical framework for the explanation and prediction of health-related behaviors. Developed in the 1950s, the HBM's original purpose was to explain why people did not participate in disease prevention and detection programs [41]. In the years since, it has continued to evolve and remains a significant tool for understanding health behaviors and designing interventions [42]. The HBM is typically applied to explain how individuals make decisions about their health in the face of possible threats. The HBM specifically posits that individuals' engagement in health-related behaviors may be predicted by their perceived susceptibility to a condition, perceived severity of the condition, perceived benefits of engaging in the behavior, and perceived barriers to engagement. Two additional constructs, cues to action and self-efficacy, may also contribute to an individual's likelihood of engaging in health behaviors under this model [43]. As such, individuals are likely to engage in health-promoting behaviors when they perceive a health threat as severe, believe they are susceptible to it, recognize the benefits of taking action, and perceive few barriers to doing so. In addition, various environmental cues may prompt their action at a specific time or place (e.g., a sign in a pharmacy advertising the availability of the influenza vaccine), as well as the individual's perception of their own self-efficacy in making the behavior change.

The HBM has been cited frequently in the literature on help-seeking behaviors among various groups, in particular the utilization of mental health services [44–47]. It has additionally served as a framework to inform digital interventions for individuals with mental health conditions [48] and to study factors in uptake and adherence to psychotropic and substance use disorder medications [49, 50]. As highlighted in case vignette 1, the BHC may consider how the patient's or parent's beliefs about their susceptibility to developing a condition, as well as the perceived severity of the condition, may impact their behaviors. The BHC may also come to understand individual beliefs about the benefits of engaging in such a behavior and help the family troubleshoot any barriers to achieving change.

A primary limitation of the HBM is its lack of inclusion of social and emotional factors that drive behavior. Furthermore, in the years since the model's proposal, the individual constructs have been found to vary in their ability to predict behavior. Of the four original constructs, perceived benefits and barriers have been found to be the strongest predictors of behavior, whereas perceived susceptibility and severity are the weakest. It is highly likely that other factors serve as mediators and moderators of behavior unaccounted for by this model [51, 52].

Theory of Planned Behavior

The third model frequently used at an individual level for behavior change is the theory of planned behavior (TPB), which is an expansion of the original theory of reasoned action. The theory of reasoned action posits that behavioral change is the result of an individual's intention to change. Intention is, in part, influenced by an individual's attitude toward the behavior and their perception of social attitudes toward the behavior [53]. TPB adds a third influence to the intention to change, an individual's perception of their control over behavioral change, which includes their self-efficacy and perceived controllability [53]. Self-efficacy is an individual's belief about their own ability to enact change. Perceived controllability, on the other hand, is typically measured based on an individual's perceived access to means of control over the behavior [54]. Furthermore, an individual's background factors, such as personality, education, demographics, and values, contribute to their beliefs, which, in turn, contribute to their attitudes, intentions, and, ultimately, their behavior.

One of the major benefits of this model is that it places an individual's intention to change within their social and cultural context. This is especially relevant for pediatric patients, as it is often the parents who are the mechanism of change in their child's health status, prioritizing relational variables as a major influence on health outcomes. Furthermore, the focus on individuals' perception of control over their own health outcomes is an important factor in understanding their health-related behaviors.

This model has a few major limitations. A primary limitation is that intention can be a poor predictor of actual behavior, a phenomenon termed the intention–behavior gap [55, 56]. Furthermore, when applying the TPB, there is a focus on a patient's perception of their situation, without acknowledgement of the reality of the situation. In contrast to the socioecological model, this leads to the possibility of underappreciation of a patient's real-world barriers to behavioral control. For example, the TPB accounts for a patient's attitudes in their patterns of fruit and vegetable consumption, but it may not account for them living in a food desert. This is also a limitation of the other three models discussed in this section, which do not robustly address macro-level barriers.

Social Cognitive Theory

A main assumption in Social Cognitive Theory (SCT) is that behavior is dependent on the constantly evolving interactions between a person and their environment and that such interactions can be both structural and social [57]. According to this theory, three main factors drive human behavior: environmental factors (social and structural), cognitive or personal factors (knowledge, expectations, and attitudes), and behavioral factors (skills, practice, and self-efficacy). For an individual to engage in health-related behavior according to SCT, they must (1) have the basic knowledge and skills required to make the behavior change, (2) witness others successfully model the behavior, (3) have the expectation that the behavior change has value, and (4) believe that they have the ability to successfully change a behavior (self-efficacy).

Learning from the social environment is a large component of social cognitive theory. This includes learning behaviors from others and observing the outcomes of these behaviors. SCT emphasizes the importance of social learning through observation and modeling. This allows individuals to acquire new behaviors without directly experiencing the consequences themselves. Additionally, SCT recognizes the role of reinforcement in shaping behavior, suggesting that individuals are more likely to adopt and maintain behaviors that are positively reinforced by their environment.

An example of an SCT-related behavioral change tool that BHCs may help their patients employ is self-monitoring. This involves tracking a behavior targeted for change [58]. SCT posits that the awareness of engagement or disengagement in a target behavior precedes change. Self-monitoring enhances awareness of current behaviors, and along with setting realistic goals for behavior change, learning and practicing new skills, it enhances self-efficacy through progress monitoring toward a goal and tying it to an expected outcome. IBH-relevant self-monitoring applications may be incorporated into the treatment protocol for adolescents undergoing habit reversal therapy (e.g., for nail-biting), caregivers aiming to increase their use of labeled praise to reinforce appropriate behavior in their child, and youth experiencing depression who are engaged in behavioral activation and monitoring their mood and activity levels.

SCT has been applied in many primary care interventions [59], demonstrating its versatility in addressing health-related behaviors. It has been widely applied to interventions for smoking cessation, dietary changes, physical activity, and other health outcomes, with good effect [60]. However, when structural barriers exist at higher levels of the socioecological model, such as policy constraints or community-level issues, or when the behavior change goes against social norms, SCT applications can be less effective. For example, some behaviors with a perceived positive social value may have negative health outcomes (e.g., drinking alcohol). In these cases, social reinforcement may outweigh perceived health risks. Additionally, individuals frequently do not observe positive or negative outcomes of health-related behavior, given the delay between behavior change and health outcomes (e.g., dietary intake and stroke risk later in life).

Considerations for Behavior Change in Pediatric Patients

BHCs embedded in pediatric practices play a crucial role in providing comprehensive care for children and adolescents, including screening, prevention, health promotion, mental health interventions, and referral [61]. The identification and treatment needs in pediatric primary care are especially broad, considering the rapid physical, social, and mental development that occurs during childhood and adolescence. BHCs must be adept at treating the range of problems that are commonly present in pediatric primary care. This includes but is certainly not limited to, anxiety disorders, depression or other mood disorders, adjustment and coping, trauma- and stressor-related disorders, dietary intake, physical activity, chronic illness management, sleep hygiene, bedtime problems, academic, behavioral, and social problems at school, behavior therapy for ADHD, developmental concerns, somatic complaints, child discipline, picky eating, repetitive behaviors, habit reversal training, procedural distress, organizational skills training, and toileting/elimination problems. This broad scope of practice allows BHCs to offer holistic support to pediatric patients and their families, addressing both physical and mental health needs within the primary care setting.

For children and adolescents, the caregiver–child relationship is an important sphere of influence on well-being. Treatment of behavioral disorders and promotion of health-related behaviors often include consideration of caregivers' roles in shaping pediatric patients' beliefs and behaviors. Particularly for young patients, parents are the agents of behavioral change and are often the target of health-related behavioral modification. This family-centered approach acknowledges the critical role that the home environment and parental practices play in a child's behavioral and emotional development.

The role of parents and caregivers is particularly evident in the treatment of externalizing behaviors in young children, where evidence-based interventions focus on parent training [62, 63]. In behavioral parent management training, parents are taught how to encourage appropriate behaviors and discourage inappropriate ones. These programs typically cover a range of topics, including effective communication, positive reinforcement, limit setting, and implementing consistent disciplinary strategies. By delivering these interventions in pediatric primary care, BHCs can promote positive child development. This approach is especially relevant given that externalizing disorders are among the most frequently treated behavioral health concerns in pediatric populations, highlighting the importance of parent- and caregiver-based interventions for pediatric behavioral health [64].

Adolescent patients also present with unique challenges in encouraging health-related behavior changes. While the foundation of health habits arguably starts to take shape in childhood, it is in adolescence that youths start to take on more responsibility for their own healthcare, beginning the transition from parent-managed care to self-managed care. Adolescence is also a distinct developmental stage, characterized by risk-taking, peer influence, and independence-seeking. For example, common considerations among adolescents regarding their food choices include social desirability and norms, the potential impact of food on their physical appearance, and practical concerns such as convenience, cost, and taste [65]. Among adolescents with mental health concerns, important considerations for seeking treatment include stigma or other negative attitudes toward mental health, family beliefs about treatment, low mental health literacy, and autonomy, including confidentiality concerns [66].

Thus, pediatric populations may add another layer in that it is often the parent(s) or caregiver(s) who are the agents of change and to whom behavioral strategies may be directed, not the referred child themselves. However, parents or caregivers may not always be able to be included in plans for behavior change for a variety of reasons or may actually be a hindrance to behavior change. It is always best to consider on a case-by-case basis if or how parents and/or caregivers can or should be involved.

Models of Change: Case Vignettes

The following case vignettes apply different models of change to the conceptualization and management of two common presenting problems in IBH: child discipline and improved dietary intake.

Case Vignette 1: Health Belief Model and Child Discipline

A common question in pediatric primary care is how to discipline children to achieve desired behavioral changes. While losing favor among contemporary parenting practices, corporal punishment, including spanking, has been a mainstay of child discipline strategies for generations [67, 68]. Factors influencing the use of corporal punishment include cultural norms, religious beliefs, parental stress, poverty, and the belief that control over children requires spanking [69]. However, corporal punishment is associated with detrimental outcomes to child behavior and mental health, and to the parent–child relationship [70]. The HBM has been applied to interventions to reduce corporal punishment and promote the uptake of evidence-based parenting interventions [71–73], but overall, the model's application to parent discipline practices is relatively novel. The following case vignette illustrates the HBM's application to the uptake of evidence-based behavioral management strategies in an integrated setting.

Noah, a 4-year-old boy, presented to his pediatrician for his annual well-child exam. He was accompanied by his mother, Ms. Parker, who provided the history. He is a healthy child with no acute or chronic health conditions and was found to be growing and developing appropriately. When his pediatrician reviewed his behavioral screening questionnaire prior to stepping into the exam room, she noted his significant externalizing score and requested the clinic's BHC, Dr. Williams, to accompany her during this portion of Noah's visit.

Ms. Parker reported difficulty controlling Noah's behavior at home, stating he defied her instructions nearly every day. This resulted in dangerous situations on a few occasions, such as walking into the street or running away from her in parking lots. Ms. Parker said that to correct his behavior, she tried timeouts, privilege restriction, yelling, and spanking, but stated "nothing worked" to correct Noah's behavior.

She said that his behavior was a significant source of distress for herself, and endorsed significant difficulties with public outings.

Noah's pediatrician and Dr. Williams listened to his mother's concerns and provided support. Recognizing his mother's distress and how Noah's behaviors have put him in danger, Dr. Williams offered Ms. Parker a brief course of behavioral parent management training, explaining that it would help equip her with some additional tools to increase Noah's compliance and reduce his unsafe and aggressive behaviors. Ms. Parker accepted. They immediately worked together to create an initial safety plan for public outings with Noah and scheduled additional appointments.

Over the course of a few months and several more appointments, Dr. Williams reviewed strategies for encouraging appropriate behavior, such as child-directed interaction, differential attention, and labeled praise, and strategies for discouraging inappropriate behavior, such as planned ignoring and effective timeouts. After building trust and rapport with Ms. Parker, Dr. Williams also shared with her some of the research findings regarding the impact of spanking. After a few months, Ms. Parker reported significant improvement in Noah's listening and said there had been no additional incidents of him darting into the street or parking lots. She said that after reflecting and learning about the detrimental effects of spanking, she had also ceased this practice.

Viewing this case through the lens of the HBM shows how each factor—perceived severity, susceptibility, benefits, barriers, cues to action, and self-efficacy—influenced Ms. Parker's uptake of Dr. Williams' treatment recommendations (Table 5.4).

Case Vignette 2: Transtheoretical Model and Dietary Intake Intervention

BHCs are crucial partners for pediatricians in enhancing patient health. Pediatricians regularly advise families on lifestyle modifications, such as diet, exercise, and sleep. Despite the widespread dissemination of recommendations like the USDA's MyPlate graphic, knowledge and adherence to dietary guidelines vary. Changes occur when patients are ready, moving through different stages of readiness, which is central to the transtheoretical model. This model has specifically been applied to adolescent populations, including increasing fruit and vegetable intake, and has been shown to be successful in creating behavior change [74, 75]. The following is a case vignette applying this model to an adolescent patient wishing to increase her fruit and vegetable intake.

Ailani is a 16-year-old cis-gender female (she/hers). At her yearly well-child visit, her pediatrician conducted routine nutrition and activity screening. Ailani reported that she ate fruits and vegetables, "every once in a while, maybe like a can of corn with dinner sometimes or an apple at lunch at school if it's not gross, or

Table 5.4 Health belief model applied to corporal punishment

HBM factor	Application to Noah's treatment
Perceived severity	Noah's defiant actions, like running into the street despite being told to stay in the yard, often endangered him, causing great concern for Ms. Parker. This led her to seek treatment with Dr. Williams, fearing severe consequences such as Noah being struck by a vehicle. This perception increased the likelihood that Ms. Parker would consider alternative discipline methods.
Perceived susceptibility	Ms. Parker deemed her son at risk of injury due to his past behavior and did not expect immediate changes without further intervention. She acknowledged Noah's susceptibility to future dangerous behaviors, leading her to seek alternative behavior management strategies beyond spanking.
Perceived benefits	Dr. Williams and Ms. Parker discussed her views on spanking. She shared that she and her siblings were spanked, and many of her friends and family still practiced it. Dr. Williams provided nonjudgmental counsel on spanking's negative impacts. Ms. Parker was ambivalent, stating that spanking didn't harm her but acknowledging its ineffectiveness on Noah. She enjoyed using positive reinforcement and child-directed interaction, which improved their bond and increased her positive feelings toward Noah. Initially doubtful, she found these methods effectively improved Noah's behavior and continued using them.
Perceived barriers	Initially, Ms. Parker felt overwhelmed by the new strategies. She worked long hours and was not sure how she would find time for one-on-one engagement with Noah. She stumbled over some aspects of child-directed interaction, such as avoiding questions, which felt unnatural to her. She and Dr. Williams problem-solved to find time in her busy schedule and pace her uptake of the strategies. It helped that the interventions were not financially burdensome. Ms. Parker's comfort increased over time, especially after observing Dr. Williams' demonstrations.
Cues to action	Ms. Parker deliberately increased her use of labeled praise until it became habitual. She and Dr. Williams considered using environmental cues to prompt her to praise Noah's appropriate behavior, such as identifying three behaviors to praise during dinner and bedtime routines. Gradually, she found it easier to notice and praise even minor appropriate behaviors. Regular appointments with Dr. Williams kept her accountable for these changes.
Self-efficacy	Dr. Williams shored up Ms. Parker's self-efficacy through non-judgmental supportive listening, problem-solving perceived barriers, unconditional positive regard, and praise for practicing strategies between sessions. These factors helped her be confident that she could try out new discipline strategies.

whatever." Her pediatrician counseled her on the benefits of increasing fruits and vegetables in her diet. Ailani shared that her parents both have type 2 diabetes and hypertension, and she is afraid of developing these conditions as she ages. Ailani agreed to a warm hand-off with the clinic's BHC, Dr. Garcia. Ailani's pediatrician introduced Dr. Garcia as an important team member who could help Ailani meet health-related goals. Dr. Garcia met with Ailani for about 20 min as part of her well-child exam to discuss her readiness to make dietary changes. According to the trans-theoretical model, Ailani's thoughts and behaviors would appear different depending on her readiness to make changes at this point. Table 5.5 identifies what Ailani would likely think and do at each of the stages of change.

Table 5.5 Transtheoretical model applied to dietary changes

	Thoughts	Behaviors
Precontemplation	Ailani has not given much thought to her fruit and vegetable intake. Like many adolescents, she does not consider how her behavior now will impact her long-term health.	Ailani has not taken any steps to increase her fruit and vegetable intake.
Contemplation	Ailani is ambivalent about increasing her fruit and vegetable intake. She is considering the benefits and drawbacks of making this change.	Ailani tells Dr. Garcia, "I know fruits and vegetables are good for me," but also, "I don't really like them and it doesn't seem like a big deal—I'm pretty healthy."
Preparation	Alaini has decided that she wants to eat more fruits and vegetables, and is considering how to do this.	Ailani tells Dr. Garcia, "I want to be healthier than my parents when I'm their age." She has been watching healthy cooking videos on TikTok.
Action	Ailani commits to her decision and sets a goal to eat one fruit or vegetable with dinner every day for the next week.	Ailani goes grocery shopping with her parent to choose some fruits and vegetables for her meals and starts to incorporate the foods into her dinner as she planned.
Maintenance	Ailani notices that she has been feeling better, and is happy about making a change that will improve her health now and in the future. She may re-enter the contemplation stage when she considers increasing her fruit and vegetable intake again.	Ailani has been eating one fruit or vegetable at every meal for the last 6 months. She tells Dr. Garcia "I'm glad I did this, and I want to do even better."

During their first appointment and at subsequent follow-up visits, Dr. Garcia used motivational interviewing (MI) to help Ailani progress through each stage of change so she could be successful in meeting her goal of increasing fruit and vegetable intake. MI is a patient-centered approach to facilitating behavior change, where the patient is viewed as the expert and the health provider's role is to support them by engaging in active listening and getting them to engage in "change talk," while giving minimal advice [76]. Through this process, Dr. Garcia assisted Ailani in identifying internal sources of motivation (e.g., "I want to be healthier than my parents at their age"). It is noteworthy that brief MI of even a single session within the medical context has been shown to have beneficial effects on behavior change [77]. Consequently, the implementation of MI in primary care settings, even for short durations, can yield significant effects on both individual and population scales.

During their initial consultation, Dr. Garcia determined that Ailani was in the *contemplation stage*. Following a consultation with her pediatrician, Ailani considered modifying her dietary habits. Dr. Garcia assisted Ailani in identifying her intrinsic motivation to increase her consumption of fruits and vegetables. Ailani cited her parents' compromised health status, both having diabetes and hypertension, which restricted their family activities like hiking. Dr. Garcia inquired about how this circumstance influenced her view of her own health. Ailani expressed a desire to maintain her physical activity at an advanced age, recognizing that an improved diet would support this goal. Dr. Garcia empathized with Ailani, acknowledging the difficulty of observing her parents' reduced activity levels. Although Ailani was contemplating dietary modifications, she was ambivalent about making the change due to her dislike for many fruits and vegetables. Dr. Garcia provided encouragement, recognizing the challenge while emphasizing the significance of the change for her long-term goals.

After this discussion, Ailani decided to start with a small change in her dietary intake. She entered the *preparation stage* with a broad goal of maintaining her activity level as she ages. Dr. Garcia explained that sustainable behavior change is best achieved incrementally through small, realistic, and achievable adjustments. At baseline, Ailani consumed about two servings of vegetables and three servings of fruits per week. She set a goal of adding one serving of fruit or vegetables per day until her next appointment with Dr. Garcia. Using open-ended questions, Dr. Garcia helped her plan, and Ailani decided dinner would be the easiest time to incorporate fruits or vegetables. She also created a grocery list and, along with Dr. Garcia, identified potential barriers, such as her parents cooking instead of her, and discussed solutions. In doing so, Dr. Garcia relied on Ailani's expertise of her own life.

At their next appointment, Ailani informed Dr. Garcia that she had begun eating a fruit or vegetable with dinner, moving into the *action stage*. She admitted she did this most of the time but missed some days due to working at the diner over the weekend. To compensate, she ate a banana with breakfast the next morning. Dr. Garcia praised her for achieving her goal on 5 days and for problem-solving by eating fruit at breakfast. Ailani identified the lack of fruits and vegetables at work as a barrier. Together, they strategized that Ailani could bring a banana or canned peaches from home. Dr. Garcia encouraged her to find solutions, offering advice only when necessary and with permission. They scheduled monthly appointments for ongoing support.

A month later, Ailani proudly reported eating a fruit or vegetable with dinner every night, indicating she was in the *maintenance stage*. Dr. Garcia's role was to help her anticipate barriers to long-term success and ensure accountability. After a few more months of achieving her goal, Ailani set a new objective: eating a serving of fruit every morning for breakfast. She re-entered the *preparation stage* for this new goal while remaining in the *maintenance stage* for her original goal.

Summary

This chapter has provided an overview of behavioral change theories, termed models of change, and their practical applications in integrated pediatric medical settings. The application of these frameworks enhances practitioners' ability to provide effective patient care. Through an examination of the socioecological model and four others, this chapter highlights the complex interplay between the factors influencing health behaviors and outcomes. By considering the multiple levels of influence on health behaviors and tailoring approaches accordingly, healthcare professionals can develop more targeted and effective strategies to promote positive change.

The integration of Behavioral Health Consultants into primary care has the potential to improve population- and individual-level health outcomes. This may be achieved through improved access to mental health services, enhanced patient–provider relationships, and collaboration between physicians and psychologists. Furthermore, the promotion of policies directed at implementing primary care behavioral health integration, as well as the practice of IBH itself, may constitute a systems-level influence with cascading effects to benefit individual patients.

References

1. Reiter JT, Dobmeyer AC, Hunter CL. The primary care behavioral health (PCBH) model: an overview and operational definition. J Clin Psychol Med Settings. 2018;25. Springer New York LLC:109–26.
2. Mancini MA. Models of change and well-being from behavioral health disorders. In: Integrated behavioral health practice. Springer International Publishing; 2021. p. 59–84.
3. McLeroy KR, Bibeau D, Steckler A, Glanz K. An ecological perspective on health promotion programs. Health Educ Q. 1988;15(4):351–77.
4. Golden SD, Earp JAL. Social ecological approaches to individuals and their contexts: twenty years of health education & behavior health promotion interventions. Health Educ Behav. 2012;39(3):364–72.
5. Frieden TR. A framework for public health action: the health impact pyramid. Am J Public Health. 2010;100(4):590–5.
6. Beronio K, Glied S, Frank R. How the affordable care act and mental health parity and addiction equity act greatly expand coverage of behavioral health care. J Behav Health Serv Res. 2014;41(4):410–28.
7. Bagalman E, Dey J, Jacobus-Kantor L, Stoller B, West KD, Radel L, et al. HHS roadmap for behavioral health integration | ASPE [Internet]. 2022 [cited 2024 Oct 1]. Available from: https://aspe.hhs.gov/reports/hhs-roadmap-behavioral-health-integration.
8. Centers for Medicare & Medicaid Services. Frequently asked questions about billing medicare for Behavioral Health Integration (BHI) Services [Internet]. 2023 [cited 2024 Oct 8]. Available from: chrome-extension://efaidnbmnnnibpcajpcglclefindmkaj/https://www.cms.gov/medicare/medicare-fee-for-service-payment/physicianfeesched/downloads/behavioral-health-integration-faqs.pdf.
9. Centers for Medicare & Medicaid Services. Calendar Year (CY) 2023 medicare physician fee schedule final rule | CMS [Internet]. 2022 [cited 2024 Oct 8]. Available from: https://www.cms.gov/newsroom/fact-sheets/calendar-year-cy-2023-medicare-physician-fee-schedule-final-rule.
10. Rowan AB, Grove J, Solfelt L, Magnante A. Reducing the impacts of mental health stigma through integrated primary care: an examination of the evidence. J Clin Psychol Med Settings. 2021;28(4):679–93.
11. Bridges AJ, Andrews AR, Villalobos BT, Pastrana FA, Cavell TA, Gomez D. Does integrated behavioral health care reduce mental health disparities for Latinos? Initial findings. J Lat Psychol. 2014;2(1):37–53.

12. Hodgkinson S, Godoy L, Beers LS, Lewin A. Improving mental health access for low-income children and families in the primary care setting. Pediatrics (Evanston). American Academy of Pediatrics. 2017;139:e20151175.
13. Zubatsky M, Pettinelli D, Salas J, Davis D. Associations between integrated care practice and burnout factors of primary care physicians. Fam Med. Society of Teachers of Family Medicine. 2018;50:770–4.
14. Njoroge WFM, Hostutler CA, Schwartz BS, Mautone JA. Integrated behavioral health in pediatric primary care. Curr Psychiatry Rep. Current Medicine Group LLC. 2016;18:1–8.
15. Torrence ND, Mueller AE, Ilem AA, Renn BN, DeSantis B, Segal DL. Medical provider attitudes about behavioral health consultants in integrated primary care: a preliminary study. Fam Syst Health [Internet] 2014 [cited 2024 Dec 4];32(4):426–32. Available from: https://pubmed.ncbi.nlm.nih.gov/25329753/.
16. Corso KA, Bryan CJ, Corso ML, Kanzler KE, Houghton DC, Ray-Sannerud B, et al. Therapeutic alliance and treatment outcome in the primary care behavioral health model. Fam Syst Health. 2012;30:87–100.
17. Misra S, Jackson VW, Chong J, Choe K, Tay C, Wong J, et al. Systematic review of cultural aspects of stigma and mental illness among racial and ethnic minority groups in the United States: implications for interventions. Am J Community Psychol. John Wiley and Sons Inc. 2021;68:486–512.
18. Patel AR, Hall BJ. Beyond the DSM-5 diagnoses: a cross-cultural approach to assessing trauma reactions. Focus (Madison). 2021;19(2):197–203.
19. Patel A, Hinton D. Two peas in a pod? Understanding cross-cultural similarities and differences in anxiety disorders. In: Bui E, Charney ME, Baker AW, editors. Clinical handbook of anxiety disorders. Humana Cham; 2020. p. 59–75.
20. Robinson PJ, Reiter JT. Behavioral consultation and primary care: a guide to integrating services. 2nd ed. Springer International Publishing; 2016. p. 18.
21. Cutler DM. Behavioral health interventions: what works and why? In: Anderson NB, Bulatao RA, Cohen B, editors. Critical perspectives on racial and ethnic differences in health in late life [Internet]. Washington: National Academies Press (US); 2004 [cited 2024 Oct 8]. p. 643–76. Available from: https://www.ncbi.nlm.nih.gov/books/NBK25527/.
22. Varghese J, Gharde PM. A comprehensive review on the impacts of smoking on the health of an individual. Cureus [Internet]. 2023 [cited 2024 Oct 6];15(10). Available from: /pmc/articles/PMC10625450/.
23. Public Health Strategies for Tobacco Prevention and Control | REACH | CDC [Internet]. [cited 2024 Oct 6]. Available from: https://www.cdc.gov/reach/php/strategies/tobacco-prevention-control.html.
24. Zhang X, Cowling DW, Tang H. The impact of social norm change strategies on smokers' quitting behaviours. Tob Control [Internet]. 2010 [cited 2024 Oct 6];19(Suppl 1):i51–5. Available from: https://tobaccocontrol.bmj.com/content/19/Suppl_1/i51.
25. Pierce JP, White VM, Emery SL. What public health strategies are needed to reduce smoking initiation? Tob Control [Internet]. 2012 [cited 2024 Oct 6];21(2):258–64. Available from: https://tobaccocontrol.bmj.com/content/21/2/258.
26. García MC, Rossen LM, Matthews K, Guy G, Trivers KF, Thomas CC, et al. Preventable premature deaths from the five leading causes of death in nonmetropolitan and metropolitan counties, United States, 2010–2022. MMWR Surveill Summ [Internet]. 2024 [cited 2024 Oct 29];73(SS-2):1–11. Available from: https://www.cdc.gov/mmwr/volumes/73/ss/pdfs/ss7302a1-H.pdf.
27. Cunningham RM, Walton MA, Carter PM. The major causes of death in children and adolescents in the United States. N Engl J Med. 2018;379(25):2468–75.
28. Buchholz M, Talmi A. What we talked about at the pediatrician's office: exploring differences between healthy steps and traditional pediatric primary care visits. Infant Ment Health J. 2012;33(4):430–6.

29. Norcross JC, Krebs PM, Prochaska JO. Stages of change. J Clin Psychol [Internet]. 2011 [cited 2024 Oct 10];67(2):143–54. Available from: https://pubmed.ncbi.nlm.nih.gov/21157930/.
30. Krebs P, Norcross JC, Nicholson JM, Prochaska JO. Stages of change and psychotherapy outcomes: a review and meta-analysis. J Clin Psychol [Internet] 2018 [cited 2024 Oct 10];74(11):1964–79. Available from: https://pubmed.ncbi.nlm.nih.gov/30335193/.
31. Nitzke S, Kritsch K, Boeckner L, Greene G, Hoerr S, Horacek T, et al. A stage-tailored multi-modal intervention increases fruit and vegetable intakes of low-income young adults. Am J Health Promot [Internet] 2007 [cited 2024 Oct 10];22(1):6–14. Available from: https://pubmed.ncbi.nlm.nih.gov/17894257/.
32. Richards A, Kattelmann KK, Ren C. Motivating 18- to 24-year-olds to increase their fruit and vegetable consumption. J Am Diet Assoc [Internet] 2006 [cited 2024 Oct 10];106(9):1405–11. Available from: https://pubmed.ncbi.nlm.nih.gov/16963345/.
33. Brinley C, Barrar C, Cotugna N. Stages of change tools to increase fruit and vegetable consumption in high school students. J Nutr Educ [Internet] 2001 [cited 2024 Oct 10];33(1):57–8. Available from: https://pubmed.ncbi.nlm.nih.gov/12031208/.
34. Schwarzer R, Cao DS, Lippke S. Stage-matched minimal interventions to enhance physical activity in Chinese adolescents. J Adolesc Health [Internet] 2010 [cited 2024 Oct 10];47(6):533–9. Available from: https://pubmed.ncbi.nlm.nih.gov/21094429/.
35. Frenn M, Malin S, Bansal NK. Stage-based interventions for low-fat diet with middle school students. J Pediatr Nurs [Internet] 2003 [cited 2024 Oct 10];18(1):36–45. Available from: https://pubmed.ncbi.nlm.nih.gov/12610786/.
36. Md Yusop NB, Mohd Shariff Z, Hwu TT, Abd Talib R, Spurrier N. The effectiveness of a stage-based lifestyle modification intervention for obese children. BMC Public Health [Internet]. 2018 [cited 2024 Oct 15];18(1). Available from: https://pubmed.ncbi.nlm.nih.gov/29490648/.
37. Wright JA, Whiteley JA, Laforge RG, Adams WG, Berry D, Friedman RH. Validation of 5 stage-of-change measures for parental support of healthy eating and activity. J Nutr Educ Behav [Internet]. 2015 [cited 2024 Oct 15];47(2):134–42.e1. Available from: https://pubmed.ncbi.nlm.nih.gov/25579067/.
38. Crabtree VM, Moore JB, Jacks DE, Cerrito P, Topp R V. A transtheoretical, case management approach to the treatment of pediatric obesity. J Prim Care Community Health [Internet] 2010 [cited 2024 Oct 15];1(1):4–7. Available from: https://pubmed.ncbi.nlm.nih.gov/23804060/.
39. Reimer K, Smith C, Reicks M, Henry H, Thomas R, Atwell J. Child-feeding strategies of African American women according to stage of change for fruit and vegetable consumption. Public Health Nutr [Internet]. 2004 [cited 2024 Dec 3];7(4):505–12. Available from: https://pubmed.ncbi.nlm.nih.gov/15153256/.
40. Toral N, Slater B. Intervention based exclusively on stage-matched printed educational materials regarding healthy eating does not result in changes to adolescents' dietary behavior. Sci World J [Internet]. 2012 [cited 2024 Oct 15];2012. Available from: https://pubmed.ncbi.nlm.nih.gov/22545007/.
41. Rosenstock IM. Historical origins of the health belief model. Health Educ Behav. 1974;2(4):328–35.
42. Alamer AS. Behavior change theories and models within health belief model research: a five-decade holistic bibliometric analysis. Cureus. 2024;16(6) https://doi.org/10.7759/cureus.63143.
43. Alyafei A, Easton-Carr R. The health belief model of behavior change. StatPearls [Internet] 2024 [cited 2024 Dec 4]. Available from: https://www.ncbi.nlm.nih.gov/books/NBK606120/.
44. Kim SB, Lee YJ. Factors associated with mental health help-seeking among Asian Americans: a systematic review. J Racial Ethn Health Disparities [Internet] 2022 [cited 2024 Dec 4];9(4):1276–97. Available from: https://pubmed.ncbi.nlm.nih.gov/34076864/.
45. Kunyahamu MS, Daud A, Tengku Ismail TA, Md Tahir MF. PsyHELP pocket guide: development of an educational tool to promote professional mental health help-seeking among the health workforce. PLoS One [Internet] 2024 [cited 2024 Dec 3];19(10):e0309224. Available from: https://pubmed.ncbi.nlm.nih.gov/39365788/.

46. Fong HF, Bennett CE, Mondestin V, Scribano PV, Mollen C, Wood JN. Caregiver perceptions about mental health services after child sexual abuse. Child Abuse Negl [Internet]. 2016 [cited 2024 Dec 3];51:284–94. Available from: https://pubmed.ncbi.nlm.nih.gov/26602155/.
47. Henshaw EJ, Freedman-Doan CR. Conceptualizing mental health care utilization using the health belief model. Clin Psychol Sci Pract. 2009;16(4):420–39.
48. Naslund JA, Aschbrenner KA, Kim SJ, McHugo GJ, Unützer J, Bartels SJ, et al. Health behavior models for informing digital technology interventions for individuals with mental illness. Psychiatr Rehabil J [Internet] 2017 [cited 2024 Dec 4];40(3):325–35. Available from: https://pubmed.ncbi.nlm.nih.gov/28182469/.
49. De las Cuevas C, de Leon J. Reviving research on medication attitudes for improving pharmacotherapy: focusing on adherence. Psychother Psychosom [Internet]. 2017 [cited 2024 Dec 4];86(2):73–9. Available from: https://pubmed.ncbi.nlm.nih.gov/28183085/.
50. Bromley E, Tarn DM, McCreary M, Hurley B, Ober AJ, Watkins KE. Attitudes about medications for alcohol use disorder among individuals with serious mental illness: a health belief model analysis. J Subst Abuse Treat [Internet] 2020 [cited 2024 Dec 4];114. Available from: https://pubmed.ncbi.nlm.nih.gov/32527506/.
51. Carpenter CJ. A meta-analysis of the effectiveness of health belief model variables in predicting behavior. Health Commun. 2010;25(8):661–9.
52. Sulat JS, Prabandari YS, Sanusi R, Hapsari ED, Santoso B. The validity of health belief model variables in predicting behavioral change: a scoping review. Health Educ. Emerald Group Holdings Ltd. 2018;118:499–512.
53. Ajzen I. The theory of planned behavior. Organ Behav Hum Decis Process. 1991;50(2):179–211.
54. Hagger MS, Chatzisarantis NLD. First- and higher-order models of attitudes, normative influence, and perceived behavioural control in the theory of planned behaviour. Br J Soc Psychol. 2005;44(4):513–35.
55. Sheeran P, Webb TL. The intention–behavior gap. Soc Personal Psychol Compass. Wiley-Blackwell. 2016;10:503–18.
56. Conner M, Norman P. Understanding the intention-behavior gap: the role of intention strength. Front Psychol [Internet]. 2022 [cited 2024 Dec 3];13. Available from: https://pubmed.ncbi.nlm.nih.gov/35992469/.
57. Bandura A. Social cognitive theory: an agentic perspective. Annu Rev Psychol. 2001;52:1–26.
58. Bandura A. Social cognitive theory of self-regulation. Organ Behav Hum Decis Process. 1991;50:248–87.
59. Islam KF, Awal A, Mazumder H, Munni UR, Majumder K, Afroz K, et al. Social cognitive theory-based health promotion in primary care practice: a scoping review. Heliyon. Elsevier Ltd. 2023;9:e14889.
60. Islam KF, Awal A, Mazumder H, Munni UR, Majumder K, Afroz K, et al. Social cognitive theory-based health promotion in primary care practice: a scoping review. Heliyon [Internet]. 2023 [cited 2024 Dec 6];9(4):e14889. Available from: https://pmc.ncbi.nlm.nih.gov/articles/PMC10070720/.
61. Talmi A, Muther EF, Margolis K, Buchholz M, Asherin R, Bunik M. The scope of behavioral health integration in a pediatric primary care setting. J Pediatr Psychol [Internet]. 2016 [cited 2024 Oct 1];41(10):1120–32. Available from: https://doi.org/10.1093/jpepsy/jsw065.
62. Sanders MR, Kirby JN, Tellegen CL, Day JJ. The triple P-positive parenting program: a systematic review and meta-analysis of a multi-level system of parenting support. Clin Psychol Rev [Internet] 2014 [cited 2024 Oct 1];34(4):337–57. Available from: https://pubmed.ncbi.nlm.nih.gov/24842549/.
63. Evans SW, Owens JS, Wymbs BT, Ray AR. Evidence-based psychosocial treatments for children and adolescents with attention deficit/hyperactivity disorder. J Clin Child Adolesc Psychol [Internet]. 2018 [cited 2024 Oct 1];47(2):157–98. Available from: https://pubmed.ncbi.nlm.nih.gov/29257898/.
64. Costello EJ, He JP, Sampson NA, Kessler RC, Merikangas KR. Services for adolescents with psychiatric disorders: 12-month data from the National Comorbidity Survey-Adolescent.

Psychiatr Serv [Internet]. 2014 [cited 2024 Oct 1];65(3):359–66. Available from: https://pubmed.ncbi.nlm.nih.gov/24233052/.

65. Daly AN, O'Sullivan EJ, Kearney JM. Considerations for health and food choice in adolescents. Proc Nutr Soc [Internet]. 2022 [cited 2024 Dec 10];81(1):75–86. Available from: https://pubmed.ncbi.nlm.nih.gov/35039094/.
66. Aguirre Velasco A, Cruz ISS, Billings J, Jimenez M, Rowe S. What are the barriers, facilitators and interventions targeting help-seeking behaviours for common mental health problems in adolescents? A systematic review. BMC Psychiatry. 2020;20(1):1–22.
67. Straus MA. Prevalence, societal causes, and trends in corporal punishment by parents in world perspective. Law Contemp Probl. 2010;73(2):1.
68. Finkelhor D, Turner H, Wormuth BK, Vanderminden J, Hamby S. Corporal punishment: current rates from a National Survey. J Child Fam Stud. 2019;28(7):1991–7.
69. Chiocca EM. American parents' attitudes and beliefs about corporal punishment: an integrative literature review. J Pediatr Health Care [Internet] 2017 [cited 2024 Oct 1];31(3):372–83. Available from: https://pubmed.ncbi.nlm.nih.gov/28202205/.
70. Gershoff ET, Goodman GS, Miller-Perrin CL, Holden GW, Jackson Y, Kazdin AE. The strength of the causal evidence against physical punishment of children and its implications for parents, psychologists, and policymakers. Am Psychol. 2018;73(5):626–38.
71. Javier JR, Deavenport-Saman A, Florendo E, Bantol KEA, Palinkas LA. Health equity and enrollment in preventive parenting programs: a qualitative study of Filipino parents. Evid Based Pract Child Adolesc Ment Health [Internet]. 2022 [cited 2024 Oct 1];7(2):245–59. Available from: https://pubmed.ncbi.nlm.nih.gov/35783995/.
72. Salari R, Filus A. Using the health belief model to explain mothers' and fathers' intention to participate in universal parenting programs. Prev Sci [Internet] 2017 [cited 2024 Oct 1];18(1):83–94. Available from: https://pubmed.ncbi.nlm.nih.gov/27638427/.
73. Walsh W. Spankers and nonspankers: where they get information on spanking. Fam Relat. National Council on Family Relations. 2002;51:81–8.
74. Di Noia J, Contento IR, Prochaska JO. Computer-mediated intervention tailored on transtheoretical model stages and processes of change increases fruit and vegetable consumption among urban African-American adolescents. Am J Health Promot. 2008;22(5):336–41.
75. Gur K, Erol S, Kadioglu H, Ergun A, Boluktas R. The impact on adolescents of a transtheoretical model-based programme on fruit and vegetable consumption. Public Health Nutr. 2019;22(13):2500–8.
76. Miller W, Rollnick S. Motivational interviewing: helping people change. 3rd ed. New York: Guilford Publications; 2012.
77. Bischof G, Bischof A, Rumpf HJ. Motivational interviewing: an evidence-based approach for use in medical practice. Dtsch Arztebl Int [Internet]. 2021 [cited 2024 Oct 1];118(7):109. Available from: /pmc/articles/PMC8200683/.

Chapter 6
Empowering Care: Crafting Patient-Centered Treatment Plans for Optimal Outcomes

Summer Chahin, Lauren Wruble, and Pradnya Joshi

The Importance of Treatment Planning

Treatment planning occurs when a patient and/or family is establishing care with a clinician or interdisciplinary team with the goal of meeting shared, agreed upon treatment goals and decisions. Treatment planning in integrative behavioral health aims to improve the effectiveness of the intervention(s) by modifying them to the specific circumstances of the individual (e.g., culture, environment, poverty, access to resources, social drivers of health [SDoH], etc.), while also designing goals that are specific, measurable, actionable/achievable, relevant, and time-limited. Treatment planning functions as a roadmap for helping patients improve health and well-being by not only tailoring interventions and treatments, but also identifying areas in which to build coping skills and improve functioning. Furthermore, treatment plans can also serve as a way for patients and providers to regroup when treatment plateaus or parties involved are experiencing confusion or frustration related to progress, or lack thereof. In this chapter, treatment planning is discussed through the lens of person-centered and motivational interviewing (MI) techniques with the purpose of enhancing the therapeutic alliance and ultimately improving patient buy-in, engagement, and outcomes.

S. Chahin (✉) · P. Joshi
Western Michigan University Homer Stryker M.D. School of Medicine, Kalamazoo, MI, USA
e-mail: Summer.chahin@wmed.edu; Pradnya.joshi@wmed.edu

L. Wruble
Michigan Medicine/C.S. Mott Children's Hospital, Kalamazoo, MI, USA
e-mail: lwruble@med.umich.edu

R. W. Apple et al. (eds.), *Using Integrated Behavioral Health in Pediatric Practice*, https://doi.org/10.1007/978-3-031-85784-3_6

Transitioning from Patient-Centered Care to Person-Centered Care

In the evolving landscape of healthcare, the shift from patient-centered care to person-centered care marks a significant paradigm change. This transition recognizes that an individual is more than just a patient; they are a person with multifaceted roles, needs, and experiences that extend beyond their health conditions. Embracing this broader perspective not only enriches the treatment process but also fosters a more holistic and empathic approach to healthcare. The person-centered treatment planning is ideal as it focuses on an individual's strengths while guiding the treatment and therapeutic process [1, 2].

The Person-Centered Approach

Person-centered care transcends the traditional hierarchical relationship between healthcare providers and patients, emphasizing mutual respect, empathy, and collaboration. In this model, patients are viewed as experts in their own lives, possessing unique perspectives, values, and goals that shape their healthcare decisions. By actively involving patients in the decision-making process, healthcare providers honor their autonomy and promote a sense of agency.

A person-centered care framework allows for a broader inclusion of individuals who can play a crucial role in the treatment planning process. For instance, family members and caregivers often have insights and observations that can be vital for creating an effective care plan. Their involvement ensures that the treatment plan is not only clinically sound but also practical and supportive of the person's everyday life (e.g., relief of acute symptoms vs. health promotion).

Moreover, this framework emphasizes the importance of relationship building within the healthcare system. When healthcare providers view their patients as whole persons, it fosters a more empathetic and trust-based relationship. This shift enhances communication, encourages mutual respect, and empowers individuals to be active participants in their own healthcare. Furthermore, the process of building relationships through person-centered approaches allows providers to better understand how their patient's health and well-being may be impacted by factors such as housing instability, food insecurity, neighborhood violence, and generational trauma. With this information, providers can call upon other members of the integrated care team (e.g., social workers, patient advocates, etc.) or specialty providers to provide additional resources and advocacy aligning with holistic health and well-being.

Creating and Reviewing Models of Care

Developing effective models of care is crucial in the transition from patient-centered to person-centered care. Initially, models focused on patient-centered care were designed to ensure that healthcare services were tailored to the individual needs and preferences of patients. These models emphasized the importance of understanding patients' medical histories, their symptoms, and their treatment preferences.

However, as we move toward person-centered care, these models require significant re-evaluation and re-design. A person-centered care model must consider the whole person, including their social, emotional, and psychological well-being. This comprehensive approach involves recognizing the various roles an individual plays in their daily life—such as being a parent, employee, or caregiver—and how these roles impact their health and well-being.

In creating these models, healthcare providers need to integrate multiple dimensions of a person's life into the treatment planning process. This involves the inclusion of family members, caregivers, and other support systems in the planning and implementation of care strategies. By doing so, the healthcare system can build stronger, more supportive relationships that contribute positively to the person's overall health outcomes.

Person-Centered Care Within Integrated Behavioral Health Services

Integrated behavioral health has become the gold standard for medical care [3]. The integration of mental health providers (psychologists, social workers, other behavioral health support) in the medical setting has helped to improve overall patient outcomes making these services more accessible for both patients and providers. Medical providers also benefit from a fully integrated model as they are able to save time during visits by utilizing behavioral health consultants and can spend more time on other tasks. Behavioral health consultants can support medical providers by addressing the psychological aspects of mental health presentations and help gather information so that the provider team has a better understanding of racial and health disparities that often accompany mental and behavioral health concerns.

Integrating mental health providers into medical care strengthens the conceptualization of the presenting concern in the context of the individual as a whole. This allows for a better understanding of the psychological aspects of conditions, which also better helps medical providers understand the intricate mind–body connection while emphasizing culturally sensitive care. Medical providers, students, and trainees all benefit from interactions with mental health providers and end up being better equipped with the skills to recognize and address disparities and support their learning related to the impact of mental health on physical health. Medical students and residents are provided with the opportunity to have hands-on experiences in addressing behavioral health issues by observing medical providers and mental health providers, which strengthens their training. This integration not only prepares them for the complexities of modern medicine but also promotes empathy, awareness, and comprehensive care, ultimately improving patient outcomes and advancing health equity.

Building Blocks of Person-Centered Care (Contextual Model and Common Factors)

Common factors (e.g., patient characteristics, unconditional positive regard, acceptance, trust, empathy, genuineness, etc.) are often interpreted as being therapeutic elements that are consistent across most therapeutic approaches. While this may be true, it must not be overlooked that these elements also influence the mechanisms of change in therapy. Despite the proposal of common factors models for differing theoretical orientations, little difference has been found regarding the importance and impact of such factors. One model consistent with the movement to person-centered care is the contextual model [4], which suggests therapy is beneficial by way of three pathways: (1) the real relationship, (2) development of expectations via discussion of disorder and treatment plan, and (3) adaptation of health promotion behaviors and actions [4]. The contextual model posits social characteristics of humans as change agents and therapy as a social healing practice [5, 6]. As such, it is imperative for the therapeutic relationship, or therapeutic alliance, to be established early on as the relationship serves as the activator for the pathways.

Caregiver Experiences and the Impact on the Patient

In order to build an appropriate model of person-centered care, one must consider the various components necessary to implement this effectively. Beyond the common factors one considers, providers should also think about the various members of a household and stakeholders in the patient's care. In this, providers must consider the impact of caregiver experiences, perceptions, and how this may impact a patient's environment, ability to access support and resources, and ability and willingness to engage, and barriers to engagement. For example, caregivers' experiences significantly shape what children are exposed to. Decades of research have showcased that stable, reliable, and nurturing caregiving leads to healthy social development and emotional regulation in children [7]. This impact is relevant for both the short and long term, as demonstrated by the Bucharest Early Intervention Project (BEIP). In this randomized controlled trial, children were randomly assigned to high-quality foster care or remained in institutional care. The results showed that receiving developmentally appropriate caregiving during critical periods of childhood translated into positive developmental outcomes in both the short and long term [8]. The children that remained in institutional care exhibited profound deficits in IQ scores, socio-emotional behaviors, and a greater incidence of psychiatric disorders, among many other adverse findings [8].

There are several examples of psychiatric disorders that can result from insufficient and unreliable care including reactive attachment disorder (RAD) and disinhibited social engagement disorder (DSED). The DSM-5 characterizes RAD as a consistent pattern of inhibited and emotionally withdrawn behavior toward adult caregivers. The current incidence is estimated to be 1.4% in the adolescent and pediatric populations [9]. RAD is more prevalent in young children who have been exposed to severe neglect prior to being placed in foster care or institutionalized care. DSED is another disorder rooted in the same etiology of social neglect and inconsistent parenting. DSED is characterized by an overly friendly demeanor with strangers and a complete lack of hesitation when approaching and interacting with strangers [10]. Additionally, DSED is associated with deficits in cognitive control, increased impulsivity and hyperactivity, poor socialization, and poor motor skills [11]. In summary, a stable caregiver environment and relationship is essential for childhood emotional, social, and psychological development, and lack of support from a caregiver can result in many adverse conditions including RAD and DSED. When crafting a patient-centered treatment plan, consideration for the impact of early caregiver experience and the current environment must be taken into account to provide holistic and comprehensive care to pediatric and adolescent patients.

In addition, caregiver stress and environment should be taken into account when assessing the impact of child behavior and function. Socioeconomic factors and family factors play a significant role in the health of children [12]. For example, economic stress is a socioeconomic factor that can affect caregiving [13]. A 2014 study investigated 124 culturally diverse parents with young children and studied the relationship between different types of economic and parent stress and how it influenced behavioral issues in children [13]. Interestingly, the study stated that different types of caregiver stressors manifested in different behavioral problems in children. Increasing levels of parenting and life stressors strongly predicted externalizing behavior problems in children, whereas negative economic stress and parenting stress correlated to internalizing behavioral issues in children [13]. In addition to economic stress and financial stability, other important factors to consider include parental mental health, education level, access to healthcare, family dynamics, etc. These showcase the wide variety of factors that affect caregivers and subsequently show how these same factors play a role in a child's environment and behaviors. Medical providers and healthcare workers should always view each patient in an individual light and incorporate all these socioeconomic and parental factors when tailoring a treatment plan.

Building a Therapeutic Alliance

A component of building a healthy and strong therapeutic relationship includes taking into consideration prior caregiver experiences, previous patient experiences, and experiences of the family as a whole. When patients initially present to therapy, they are consciously, unconsciously, overtly, and/or covertly bringing their beliefs, expectations, values, culture, prior experiences, and more along with them. Finding common ground and focusing on building a strong therapeutic alliance is imperative as the relationship has consistently been linked to therapy outcomes regardless of presenting problems, treatment modalities, and contexts. Frankly, the alliance is a critical component for therapeutic treatment and successful outcomes. Three primary characteristics of the therapeutic alliance have consistently been identified across theoretical approaches: (1) the collaborative nature of the relationship, (2) the affective bond between the patient and provider, and (3) the agreement between patient and provider on treatment plans and goals [14]. The therapeutic alliance is also often referred to as a "working alliance" due to the nature of the relationship changing over time (i.e., building, maintaining, and terminating). Prior to engaging patients in interventions, providers should prioritize building rapport with patients through collaborative conversations and the development of a treatment plan. If integrated healthcare providers rely solely on diagnostic symptoms for treatment planning, suboptimal outcomes and/or high dropout rates may result. Alternatively, if providers meet patients and family where they are and patients actively participate in their treatment planning so they see their own language reflected in the plan, it is likely they will feel more aligned with the provider and the plan, leading to increased engagement in services.

Meeting Individuals and Families Where They Are

The idea of meeting individuals and families where they are has been a common topic within healthcare communities. One of the most challenging parts of being in the healthcare field is meeting families where they are, yet it's one of the most essential pieces of building trust within the provider–patient relationship. This concept is a means to collaborate with patients and families in learning their goals and needs. Providers should illustrate respect for the patients and families that they work with as well as respect for their cultures, choices, and factors that lead to their lifestyles, and specific contextual factors within families' lives. As healthcare providers, we value the diversity, individuality, and uniqueness of each and every patient and family we interact with. It's imperative to assess the strengths, limitations, and unique factors within the individuals and families we work with in order to best support the collaborative development of an effective treatment plan and to provide treatment options and choices when possible. The rest of this section will further highlight strategies providers can utilize to assess family and individual strengths, limitations, and unique factors.

Exploration of Individual and Familial Strengths

An important aspect of meeting families where they are and engaging in client-centered treatment is a thorough exploration of the strengths of the individual patient as well as the strengths of the family as a whole. It is essential to understand various factors, including—but not limited to—the abilities, talents, competencies, and accomplishments of the individual and family across different settings, such as home, school, work, social environments, and any other contexts that hold significance for the family. It's also important to explore the values and traditions that each individual or family practices as this can play a significant role in treatment planning. Values and traditions can also present as barriers to adherence for families. For example, individuals and families who observe Ramadan may not be able to fully engage in all medical recommendations, dietary plans and needs, or procedures. Families who observe Ramadan engage in fasting (no food or water) from dawn until dusk. Ramadan celebration often involves prayer late into the night where it is not unusual to be up past midnight for prayers and then get up around 5 am to eat before dawn and prayer. Patients and their families may be tired, hungry, and thirsty—especially later in the day. These families may also require flexibility and accommodation whenever possible and it's important to recognize the importance of values and traditions such as these to families and the impact they have on family functioning. Providers who take the time to query about these values and traditions tend to have more success when collaborating with families to find ways for them to observe Ramadan while adhering to medical care and needs safely.

Another example comes from the ancient Asian dermabrasion therapy practice known as "coining." Coining is performed by applying pressured strokes along a patient's skin via some hard object, often a coin [15]. The technique is widely practiced among various Asian countries, including China and Southeast Asian countries, for the purpose of treating a wide variety of medical illnesses including chronic pain, fever, flu, headaches, heatstroke, and upper respiratory infections [16]. One intentional side effect of coining is ecchymosis, which practitioners believe are negative energies leaving the body [15]. This practice is still widely utilized despite more well-documented treatments for the above-mentioned medical ailments. However, when patients who receive coining visit physicians that are unfamiliar with the therapy, the physicians can wrongfully assume that the patients are victims of physical abuse, as the practice often leaves many linear abrasions on the skin that can appear medically alarming. There is the potential for a serious misdiagnosis or misunderstanding from physicians unfamiliar with coining, especially since there is no standardized medical education curriculum that informs physicians about medical treatments and therapies practiced in various cultures.

In the event that physicians or caregivers are unsure of a cultural practice, the most effective and direct communication would be to ask open-ended questions in a non-judgmental manner. This allows the patient to provide context for the physicians without the fear of judgment. The physicians in turn should also strive to understand the cultural context in which the patient presents. The practice of collecting a full medical history along with cultural practices will help the physicians understand a holistic picture of the patient and this will strengthen the patient–physician relationship by building trust. There is a plethora of medical treatments that people participate in, and not all of them are well documented in the medical literature, hence it is vital that physicians showcase empathy and understanding when encountering patients who practice less common non-western practices and therapies that are not well known.

Further exploration of individual and family interests, cultures, hopes, dreams, aspirations, and motivations can be helpful in determining how treatment recommendations may fit into an individual or family's lifestyle. This knowledge would allow providers to tailor treatment planning and recommendations to fit around the activities that families engage in on a normal basis. This method of questioning would also allow providers to help build rapport with families and potentially have more buy-in from families into the treatment planning process, which showcases to the families that they are heard and that all parts of the individual and family functioning are being considered. This is especially the case in culturally aware physicians, as it is documented that many non-Western cultures have a distrust for Western medicine. It is worth pursuing anything that can help bridge these gaps and earn back this trust, starting in hospitals and primary care clinics [17, 18].

Beyond these important individual, familial, and cultural factors, it is imperative to explore where a family falls within the SDoH. The SDoH are non-medically related factors that impact individual and family functioning and represent five major environmental contributors to family functioning, health, and quality of life. The factors include economic stability, access to education and quality of education, access to healthcare and quality of the healthcare, the neighborhood one lives in and the environment they live in, and finally one's social and community context. In order to truly understand and appreciate the strengths of an individual and family, it's important to explore the family's full context including the hardships they may experience (Fig. 6.1).

When exploring the SDoH with families, providers should ask about the resources and assets available to them, including their economic situation (socioeconomic status) as well as both their social and interpersonal resources and support. These factors can significantly impact a family's ability to successfully implement and engage in a treatment plan. Furthermore, to get a comprehensive understanding of a family's functioning, providers should ask about the unique individual and familial attributes that exist in the family unit. These attributes can include physical, psychological, performance-based characteristics, as well as unique capabilities and preferred coping methods (using humor to cope, spending time together as a family, etc.). In addition, providers should discuss with families what strategies they have tried in the past to overcome hardships that have worked in the past. This

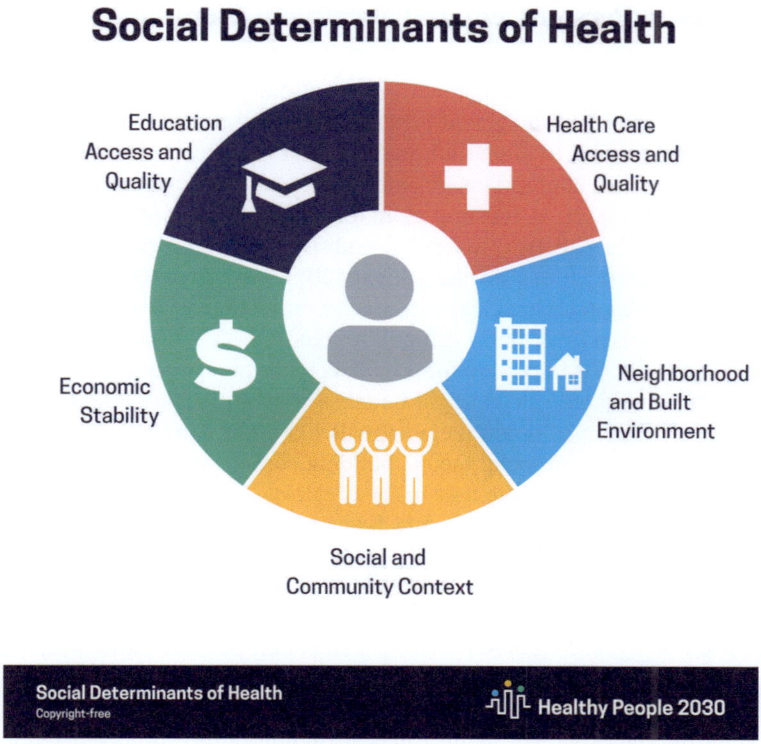
Social Determinants of Health
Education Access and Quality
Health Care Access and Quality
Economic Stability
Neighborhood and Built Environment
Social and Community Context
Social Determinants of Health
Copyright-free
Healthy People 2030

Fig. 6.1 Social determinants of health—Healthy People 2030 [19]

information can help providers learn how to communicate and support families throughout the process of treatment planning, help providers come up with better solutions for families when barriers arise, and help providers know how to support individuals and families when things become challenging. Lastly, providers should assess these factors in all areas of an individual or family's life including how these factors exist in their home, school, and work lives as well as other spaces they engage in within the community. Another significant factor that should be thoroughly explored includes the individual's and family's experience with bias, discrimination, racism, and stigma and how this has impacted their worldview as well as their past experiences within healthcare.

Assessing individual and family strengths can look many different ways. One way is to have an open discussion with the individual or family and encourage members to speak openly about their own strengths, the strengths of other family members, and the strengths of the family unit. Another way to explore strengths may be to have each member write down their strengths and share them with each other afterward. Exploration of strengths can take place over time over several interactions with individuals and the family unit. Providers can also identify additional strengths just by pure observation during one's interactions with the family unit.

Challenges in Person-Centered Treatment Planning

Despite collaborative, person-centered treatment planning being the ideal method for treatment planning in integrated behavioral health settings, providers may face challenges while trying to align with patients. For example, what a provider may deem to be realistic, appropriate, or achievable may look significantly different from a patient's perspective. It is important for providers to ensure they are developing goals through the patient's lens and not substituting their own goals or imposing their beliefs or expectations on the patient [20]. Another challenge in treatment planning is ensuring goals are clear and concise rather than vague and abstract [20]. If a patient presents a goal that is difficult to measure ("I want to feel better" or "I want to be happy"), it is important for providers to encourage patients to think about what specific, measurable steps might be taken to work toward "feeling better" or "being happy." Examples might include goals like improving sleep, spending less time "doom-scrolling" on social media, building coping skills to reduce symptoms of depression, or spending more time in social settings. These goals are specific, can be measured throughout treatment, and focus on positive, growth, and recovery-oriented tasks. Therefore, patients and providers can evaluate progress consistently between sessions and determine whether adjustments need to be made. Similarly, if goals and objectives become too detailed, they can become overwhelming and confusing [20]. Finally, pacing is important. Patients may become either overwhelmed or bored if their goals and progress are set at a pace that is too fast or too slow, respectively. Therefore, providers checking in consistently about patient progress and pacing through a variety of measures including observation, self-report, collaborative conversation, and collateral information can help to determine whether the pacing is appropriate [20].

When going through treatment, setbacks occur often for a variety of reasons. Because this is part of the therapeutic process, it is imperative that providers prepare their patients for the possibility of setbacks, but also that providers are mindful of how they are responding when setbacks inevitably happen. When setbacks occur, providers should be genuine and supportive, while also working with the patient to determine what led to the setback, if or how the plan needs to be adjusted, what the next steps look like, and supporting the patient in moving forward [20].

Utilizing Motivational Interviewing Techniques in the Context of Person-Centered Treatment Planning

The integration of MI into person-centered treatment planning represents a symbiotic relationship that enhances patient engagement and facilitates meaningful outcomes. Through empathetic listening and reflective questioning, healthcare providers employing MI techniques create a safe and supportive environment conducive to honest self-reflection and exploration. By affirming patients' strengths and highlighting their intrinsic motivations, providers empower individuals to envision a future aligned with their values and aspirations.

Incorporating MI into person-centered treatment planning represents a paradigm shift toward a more collaborative and empowering approach to healthcare. By honoring patients' autonomy, fostering intrinsic motivation, and tailoring interventions to individual needs, providers can cultivate meaningful partnerships that facilitate sustainable behavior change and promote holistic well-being. As medicine continues to evolve, embracing the strong relationship between MI and person-centered care holds the promise of transformative outcomes for both patients and providers alike.

Motivational interviewing (MI) is a powerful technique that aligns with the principles of person-centered treatment planning. At its core, MI is a collaborative, goal-oriented style of communication designed to strengthen an individual's motivation to change. This method respects the client's autonomy and emphasizes their intrinsic ability to make positive changes on their own, making it an invaluable tool in person-centered care.

In the realm of modern medicine, the ethos of person-centered care has become a cornerstone of effective patient management. Recognizing patients as partners in their own health journey, healthcare providers are increasingly embracing collaborative approaches that empower individuals to take ownership of their well-being. At the heart of this paradigm shift lies the art of motivational interviewing, a communication style that fosters intrinsic motivation and promotes positive behavioral change.

Understanding Motivational Interviewing

MI, rooted in the principles of humanistic psychology, operates on the belief that individuals possess the capacity for change and growth. Rather than imposing directives or judgments, MI practitioners engage patients in a non-confrontational dialogue aimed at exploring their ambivalence toward change and eliciting their intrinsic motivations. Central to MI is the concept of "change talk"—statements made by patients that reflect their desire, ability, reasons, and need for change.

Providers play a unique role in that they can use MI as a tool to assess the stage of change a person or family is in terms of making a change to their health and meeting families where they are at in the treatment planning process as well. Assessing the stage of change an individual or family is in allows providers to learn more about the mindset of the individual. Understanding a person's readiness for change allows providers to gain insight into their mindset, assess potential barriers and uncertainties, and collaboratively problem-solve. By addressing these concerns, providers can help individuals and families progress toward greater readiness for change.

Within this approach, there are six stages of change that an individual may vacillate between. It's important to remember that this process can be bi-directional and individuals and families can move back and forth between these stages, so frequent assessment of the stage of change one is in is necessary especially when you sense changes in how an individual or family is discussing their health goals, needs, and understanding of the treatment plan.

Stages of Change Within the Context of Patient-Centered Care and Treatment Planning

The stages of change are an integral part of the process of motivational interviewing. Identifying the stage an individual or family is in is paramount to understanding the desire or ambivalence to change [21]. The conceptualization and understanding of these stages have changed over time. At first, providers need to identify where the individual or family lands on their understanding of the status of the health problem, their acceptance of the health problem and need to make changes, and their willingness to engage in a solution-focused action plan to make the appropriate changes to improve the health issue. Once a provider has accurately identified the stage of change an individual or family is in, then they can collaborate with the family in creating and adjusting a treatment plan that suits the needs of the family and meets them where they are in that particular moment (Table 6.1). Over time, the provider should work with the family and conduct an ongoing assessment of the stage of change they are in and adapt the treatment plan accordingly.

In the most recent version of the adaptation, there are six stages of change. The first and lowest stage, known as the *Precontemplation Stage*, involves individuals or families experiencing negative consequences related to a problem (e.g., drug use, health issues) but not perceiving it as a significant concern. At this stage, they lack motivation to change their behavior and do not recognize the presence of a problem.

The second stage is called the *Contemplation Stage*. During this stage, individuals or families may recognize that a problem does indeed exist but they are unsure whether they want to or should make a change. Individuals in this stage may have even considered making a change at some point, but despite this, they have not made an effort to attempt to make changes to their behavior or fix the problem.

The next stage is called the *Preparation Stage*. During this stage, the individual or family recognizes that there is an issue, wants to change the behavior to fix the problem, and has made some commitment to changing the behavior and taking on the responsibility to engage in strategies to fix the problem. In order to get to this stage, many individuals have thought out the benefits versus consequences of maintaining the behavior. Individuals quickly realize that the consequences of the behavior or problem outweigh any positives they are getting from the behavior. During this stage, it's possible that one has attempted to create a plan to fix the problem or change the behavior, but has not yet taken any actions toward implementing the plan or making an actual change.

Table 6.1 Applied example of the stages of change

Stage of change	Example
Precontemplation	Parents of a 10-year-old child who is overweight are not aware of or are in denial about the health risks associated with their child's weight. They may believe that their child's weight is just a phase or that they will naturally grow out of it. They may not see the need for any changes in diet or physical activity and may resist suggestions from healthcare professionals to address their child's weight. They might attribute their child's weight to genetics or other factors beyond their control, rather than acknowledging the role of diet and lifestyle choices. In this stage, the focus may be on raising awareness and providing education to help parents recognize the importance of addressing their child's weight for their long-term health and well-being.
Contemplation	Parents acknowledge that their child is overweight and may be considering making changes to their diet and lifestyle but haven't taken any concrete steps yet. They are weighing the pros and cons of making changes.
Preparation	Parents have decided to take action and are gathering information about healthy eating habits, seeking advice from healthcare professionals, and planning how to implement changes in their child's diet and physical activity.
Action	Parents have started making changes in their child's diet and lifestyle, such as cooking healthier meals, reducing portion sizes, and encouraging physical activity. They are actively implementing their plan to help their child achieve a healthier weight.
Maintenance	Parents have successfully implemented changes in their child's lifestyle and are working to sustain these changes over the long term. They continue to monitor their child's diet and physical activity, adjust their approach as needed, and seek support from healthcare professionals and other resources.
Relapse	Despite their efforts, the child's weight begins to increase again due to factors such as returning to old habits, lack of support, or external stressors. The parents may feel discouraged but can use this experience to learn from mistakes and recommit to making healthy changes.

In the fourth stage, individuals tend to be more actively involved and engaged in strategies and implementing plans to change their behavior. There is no set definition about how much effort or action is required to be placed in this stage of change, but one can be considered to be in the aptly named, *Action Stage*, with any amount of effort or action toward behavior change. During this stage, individuals are able to understand that they are responsible for their actions and behaviors. Although people in this stage are ready to make a change, they typically benefit from having additional support to implement and maintain the change behavior.

During the *Maintenance Stage*, individuals have developed and implemented a plan with some success and have found efficient methods to change the behavior or work toward fixing the problem. Although behavior changes take time, individuals can use this initial momentum to help them continue working on change and work toward repairing the issue. In order to qualify for this stage of change, one must have implemented and maintained these change behaviors for at least 6 months.

Finally, in the last stage, the *Termination Stage*, the individual or family has made all of the changes necessary for them to change their behavior or fix the problem completely and maintain the reparations. Although the name of this stage signals the end of the process, many individuals need continued support to maintain these changes over a longer period of time. In this stage, individuals and families have successfully made positive changes, have fixed or overcome their problems, learned and developed new habits that are maintainable, and continue to improve in this pattern and trajectory.

As discussed above, there is a high level of variety in the way individuals and families progress through these stages of change. There are some individuals who progress in a much more linear direction through the stages, while others vacillate between their readiness for change and the effort they put into making changes. It is integral to periodically assess the stage of change throughout treatment planning and the treatment process to support families in assessing barriers to change and maintaining the progress they have made. It is to be expected that adaptations to treatment plans will need to be made through providers working with families.

Maximizing Potential: Utilizing SMART Goals Framework for Success

Goal setting is an incredibly powerful tool for starting to take steps toward achieving one's goals. However, not all goals are created in an equal achievable fashion. There are several frameworks that have been created for setting appropriate, effective, and achievable goals for all areas of one's life. We will focus on the SMART goals framework in this chapter, which is defined as specific, measurable, achievable, relevant, and time-bound goals [22]. This specific goal-setting framework provides a structured approach to goal-setting that enhances clarity and motivation. The SMART goals framework is also ideal for use in the integrated behavioral health setting given the brief intervention solution focus of the IBH model. Similarly, the SMART goals framework is a brief solution-focused strategy that can be utilized when working on goal setting with patients and their families. This format of goal setting is also beneficial when working on specific health-related goals (e.g., losing weight, increasing exercise, increasing water intake, increasing intake of fruits and vegetables, increasing adherence with medications, etc.).

The first element of a SMART goal emphasizes the importance of making goals clear and precise. A specific goal answers the questions of what, why, and how. Instead of saying, "I want to get fit," a more specific goal would be, "I will exercise for 30 minutes, 5 days a week, to improve my overall health." This clarity helps one understand exactly what needs to be done and eliminates any confusion.

Furthermore, when goals are set, one should track goal-relevant data to know whether one is making progress toward their goals. One feature of effective goals that individuals often miss is that goals must be measurable. In making goals measurable, it allows one to monitor their progress and stay motivated. For example, using the previous example, one can measure their progress by tracking the number of workout sessions one completes each week and for how long one exercises per workout session. This step makes goals quantifiable, which further allows for a sense of accomplishment and can highlight barriers so one can address any areas of improvement.

Additionally, goals are meant to be achievable. Although some individuals aim high, some goals become unrealistic and unachievable due to the way the goal is set up, which ultimately leads to frustration and disappointment and individuals deciding to give up. Goals that are achievable are a good balance between being challenging and attainable. For example, if you are new to exercise, setting a goal to run a marathon in 1 month may not be realistic. Instead, setting a goal to run a 5 K in 3 months is much more realistic and attainable. In focusing on making goals more achievable in this way, it more likely ensures that one is pushing their own limits without setting oneself up for failure.

Goals should also be relevant. One's goals should align with one's broader life objectives and values. A relevant goal resonates with one's long-term vision and contributes to their overall fulfillment. For example, if one's physician expresses that they should lose weight, a relevant goal may be to incorporate exercise into a daily routine. This alignment fosters a sense of purpose and motivation especially when one can see exactly how a goal fits into their overall vision for their life.

Finally, goals should be time-bound and have some type of deadline associated with them. This is another reason why the SMART goals framework may be a good strategy to implement during integrated behavioral health visits as the IBH model is also time limited and focused. Time-bound goals also create a sense of urgency and help one prioritize their time and effort. For example, instead of saying, "I want to lose weight," a more time-bound goal would be, "I will lose 10 pounds in six months." This clear timeframe encourages consistent action and helps one stay focused on their objectives.

Incorporating the SMART goal framework into one's goal-setting process enhances clarity and motivation and also paves the way for tangible success. In defining goals that are specific, measurable, achievable, relevant, and time-bound, one can effectively navigate challenges and celebrate milestones along the journey. Embracing SMART goals transforms aspirations into actionable plans and empowers one to unlock their full potential and health goals.

Whole-Health Focus

The shift to person-centered care also brings a focus on whole health. This means considering not just the physical aspects of health but also mental, emotional, and social factors. A whole-health focus recognizes that various elements of a person's life are interconnected and that true health can only be achieved by addressing all these components comprehensively.

By integrating this whole-health perspective, healthcare providers can develop more holistic care plans that support the overall well-being of the person. This approach can lead to more sustainable health outcomes and improve the quality of life for individuals, as it ensures that all aspects of their health are addressed in a coordinated and supportive manner.

The transition from patient-centered care to person-centered care is a crucial development in modern healthcare. It emphasizes the need to see individuals as more than just patients, incorporating their full range of experiences, roles, and needs into the care process. By creating and reviewing models that support this holistic approach, healthcare providers can build stronger relationships, foster greater trust, and ultimately deliver more effective and compassionate care.

Person's Experiences and Their Role in Healthcare

Person-centered care places significant value on the individual's experiences and their active role in healthcare. By understanding the unique experiences of each person, healthcare providers can tailor treatments that are more aligned with their personal needs and preferences. This approach acknowledges that individuals are experts in their own lives and can offer invaluable insights into their health and well-being.

Furthermore, recognizing the person's role in treatment planning leads to more personalized and effective care. It moves beyond the one-size-fits-all approach, allowing for adjustments that accommodate the person's lifestyle, cultural background, and personal goals. This personalization helps in achieving better adherence to treatment plans and ultimately improves health outcomes.

Tailoring Treatment Plans

Central to person-centered treatment planning is the customization of interventions to meet the unique needs and preferences of each individual. MI provides a framework for collaboratively setting realistic and attainable goals that resonate with the patient's values and priorities. By acknowledging the complexity of behavior change and addressing ambivalence with empathy and understanding, providers can co-create actionable strategies that empower patients to take meaningful steps toward their desired outcomes.

Writing the Treatment Plan

Components: Case Conceptualization & Treatment Plan

Case conceptualization is the synthesis of patient information that may include some or all of the following information: patient strengths and resources, presenting concern(s), a brief summary of historical and current physical and behavioral health symptoms, diagnoses, and functioning, relevant social history, substance use history, trauma history, and social drivers of health [20].

1. Shared understanding is foundational for shared-decision making.
2. Care is not person-centered if the physician and patient have vastly differing understandings of the problem and strategies for promoting or returning to health.
3. Return to discussion of goals and barriers that may prohibit meeting goals in the setting of illness.

The treatment plan should include goals that are agreed upon by the patient and/or family as well as their provider. The written agreed-upon goals should be collaboratively written with the aim of improving the appropriate health outcomes. In addition to very specific goals, timelines, check-ins, and specific action plans should also be discussed, agreed upon, and written. Although goals are important to highlight and break down, it is hard to meet these goals, without a specific action plan and steps to take to reach these goals. As highlighted above, the utilization of a combination of a goal-setting framework as well as motivational interviewing can really help establish what actionable steps need to be taken to effectively achieve the agreed-upon goals. There are several other components that are important to have an accurate and effective treatment plan. These are highlighted below.

1. Goals: As stated above, goal setting is a foundational component of effective treatment planning. Goals should be specific, achievable, measurable, and individualized to the patient's needs.
2. Interventions: These are the actions that providers and patients/families will take to reach the goals.
3. Measurable Objectives: These are actionable and concrete steps that outline how the patient and family will reach these goals.
4. Timelines: It is important that goals have timelines or specific timeframes for checking in on the progress of the goal.
5. Frequency: An important component of treatment planning is deciding how often patients/families and providers should meet to work on and check in on goals. Frequent check-ins allow everyone to stay on track with their responsibilities related to the goal. Frequent check-ins also allow for ongoing assessment of barriers and challenges to engagement in reaching goals.
6. Progress and Tracking: Another important component of treatment planning and goal setting is tracking progress on the goal. A good way to assess progress is to track goal-specific data. The data collected is of course specific to the individual

and their goal. For example, if the goal is to lose 10 pounds, relevant data may include weight changes over time, types of exercise (e.g., cardio vs. weightlifting), the amount of weight lifted, and the duration of each workout session. Tracking this information allows for adjustments to goals, action steps, and the overall treatment plan as needed.

7. Assessment: Finally, gathering a thorough psychosocial and sociocultural history is one of the most important pieces of treatment planning.

Beyond the initial appointments with medical providers, an essential resource for ongoing follow-up is the integrated behavioral health team. These professionals are highly trained and are experts in motivational interviewing, goal setting, assessing barriers, and collaboratively problem-solving strategies to improve healthy lifestyles and goal achievement. After the initial interactions with medical providers, BHCs can take over the follow-up of these types of cases, which allows the medical providers to manage other higher-level care patients. There are times when the BHC and medical provider must collaborate to have more effective healthcare such as eating disorders or diabetes care, but ultimately these types of assessments can be conducted and managed by behavioral health teams and psychologists.

Case Example: Patient-Centered Treatment Planning for a Child Patient

Patient: Sarah, 8 years old

Chief Complaint: Anxiety and Difficulty Sleeping

Background:

Sarah is an 8-year-old girl who lives with her parents and younger brother. She was referred to the pediatric clinic by her school counselor due to complaints of anxiety and difficulty sleeping. According to her parents, Sarah has been excessively worrying about school, particularly about making friends and performing well academically. Her anxiety has escalated to the point where she often struggles to fall asleep at night and experiences frequent nightmares when she does manage to sleep.

Initial Assessment:

Upon assessment, Sarah presents as a shy and reserved child. She appears tense and frequently fidgets with her hands. During the interview, Sarah expresses her worries about school, stating that she feels lonely and overwhelmed by academic expectations. She admits to feeling scared and having trouble relaxing, especially at bedtime. Sarah's parents report similar concerns and describe her as typically well-behaved but increasingly irritable and withdrawn lately.

Patient-Centered Treatment Planning:

Establishing Trust and Rapport:

- The first priority is to establish a trusting and supportive relationship with Sarah. The healthcare provider takes time to connect with her on a personal level, engaging in age-appropriate conversation and demonstrating empathy and understanding toward her concerns.

Psychoeducation:

- Sarah and her parents are provided with psychoeducation about anxiety in children, including its common symptoms, causes, and strategies for coping. They are assured that Sarah's feelings are valid and that they are not alone in dealing with this issue.

Collaborative Goal Setting:

- Sarah, her parents, and the healthcare provider collaboratively set treatment goals based on Sarah's needs and preferences. These goals include reducing Sarah's anxiety symptoms, improving her sleep quality, and enhancing her coping skills.

Cognitive-Behavioral Techniques:

- The healthcare provider introduces Sarah to age-appropriate cognitive-behavioral techniques to manage her anxiety, such as deep breathing exercises, progressive muscle relaxation, and guided imagery. Sarah is encouraged to practice these techniques regularly, both at home and in school.

Sleep Hygiene Practices:

- Sarah's sleep hygiene practices are assessed, and personalized recommendations are provided to promote better sleep quality. This includes establishing a consistent bedtime routine, creating a calm and comfortable sleep environment, and limiting screen time before bed.

School-Based Interventions:

- Collaboration with Sarah's school is initiated to implement supportive interventions in the educational setting. This may include arranging regular check-ins with the school counselor, providing academic accommodations if needed, and facilitating peer support groups to help Sarah build social connections.

Regular Follow-Up and Monitoring:

- Sarah's progress is regularly monitored through follow-up appointments with her healthcare provider. Adjustments to the treatment plan are made as necessary based on her response to interventions and any emerging concerns or challenges.

Family Support and Involvement:

- Sarah's parents are encouraged to actively participate in her treatment plan and provide ongoing support at home. They receive guidance on how to effectively communicate with Sarah about her feelings, reinforce positive coping strategies, and foster a nurturing and supportive family environment.

By prioritizing Sarah's needs, preferences, and unique circumstances, this patient-centered treatment plan aims to empower her to overcome her anxiety and sleep difficulties while promoting her overall well-being and resilience. Ongoing collaboration and support from her healthcare provider, parents, and school community are essential components of her journey toward improved mental health.

References

1. Adams N, Grieder D. Treatment planning for person-centered care: shared decision making for whole health. 2nd ed. Amsterdam: Academic Press; 2014.
2. Tondora J, Miler R, Slade M, Davidson L. Partnering for recovery in mental health: a practical guide to person-centered planning. Hoboken: Wiley; 2014.
3. Schrager S. Integrating behavioral health into primary care. Fam Pract Manag. 2021;28(3):3–4.
4. Wampold B, Imel Z. The great psychotherapy debate: the evidence for what makes psychotherapy work. 2nd ed. Routledge/Taylor & Francis Group; 2015.
5. Wampold B, Budge S. The 2011 Leona Tyler award address: the relationship- and its relationship to the common and specific factors of psychotherapy. Couns Psychol. 2012;40(4):601–23.
6. Wampold B. How important are the common factors in psychotherapy? An update. World Psychiatry. 2015;14(3):270–7.
7. Gee D, Cohodes E. Caregiving influences on development: a sensitive period for biological embedding of predictability and safety cues. Curr Dir Psychol Sci. 2021;30(5):376–83.
8. Wade M, Parsons J, Humphreys KL, McLaughlin KA, Sheridan MA, Zeanah CH, Nelson CA, Fox NA. The Bucharest Early Intervention Project: adolescent mental health and adaptation following early deprivation. Child Dev Perspect. 2022;16(3):157–64.
9. Pritchett R, Pritchett J, Marshall E, Davidson C, Minnis H. Reactive attachment disorder in the general population: a hidden ESSENCE disorder. Sci World J. 2013;2013:818157.
10. American Psychiatric Association. Diagnostic and statistical manual of mental disorders. 5th ed. Washington: American Psychiatric Association.
11. Guyon-Harris K, Humphreys K, Miron D, Gleason M, Nelson C, et al. Disinhibited social engagement disorder in early childhood predicts reduced competence in early adolescence. J Abnorm Child Psychol. 2019;47(10):1735–45.
12. Smiley K, Noy I, Wehner M, Frame D, Sampson C, Wing O. Social inequalities in climate change- attributed impacts of hurricane Harvey. Nat Commun. 2022;13:3418.
13. Puff J, Renk K. Relationships among parents' economic stress, parenting, and young children's behavior problems. Child Psychiatry Hum Dev. 2014;45(6):712–27.
14. Horvath A, Symonds D. Relation between working alliance and outcome in psychotherapy: a meta-analysis. J Couns Psychol. 1991;38(2):139–49.
15. Tan A, Mallika P. Coining: an ancient treatment widely practiced among Asians. Malays Fam Physician. 2011;6(2):97–8.
16. Darsha A, Cohen P. New onset of linear purpura on the back: coining therapy-associated ecchymoses. Cureus. 2020;12(6):e8833.
17. Sung C. Asian patients' distrust of western medical care: one perspective. Mt Sinai J Med. 1999;66(4):259–61.
18. Thorburn S, Kue J, Keon K, Lo P. Medical mistrust and discrimination in health care: a qualitative study of Hmong women and men. J Community Health. 2012;37(4):822–9.
19. Social Determinants of Health- Healthy People 2030 (DHHS, 2022).
20. Mancini M. Person-centered treatment planning. In: Manicini MA, editor. Integrated behavioral health practice. Springer; 2021.
21. Hall K, Gibbie T, Lubman D. Motivational interviewing techniques: facilitating behavior change in the general practice setting. Aust Fam Physician. 2012;41(9):660.
22. Doran G. There's a S.M.A.R.T. way to write management's goals and objectives. Manag Rev. 1981;70(11):35–6.

Chapter 7
Integrated Behavioral Health in Pediatric Residency Training Programs

Theotonius J. Gomes, Lucie M. Romano, Eva Lieberman, and Thomas L. Fisher

Introduction of Integrated Behavioral Health Within Training Programs

Integrated behavioral health (IBH) in primary care settings has been well established as important in improving the quality of care and patient outcomes [1, 2]. It is without a doubt that the incorporation and education of physician trainees in integrated behavioral health becomes a necessity in the current day and age to equip physicians early in their training with the necessary tools to utilize IBH effectively. Integrated models are central to the idea of the home healthcare model, and patient-centered medical homes and IBH help to orient trainees to this care model [3, 4]. The incorporation of IBH in residency training programs may also decrease the burden on trainees to feel they alone have to address all care needs for their patients and can aid in facilitating diagnosis, interventions, and treatment [5], which can be critical to the confidence of early physician learners.

In 2015, the American Psychiatric Association (APA) Council on Medical Education and Lifelong Learning released a policy statement regarding the recommendation of teaching IBH services through integrated clinical experiences in graduate medical education (GME) as well as in continuing medical education [6].

T. J. Gomes (✉)
Department of Pediatric and Adolescent Medicine, Department of Internal Medicine-Division of Combined Internal Medicine-Pediatrics, Western Michigan University Homer Stryker MD School of Medicine, Kalamazoo, MI, USA
e-mail: theotonius.gomes@wmed.edu

L. M. Romano · E. Lieberman · T. L. Fisher
Department of Pediatric and Adolescent Medicine, Western Michigan University Homer Stryker MD School of Medicine, Kalamazoo, MI, USA
e-mail: lucie.romano@wmed.edu; eva.lieberman@wmed.edu; thomas.l65.fisher@wmich.edu

R. W. Apple et al. (eds.), *Using Integrated Behavioral Health in Pediatric Practice*, https://doi.org/10.1007/978-3-031-85784-3_7

Although teaching practices have begun to implement strategies to achieve collaboration between physicians and psychologists, co-training between primary care psychology fellows and residents within an integrated environment is rare and typically occurs without any formalized curricula [2]. Most of the research has focused on family medicine residencies with far fewer in other primary care specialties like pediatrics or internal medicine.

It has been described that academic medicine has been delayed in incorporating strategies for training that have emerged after changes in healthcare delivery [7]. Most residency programs across the country are governed by requirements as outlined by the Accreditation Council of Graduate Medical Education (ACGME). Recent research suggests that most residency programs do not incorporate access to training in integrated settings in general. Several reasons are quoted for this rationale including the funding structure and lack of sufficient providers acquainted with the knowledge to provide adequate supervision to trainees [3].

There has been a wide spectrum of how to incorporate the teaching of integrated care to physician trainees from clinical exposure to didactic and web-based learning [3]. In addition, clinical exposure to IBH appears to occur in a myriad of different training sites including community mental health centers, federally qualified health centers, and a few internal medicine, family medicine, and pediatric primary care clinics.

Although challenges to integrating behavioral health will be discussed later in this chapter, a major barrier to the widespread implementation of integrated care models for trainee exposure is the lack of specific instruction in ACGME program requirements as currently written. It has been suggested that incorporating a directive under the general program requirements, along with ACGME milestones focused on integrated care, would help to establish this training as a core competency for resident physicians and thus expand its inclusion in residency training programs nationwide [3].

Landscape of Integrated Behavioral Health in Pediatric Residency Training

Considering the high prevalence of behavioral health conditions in the pediatric population that present for treatment in pediatric offices and the lack of follow-through when these patients are referred to behavioral health providers, pediatric offices, including primary care residency clinics, often become the primary providers managing these issues [8]. In 1997, the ACGME indicated a required 4-week developmental-behavioral pediatrics (DBP) rotation and embedded DBP training throughout pediatric residency programs to ensure future pediatricians are better equipped to address behavioral health concerns. Despite these requirements, many pediatricians feel inadequately trained in managing behavioral health issues [9]. The American Academy of Pediatrics (AAP) has also advocated for better behavioral health training. A 2009 AAP policy statement emphasized the need for improved behavioral health competencies through innovative curricula.

In 2006, a study assessing mental health and psychiatry training in primary care residency programs found that 85% of residency program directors regarded their behavioral health training as suboptimal. By 2018, another study surveying pediatric residency program directors indicated significant improvement, with only 62.8% still considering their behavioral health training suboptimal. Notably, the suboptimal rate for the developmental-behavioral pediatric rotation was even lower, at 36.6%, demonstrating further progress in this area [8]. These findings support the belief that changes to the training curriculum made by ACGME that emphasize the importance of IBH will have downstream effects on perceived preparation to address behavioral health concerns within residency training clinics.

It was found that pediatric residents training in clinics without integrated mental health clinicians have often felt unsupported and fearful of addressing mental health concerns, sometimes leading them to ignore these issues. In contrast, those training alongside psychology trainees feel better prepared to collaborate with behavioral health providers but only somewhat more confident in handling behavioral health issues independently after graduation [10]. It is also clear from this work that behavioral health plays an integral role as an established presence in the outpatient practice setting during and after training.

Integration of IBH in Primary Care Residency Clinics

There are three prominent models used to integrate behavioral health services within primary care including (a) the Screening, Brief Intervention, and Referral to Treatment (SBIRT) model, (b) the Collaborative Care model (CoCM), and (c) the Primary Care Behavioral Health (PCBH) model [11]. The SBIRT model has been shown to be effective in identifying patients at risk for substance use disorders and linking them to treatment [12, 13]. The CoCM targets patients with anxiety and depression and typically involves using validated clinical rating scales and psychological/psychiatric consultation for patients who do not show improvement [14]. The PCBH model is a primary care approach that involves utilizing a multidisciplinary team to manage behavioral health problems and biopsychosocial health conditions [15]. This model incorporates a behavioral health consultant (BHC) as part of the primary care team who often engages as a generalist practitioner for patients of all ages and health concerns and provides consultation and psychoeducation to the team [15]. PCBH has been successfully implemented across the United States in large healthcare systems, community health organizations, university health centers, clinics for unhoused populations, and family medicine clinics [11].

Overall, IBH has been most frequently and successfully implemented within family medicine residency training programs, which are required to have behavioral health faculty and provide training in IBH [16]. These residency clinics typically provide training for physicians, nurses, social workers, psychologists, and other learners. Because of the variety of training backgrounds and the need to address patient behavioral health concerns, training program curricula must include effective models of IBH delivery [17]. The proper implementation of IBH requires specific skills and specialized training for medical and behavioral health clinicians [18].

Research on the implementation of IBH services within primary care settings has grown substantially over the last three decades [19]. Utilizing effective, evidence-based curricula and evaluating outcomes is a crucial component to implementing IBH within a primary care residency clinic. Established core competencies can guide the development of curricula. There are two current core competencies that outline the essential knowledge, skills, and attitudes for behavioral health professionals working alongside primary care clinicians [7, 20]. However, there are currently no ACGME competencies for primary care clinicians collaborating with behavioral health providers [19]. As such, there is a need for more educational and outcome research for best-practice methods of implementing IBH within primary care residency training programs.

Patient outcomes can be used as a measure of the effectiveness of a residency training program utilizing IBH. Previous research has shown that training primary care clinicians in behavioral health treatment alone is not sufficient in leading to improvements in patient outcomes [21]. Instead, targeting collaborative care when training clinicians can result in better patient outcomes [22]. Some authors have identified important strategies for training resident physicians to implement collaborative care within IBH, including the clinic huddle, shadowing, pull-ins, warm hand-offs, co-counseling, lectures, video observations, and feedback [23]. Utilizing many of these strategies, Martin et al. [24] designed a multi-modal curriculum based on established competencies to train family medicine residents on essential skills for working collaboratively in an IBH setting. Results indicated that implementation of competency-based IBH training within a residency program was feasible, desirable, and timely and improved residents' abilities in working on an IBH team. Reported challenges to implementation included scheduling constraints, motivation to complete curriculum modules outside of training time, and varying levels of resident training needs, behavioral health integration within the clinic setting, and instructor knowledge and competence for feedback. Additionally, this curriculum utilized online modules and a single, interactive workshop with faculty and other residents roleplaying and providing feedback, which does not as closely mimic a naturalistic patient encounter. One way to address this limitation is by using simulated patients.

Jones and colleagues [25] evaluated a pilot curriculum to train pediatric residents to operate in an IBH model using simulated patients with feedback from BHCs. Participation in this curriculum improved self-efficacy in patient care, indicating that training via simulated patients can improve physician's skills in IBH. Although residents' skills in IBH implementation increased, many reported discomfort or anxiety about receiving feedback from a nonpeer (i.e., a BHC or another interdisciplinary team member). To address these and other limitations of competency-based and simulated training experiences, some authors have suggested training resident physicians and behavioral health trainees in the same setting [26].

Duggan and colleagues [2] created and evaluated a co-training curriculum for family medicine resident physicians and primary care psychology post-doctoral fellows, which expanded up and enhanced existing ACGME-required components for family medicine resident training. Across the 4-year project, all trainees met the required competencies and there was a significant increase in patient access to IBH services. Trainees reported gaining the strongest IBH training from co-learning in clinical environments (e.g., co-precepting). Resident physicians reported that the integration of a BHC reduced stress and increased their skills, and many of them indicated that they would advocate for BHCs in their future practices. Psychology fellows reported some of the unique challenges of working in IBH, including serving in multiple roles on the team (e.g., provider, preceptor, and educator). Fellows also highlighted the value of team members understanding and advocating for the role of the BHC, further emphasizing the importance of training primary care teams in understanding and implementing the IBH model. The authors also stress that case identification, care coordination, and follow-up require clear structure, instructions, and feedback.

Based upon the previous literature described, we recommend the following strategies for integrating IBH in primary care residency clinics: (a) evaluate and leverage program commitment, (b) conduct a needs assessment for individual clinic settings, (c) amend and expand upon established residency curricula, (d) utilize existing competencies to evaluate training targets and outcomes, (e) utilize simulated and experiential learning and training opportunities to mimic naturalistic situations, (f) co-train residents and behavioral health providers when possible, (g) establish clear workflows, (g) foster and promote frequent communication among interdisciplinary team members, (h) recruit diverse trainees who value health equity, and (i) cultivate understanding and respect for all interdisciplinary team members and their respective individual and collaborative roles. Continued focus on these strategies may lead to increased resident skills and confidence in collaborative care, and, thus, better patient outcomes.

Identifying Patients

Approximately 70% of primary care visits involve the discussion or treatment of a behavioral health concern [11, 27]. Additionally, 75% of pediatric and adolescents with behavioral health issues first present to primary care and 40–80% may not be diagnosed that need intervention [5, 8]. Identifying patients who may benefit from behavioral health services is an essential, yet complex, initial component to successfully implementing IBH. Behavioral health needs can be structured on the following dimensions: (a) promoting healthy behaviors and wellness, (b) identifying mental health and substance use risk factors and symptoms, (c) identifying medical conditions that are complicated by behavioral health functioning and vice versa, and (d) addressing complex biopsychosocial factors that impact functioning. These dimensions are also influenced by factors such as age, gender, sexual orientation, and other demographic variables and social determinants of health [4]. Within a pediatric clinic, patient needs can include parent training and skills coaching, substance use, weight management and healthy eating, attention and behavioral concerns, sleep and toileting concerns, chronic health management and medication adherence, pain management, and many other presentations appropriate for IBH.

Identification of behavioral health concerns is often done on a case-by-case basis. This can occur when physicians or other healthcare providers or staff identify patients who require repeated visits for the same condition, frequent and lengthy visits, frequent switches from providers, or any other patient who requires more than the average patient. This can also include patients who present with symptoms that do not have apparent physical or medical origins or etiologies, patients who do not respond to typical medical interventions, patients who frequently access medical services without improvement or a medical explanation for the repeated visits, patients who have strained relationships with providers, patients who struggle with nonadherence or frequent missed visits, and patients who experience delayed recovery. Many of these individuals may have diagnosable mental health or substance use conditions, but this is not to say that any of these concerns are "all in their head" or that they are engaging in any of these behaviors with intention or malice. Rather, many patients may be experiencing distress, fear, mistrust, demoralization, hopelessness, life stressors, systemic factors, and a variety of other concerns that impact their functioning and impede their ability to interact with the medical system efficiently and effectively. Thus, the integration and coordination of care within an IBH setting can be beneficial for these individuals by addressing the emotional, behavioral, and social factors, and detection can occur through provider reports or through visit data, claims data, or other clinical indicators.

Another way to identify patients who can benefit from IBH is through psychometrically validated, norm-referenced screening tools. This can occur within the clinic setting, as well as within the larger population to identify and assess community needs. This also allows providers to identify populations and individuals who are at risk for mental health or substance use concerns. Once a screening tool identifies an individual or population, follow-up assessment, specific treatment protocols, and referrals to other providers can be implemented. However, many of the screening tools used in IBH settings are focused primarily on mental health, substance use, and chronic disease. Although there are some validated screening tools to assess quality of life, readiness to change, level of engagement in healthcare, response to treatment and treatment acceptability, optimism, and self-efficacy, these tools have not been widely used or evaluated in primary care settings. Many of these constructs may influence wellness and treatment outcomes. As such, there is a need for research and clinical application in these areas within IBH primary care settings [4].

In addition to provider reports, clinical indicators, and screening tools, BHCs can aid in the identification of patients who would benefit from IBH services. To achieve this, BHCs should be involved throughout the process of a patient visit in a variety of ways. It is crucial for BHCs to be present during the huddle or walking or table rounds when the patient list and presenting concerns are discussed. This can promote conversation about where the physicians might be struggling with patient symptom presentations, interactions, or other factors that may be influencing responses to treatment. BHCs can also help to identify biopsychosocial factors that may be impacting symptoms. Interdisciplinary huddles or rounds allow the team to coordinate the visit such that the BHC is able to be in the room as soon as they are needed and often at the start of the visit when a patient has been identified. Additionally, BHCs must have access to the electronic health record to review the chart for any potential behavioral health concerns. This can include a history of mental health or substance use concerns or other social determinants of health. This can also include previously mentioned factors such as repeated visits with no improvement or apparent physical cause. BHCs can also use the chart to help identify biopsychosocial factors that may be influencing health conditions and response to treatment, such as exposure to traumatic events (e.g., serious accidents). During precepting, BHCs should be present in the room with the attending(s) and resident physician(s) to listen for any potential concerns that may have come up during the visit that were not previously identified. For example, parents will often use visits with their child's pediatrician to inquire about strategies for remote behavioral concerns. If the BHC is present during precepting, this also allows for the residents to seek direct consultation with the BHC. Regardless of how a patient is identified, debriefing should occur with all team members to discuss the patient's subjective factors from the perspective of each provider, any objective data gathered by each provider, and for the care team to agree upon the assessment and plan.

Structure and Workflow of IBH

With a continually growing emphasis on incorporating mental and behavioral healthcare into the primary care setting, educating providers, residents, and interns on a model of integrated care has become an important part of a training curriculum. As mentioned previously, current residency training programs do not require, nor do they all have access to, implementation of integrated behavioral health in the training of residents (Reed, 2016). Inclusion of IBH is ideally an integrative process, where the role of the IBH providers and their model of care is understood to improve collaboration and promote fully integrating the IBH team into the primary care model. As mentioned, there are several models of this integration. Though there are different working models of integrated care, functional frameworks of integration share important features. To fully integrate behavioral health into residency training, it involves more than communication between providers or shared proximity. Instead, a shift in the model of resident education and staffing of primary care education is required to help the practice toward effective implementation of IBH [28, 29].

One of the initial and most important steps in the integration of behavioral health is the physical presence of the BHC within the learning environment. Consistent communication and collaboration between providers are best afforded when the BHC is sharing space with attending physicians and residents staffing their patients

[28]. The experience of the authors has been that this shared space allows residents in training to easily access BHCs and allows the BHC to appropriately provide learning experiences and input on patient care that the residents may otherwise not recognize as needed.

In addition to sharing space, further incorporating the behavioral health providers into the practice can be achieved by including them in the huddle at the start of a clinical shift. As previously discussed, integrating the BHCs into these huddles further exemplifies that they are part of the clinical team and positions the BHCs to start the clinical shift with the same information as the rest of the team to appropriately provide care [30].

Part of the workflow of a BHC as mentioned involves identifying patients who may benefit from behavioral health at their visit. This identification process may occur during team huddles, by the physician upon chart review, by the physician identifying a patient need during the visit, or by BHCs. To best optimize this identification process, it is recommended that BHCs look through the clinic schedule for the day by doing their own chart review [31]. A patient may present to their clinic with a primary presenting problem that could obviously be relevant for IBH services, like depression, anxiety, or ADHD. Alternatively, there may be a past history or note in the chart that would indicate that IBH services would be beneficial. Patient identification by the IBH team affords the team the opportunity to both identify patients who might benefit from IBH services where it may not be obvious to other providers and to identify problems where behavioral solutions may be effective but potentially unknown by resident physicians (i.e., sleep, GI concerns, smoking cessation).

Upon identification that a patient may benefit from IBH services, the BHC, resident physician, and attending physician staffing the case discuss the best way to coordinate care. These discussions may occur prior to seeing the patient that day, in the middle of the appointment when the resident staffs the case, or toward the end of the visit. In the authors' experience, conversations about including the BHC most commonly occur prior to seeing the patient, after the BHC has reviewed the chart and identified a patient need, or when the resident physician is staffing with the attending after meeting with the patient. This staffing discussion occurs in a shared location with the BHC, where the resident physician or attending can easily consult the BHC, or where the BHC can listen to the patient care discussion and consult where appropriate. These are valuable training opportunities for residents, where they discuss patient care with the attending physician and with the BHC who have more extensive background and training in behavioral health.

From this point, the resident physician, attending physician, and BHC determine the best treatment plan for the patient. Sometimes this may not include including the BHC into the patient's care plan, while other times it may mean that the most appropriate provider on the care team is the BHC. More often, in these authors' experience, the entire team works together to discuss the next steps and care for the patient. It is important that residents in training recognize the value of the IBH team, as some patients may feel stigma or be unwilling to talk with "a therapist." Identifying the BHC as a part of the patients' medical care team is crucial in forming the same trust and belief in their behavioral health provider as they feel toward their physician.

Provider Education

Appropriate education on IBH is essential for fully integrating behavioral health into a residency training clinic. To ensure effective implementation, residents must learn to recognize cases where IBH services would be beneficial, attending faculty should encourage residents to consider IBH as a treatment option, and behavioral health providers should be included as part of the care team. Education on IBH should occur both before and throughout the integration process to maximize its effectiveness.

The first point of education about IBH is simply creating an awareness of the service. This can happen during didactic training but can also occur in the clinic. Having behavioral health providers sharing space with residents and supervising physicians in and of itself affords awareness of the service. Additionally, ensuring that faculty members know about IBH and recommend the service as care options to their residents further promotes awareness. Initial training of IBH can be instructional and included in seminars, lectures, or morning reports. This achieves awareness of IBH and the on-paper understanding of IBH. Further training comes from implementation and practice. Working with attending faculty members and resident physicians, IBH providers can continue education while in the clinic. Team discussions about optimal care and when and how to best include the behavioral health team for a patient increase awareness for future cases and promote education of the integrated service. To best integrate behavioral health into a clinic, all providers need to be appropriately educated on the form and function of IBH.

Benefits of Integrated Behavioral Health in Residency Clinical Care Settings

While the advantages of integrating behavioral health into primary care for enhancing patient outcomes are widely recognized, there is currently a lack of substantial research specifically examining its benefits for physician trainees, with most insights coming from anecdotal reports.

Physician trainees, especially early post-graduate year residents, often find it challenging to adjust to the workflow of an outpatient practice. Managing the typical patient load with inherent limitations and time constraints can be difficult, even for seasoned physicians. This adjustment is further complicated by the need for precepting by a supervising physician and the discussions and education that take place before a patient is released from the office visit.

Addressing social and mental health issues tends to be particularly time-consuming and draining for providers. Integrated health offers several benefits in this context. With behavioral health providers on board, physician trainees do not feel they are solely responsible for patient care [5], which is crucial for trainees whose range of solutions to offer patients may be limited initially. Having a behavioral health provider see the patient either before, during, or after the physician visit or when the trainee is precepting helps streamline the process, reducing wait times for patients.

For physician trainees, this is especially important as delays can be more pronounced. Patients and their families also feel they receive better care with more focused attention to their concerns. Additionally, behavioral health providers can contribute to expanding the differential diagnoses and treatment plans for patients, enhancing overall care.

Another significant benefit lies in enhancing key competencies crucial to the relationship between a provider and their patient. Referred to in some studies as "common factors," these include transdiagnostic approaches that prioritize interpersonal communication skills, empathy and listening abilities, patient-centered language, partnering with families, reinforcing strengths, and utilizing motivational interviewing techniques [8, 32]. These elements often serve as foundational building blocks for effective communication. Introducing these concepts early in physician training, with real-life patient interactions, could be particularly impactful in fostering these essential skills.

Finally, integrating IBH into residency training can have a profound impact on early learners. Resident physicians will learn how to effectively collaborate with behavioral health specialists, incorporate this expertise into their workflow, and understand the dynamics of working with these professionals. Should they enter a practice where behavioral health is not yet integrated, they will be well-equipped to establish it themselves. This preparation positions them well for future roles in fellowship or private practice.

Conversely, psychology interns or fellows will gain invaluable experience in working alongside medical providers. They will develop a deeper understanding of how medical providers make management decisions, benefiting from observing resident physicians as they receive this education. They also benefit from having direct access to the interdisciplinary team to better utilize collaborative care for their patients. Conducting interventions in a medical training environment also allows psychology interns or fellows to gain more direct knowledge about the impacts of health on psychological functioning and vice versa. Thus, a holistic approach to treatment also benefits the patients. This reciprocal learning environment enriches both medical and psychological trainees, fostering comprehensive and collaborative care that may improve patient outcomes and increase access to services.

Challenges of Integrated Behavioral Health in Residency Clinical Care Settings

Integrating behavioral health into residency training environments presents both significant opportunities and notable challenges. While many organizations, such as the ACGME, the American Academy of Pediatrics, and the American Psychiatric Association, acknowledge the importance of integrating IBH (Integrated Behavioral Health) in teaching institutions, as mentioned previously there are no universal guidelines for its implementation. This often results in a lack of funding for its integration within institutions.

The Affordable Care Act has introduced policies and programs providing grants for behavioral health integration, including over 100 grants available through the Substance Abuse and Mental Health Services Administration (SAMHSA) and the Behavioral Health Homes State Plan Amendment. However, these grants are not widely implemented in training environments. Moreover, residency programs are primarily funded by Medicare at university/hospital-affiliated sites, which tend to emphasize inpatient care. Even at community sites with a greater focus on outpatient care and behavioral health, additional barriers such as billing for trainee services and the need for certification from Medicaid can hinder effective implementation. Funding becomes even more complex when multiple academic departments share resources, especially when multiple learners are involved.

Equity among medical and behavioral health providers is as crucial as funding. Equity encompasses respect, physical space, and equal access to patient electronic health records. At many institutions, many of these resources may be finite and limited. A shortage of IBH providers with an overabundance of medical providers or vice versa can create a disproportionate level of care that is insufficient to meet the needs of patients. Typically, it is usually the former that occurs more frequently given the number of physician trainees that outnumber behavioral health providers at most institutions.

A specific challenge is the staffing model, which varies across residency programs. Factors such as the structure of outpatient clinics, patient management, available resources, and the presence of supervising attendings and behavioral health psychologists can lead to inconsistency and disruption. However, a well-established structure can maximize provider exposure and collaboration.

Despite these efforts, inadequate follow-up by the same provider and potential continuity of care issues can lead to patient dissatisfaction or loss to follow-up. Additionally, training for incorporating interprofessional teams into clinical environments and developing educational programs for both resident and faculty physicians, as well as behavioral health providers, is essential but can be overwhelming. A local needs assessment may be necessary before implementing a behavioral health program, and competency targets should be established for all trainees.

Overall, while integrating IBH in residency training presents challenges, addressing these issues can lead to significant benefits for both providers and patients.

Opportunities for Integrating and Educating IBH in Novel Training Environments

The integration of behavioral health providers alongside physician trainees has predominantly occurred in family medicine and psychiatry residencies, with fewer instances in pediatric residencies and a very small minority in internal medicine residencies. Only one study in the published literature has evaluated perceptions of integrated behavioral health from attendings, residents, and behavioral health personnel, focusing on education and care coordination within Internal Medicine [33]. Notably, there is a significant overlap in the patient populations of family medicine and internal medicine, suggesting a clear opportunity to expand IBH training and service provision into internal medicine training clinics.

At the authors' home institution, behavioral health has been successfully integrated into internal medicine, pediatrics, and combined medicine-pediatrics programs, with early-stage expansion into subspecialty clinics. Programs without IBH may not be aware of their benefits or existence, reducing the speed at which IBH services are expanded. Although the reasons for consulting behavioral health providers vary based on the practice setting, population, and patient-specific factors, the need for a biopsychosocial model in primary care settings remains paramount to providing quality, holistic patient care, whether through co-location with the physician team or via a referral base.

Integrated care models with behavioral health are nearly absent in subspecialty training. However, given the medical complexity of the patients often treated in these settings, IBH services should be considered an essential component of comprehensive patient care, offering a range of benefits that enhance both medical and mental health outcomes. By embedding behavioral health professionals within specialty clinics such as cardiology, endocrinology, oncology, and others, resident training clinics can address the complex interplay between physical and mental health.

As trainees expand their comfort in addressing the medical concerns that precipitate presentation in a subspeciality clinic, the addition of IBH services to these clinics allows the overall care team to address the psychological and emotional challenges that often accompany chronic medical conditions. Patients with illnesses such as diabetes, heart disease, or cancer frequently experience anxiety, depression, or stress related to their diagnosis, treatment, or prognosis. These mental health symptoms have the potential to subsequently exacerbate physical symptoms and complicate medical management. For example, significant depressive symptoms may reduce a patient's motivation to fully engage with their provider's recommended treatment plan, leading to poorer health outcomes. By incorporating behavioral services into subspecialty treatment settings, physicians and behavioral health providers can collaborate to address the spectrum of factors that may impact chronic disease management, while signaling to the patient the importance of maintaining both their physical and mental health.

While the rollout of IBH services in this area has been slow possibly because the utility of IBH services in these settings may be less apparent, future efforts to expand the availability of IBH services in subspeciality clinics should emphasize the potentially similar impacts of IBH in these clinics as those observed in family medicine, internal medicine, and pediatric training clinics. IBH services can enhance the efficiency and effectiveness of specialty clinics as behavioral health providers assist with behavioral interventions that support disease management, such as helping patients implement lifestyle changes, manage pain, or cope with the side effects of medical treatments. They can also help medical teams navigate complex cases where psychosocial factors significantly impact the patient's health. This collaboration allows specialty physicians to focus on their areas of expertise while ensuring that patients receive the emotional and psychological support they need.

Subsequent chapters in this book aim to further showcase the impact of the integration of behavioral health in pediatric subspecialty practices. Recognizing the value within these settings, it is logical to advocate for the expansion of behavioral health into adult subspecialty practices and other medical disciplines beyond primary care, such as obstetrics, surgery, physical medicine and rehabilitation, and orthopedics.

This discussion raises the question of whether formalized training in care coordination and working with behavioral health clinicians should be included in undergraduate medical education. Medical students will work alongside residents and attending physicians in various practice settings, both community and academic. Therefore, integrating training from the formative years would be beneficial.

Conclusion

Integrated behavioral health (IBH) in primary care significantly enhances the quality of care and patient outcomes. Educating physician trainees on IBH is essential to equip them with the necessary tools early in their careers. IBH models are foundational to home healthcare and patient-centered medical homes, helping to orient trainees to this integrated care model.

Multiple governing bodies recommend teaching IBH through integrated clinical experiences in graduate and continuing medical education. Despite these recommendations, co-training between primary care psychology fellows and residents remains rare, with most research focusing on family medicine residencies.

Even with the ACGME's 1997 requirement for a 4-week developmental-behavioral pediatrics rotation, many pediatricians feel inadequately trained in behavioral health. This has prompted the American Academy of Pediatrics to advocate for improved training. Although studies showed significant improvement in behavioral health training perceptions by 2018, challenges remain.

Effective IBH implementation requires specific skills and training for both medical and behavioral health clinicians. There is a need for more educational and outcome research to establish best practices for IBH in residency programs. Strategies for training include simulated and experiential learning, co-training residents and behavioral health providers, and fostering interdisciplinary communication.

Full integration of IBH into residency training involves more than just communication and proximity. Significant changes in resident education models and primary care staffing are required for effective implementation. Key steps include the physical presence of IBH teams in the learning environment, participation in team huddles, thorough chart reviews to identify patients who might benefit from IBH, and collaborative discussions between IBH providers, resident physicians, and faculty to develop optimal treatment plans.

Continuous education through practical implementation, team discussions, and consultations within the clinic helps ensure all providers understand the role and function of IBH, leading to better patient care.

While behavioral health integration has been predominant in a few specialties, the need for a biopsychosocial model in primary care settings is crucial. This underscores its importance in graduate medical education and potentially in undergraduate medical education curricula as well.

References

1. Smith TE, Erlich MD, Sederer LI. Integrated care: integrating general medical and behavioral health care: the New York state perspective. Psychiatr Serv [Internet] 2013 [cited 2024 Dec 12];64(9):828–31. Available from: https://pubmed.ncbi.nlm.nih.gov/24026832/.
2. Duggan M, Bancroft C, Browder C, Gorski V. Advancing integrated care through cotraining of residents and psychology postdoctoral fellows. Fam Syst Health. 2022;40(4):540–51.
3. Reed E, Crane D, Svendsen D, Herman L, Evans B, Niedermier J, et al. Behavioral health and primary care integration in Ohio's psychiatry residency training. Acad Psychiatry. 2016;40(6):880–6.
4. Talen MR, Valeras AB. Integrated behavioral health in primary care: evaluating the evidence, identifying the essentials, vol. 1. Springer Science & Business Media. p. 1–354.
5. Amin S, Gibson KM, Bines D. Integrated behavioral health collaborative practice embedded within the Pediatric Residency Continuity Clinic: incorporating a multicultural lens. Pediatr Clin North Am [Internet]. 2021 [cited 2024 Dec 12];68(3):659–68. Available from: https://pubmed.ncbi.nlm.nih.gov/34044992/.
6. Moran M. APA's Education Council issues report on need for integrated care training. [Internet]. 2015 [cited 2024 Dec 12];50(5):1. Available from: https://psychiatryonline.org/doi/10.1176/appi.pn.2015.3a29.
7. Hoge MA, Morris JA, Laraia M, Pomerantz A, Farley T. Core competencies for integrated behavioral health and primary care enhanced reader [Internet]. Washington; 2014 [cited 2024 Dec 12]. Available from: https://www.thenationalcouncil.org/wpcontent/uploads/2020/01/Integration_Competencies_Final.pdf.
8. Shahidullah JD, Kettlewell PW, Palejwala MH, Forman SG, Billups A, Anismatta SL, et al. Behavioral health training in pediatric residency programs: a National Survey of training directors. J Dev Behav Pediatr [Internet] 2018 [cited 2024 Dec 3];39(4):292–302. Available from: https://journals.lww.com/jrnldbp/fulltext/2018/05000/behavioral_health_training_in_pediatric_residency.3.aspx.
9. Horwitz SMC, Storfer-Isser A, Kerker BD, Szilagyi M, Garner A, O'Connor KG, et al. Barriers to the identification and management of psychosocial problems: changes from 2004 to 2013.

Acad Pediatr [Internet] 2015 [cited 2024 Dec 6];15(6):613–20. Available from: http://www.academicpedsjnl.net/article/S1876285915002739/fulltext.

10. Kelsay K, Bunik M, Buchholz M, Burnett B, Talmi A. Incorporating trainees' development into a multidisciplinary training model for integrated behavioral health within a pediatric continuity clinic. Child Adolesc Psychiatr Clin N Am. 2017;26(4):703–15.
11. Hunter CL, Dobmeyer AC, Reiter JT. Integrating behavioral health services into primary care: spotlight on the Primary Care Behavioral Health (PCBH) model of service delivery. J Clin Psychol Med Settings [Internet]. 2018 [cited 2024 Dec 3];25(2):105–8. Available from: https://link.springer.com/article/10.1007/s10880-017-9534-7.
12. Babor TF, McRee BG, Kassebaum PA, Grimaldi PL, Ahmed K, Bray J. Screening, brief intervention, and referral to treatment (SBIRT): toward a public health approach to the management of substance abuse. Subst Abus [Internet] 2007 [cited 2024 Dec 13];28(3):7–30. Available from: https://pubmed.ncbi.nlm.nih.gov/18077300/.
13. Moyer VA. Screening and behavioral counseling interventions in primary care to reduce alcohol misuse: U.S. preventive services task force recommendation statement. Ann Intern Med [Internet]. 2013 [cited 2024 Dec 13];159(3):210–8. Available from: https://pubmed.ncbi.nlm.nih.gov/23698791/.
14. Archer J, Bower P, Gilbody S, Lovell K, Richards D, Gask L, et al. Collaborative care for depression and anxiety problems. Cochrane Database Syst Rev. 2012;2012:CD006525.
15. Reiter JT, Dobmeyer AC, Hunter CL. The primary care behavioral health (PCBH) model: an overview and operational definition. J Clin Psychol Med Settings. 2018;25(2):109–26.
16. Accreditation Council on Graduate Medical Education. ACGME Program Requirements – Family Medicine Residency [Internet]. 2024 [cited 2024 Dec 12]. Available from: https://www.acgme.org/globalassets/pfassets/programrequirements/2024-prs/120_familymedicine_2024.pdf.
17. Waxmonsky JA, Williams MD. Training primary care practitioners about integrated behavioral health: how integrated is the training? J Health Care Poor Underserved. 2020;31(4):144–53.
18. Filippi MK, Waxmonsky JA, Williams MD, Robertson E, Doubeni C, Hester CM, et al. Integrated behavioral health implementation and training in primary care: a practice-based research network study. J Am Board Fam Med. 2024;36(6):1008–19.
19. Martin MP. Integrated behavioral health training for primary care clinicians: five lessons learned from a negative study. Fam Syst Health. 2017;35(3):352–9.
20. Kinman CR, Gilchrist EC, Payne-Murphy JC, Miller BF. Provider- and practice-level competencies for integrated behavioral health in primary care: a literature review [Internet]. Rockville; 2015 [cited 2024 Dec 13]. Available from: https://integrationacademy.ahrq.gov/sites/default/files/2020-06/AHRQ_AcadLitReview.pdf.
21. Sikorski C, Luppa M, König HH, Van Den Bussche H, Riedel-Heller SG. Does GP training in depression care affect patient outcome?-A systematic review and meta-analysis [Internet]. 2012. Available from: http://www.biomedcentral.com/1472-6963/12/10.
22. Gilbody S, Whitty P, Grimshaw J, Thomas R. Educational and organizational interventions to improve the management of depression in primary care a systematic review [Internet]. Jama. 289(23):3145–51. Available from: www.jama.com.
23. Porcerelli JH, Fowler SL, Murdoch W, Markova T, Kimbrough C. Training family medicine residents to practice collaboratively with psychology trainees. Int J Psychiatry Med. 2013;45(4):357–65.
24. Martin MP, Banks E, Myerholtz L, Zubatsky M, Suri Y, Mauksch L. Preparing residents to practice integrated behavioral health care: multi-site feasibility study of a competency-based curriculum. [Internet]. 2022 [cited 2024 Dec 3];58(3):201–13. Available from: https://journals.sagepub.com/doi/10.1177/00912174221086930.
25. Jones MR, Dadiz R, Baldwin CD, Alpert-Gillis L, Jee SH. Integrated behavioral health education using simulated patients for pediatric residents engaged in a primary care community of practice. Fam Syst Health. 2022;40(4):472–83.

26. Hoover M, Andazola J. Integrated behavioral care training in family practice residency: opportunities and challenges. J Clin Psychol Med Settings. 2012;19(4):446–50.
27. Vohs JL, Shi M, Holmes EG, Butler M, Landsberger SA, Gao S, et al. Novel approach to integrating mental health care into a primary care setting: development, implementation, and outcomes. J Clin Psychol Med Settings [Internet]. 2023 [cited 2024 Dec 13];30(1):3–16. Available from: https://pubmed.ncbi.nlm.nih.gov/35543900/.
28. Heath BW, Wise Romero P, Reynolds K. A standard framework for levels of integrated healthcare. SAMHSA-HRSA Center for Integrated Health Solutions; 2013.
29. Vogel ME, Kanzler KE, Aikens JE, Goodie JL. Integration of behavioral health and primary care: current knowledge and future directions. J Behav Med. Springer New York LLC. 2017;40:69–84.
30. Kwan BM, Nease DE. The state of the evidence for integrated behavioral health in primary care. In: Integrated behavioral health in primary care: evaluating the evidence, identifying the essentials. New York: Springer; 2013. p. 65–98.
31. Butler M, Kane RL, McAlpine D, Kathol R, Fu SS, Hagedorn H, et al. Does integrated care improve treatment for depression? A systematic review. J Ambul Care Manag. 2011;34:113–25.
32. Foy JM, Health for the AA of PTF on M. Enhancing pediatric mental health care: algorithms for primary care. Pediatrics [Internet]. 2010 [cited 2024 Dec 7];125(Supplement_3):S109–25. Available from: https://publications.aap.org/pediatrics/articleabstract/125/Supplement_3/S109/29855/Enhancing-Pediatric-Mental-Health-Care-Algorithms.
33. Hemming P, Revels JA, Tran AN, Greenblatt LH, Steinhauser KE. Identifying core curricular components for behavioral health training in internal medicine residency: qualitative interviews with residents, faculty, and behavioral health clinicians. Int J Psychiatry Med [Internet] 2019 [cited 2024 Dec 3];54(3):188–202. Available from: https://pubmed.ncbi.nlm.nih.gov/30269631/.

Part II
Health Equity/Cultural Humility

Chapter 8
Improving Health Equity in Primary Care by Integrating Behavioral Health

Cheryl A. Dickson and Nickoli Nickerson

Introduction

It is important to define what the terms health equity and integrated behavioral health mean as a core fundamental foundation for the chapter discussion.

Health equity as a concept applies broadly to all aspects of healthcare, systems, policies, administration, legislature, and research [1]. How health equity is defined has varied among many different organizations. A consistent theme across all definitions of health equity is the gap between the current and ideal states and the enumeration of the factors that impede the attainment of the ideal state [2].

A widely accepted definition put forward by the National Academies of Science, Engineering, and Medicine is the following: "Health equity is the state in which everyone has the opportunity to attain their full health potential and no one is disadvantaged from achieving this potential because of social position or any other socially defined circumstance" [3]. The Robert Wood Johnson Foundation (RWJF) has recently recommended making the definition more specific by explicitly stating which populations and groups it refers to and what it means for action [4]. The definition, although longer makes it clearer, reduces ambiguity and addresses all the key determinants of health as well as provides transparency for all to understand.

> Health equity means that everyone has a fair and just opportunity to be as healthy as possible. This requires removing obstacles to health such as poverty, discrimination, power-

C. A. Dickson (✉)
Pediatrics and Adolescent Medicine, Western Michigan University, Homer Stryker M.D. School of Medicine, Kalamazoo, MI, USA
e-mail: Cheryl.dickson@wmed.edu

N. Nickerson
Western Michigan University, Homer Stryker MD School of Medicine, Kalamazoo, MI, USA
e-mail: Nikoli.nickerson@wmed.edu

R. W. Apple et al. (eds.), *Using Integrated Behavioral Health in Pediatric Practice*, https://doi.org/10.1007/978-3-031-85784-3_8

lessness, and their consequences including lack of access to good jobs with fair pay, safe environments, and quality education, housing, and health care [4].

An important aspect of the definition of health equity is the distinction between equity and equality. Equality involves providing everyone with the same resources, whereas equity acknowledges that individuals who have experienced exclusion or marginalization often require more—not the same—resources to address the impact of that exclusion and marginalization.

With regard to children, the American Academy of Pediatrics' Council on Community Pediatrics has noted that the principles of pediatric health equity include a recognition of children's rights, social justice, and ethics. In their 2010 policy statement, they emphasized that the well-being of children and their families requires the existence of equity [5].

For the purposes of measurement, health equity means reducing and ultimately eliminating disparities in health and its determinants that adversely affect excluded or marginalized groups [15]. In this statement, it is important to emphasize that health equity means more than the mere absence of disparities in health; it also implies the absence of disparities in the determinants of health, including the social determinants. Disparities in health and its key determinants are the metrics used to indicate progress toward or away from health equity [5]. This is especially important in pediatrics as health disparities have a long-term impact on the future attainment of health, including educational and economic success [6–8].

Integrated behavioral health by definition results from a practice team of primary care and behavioral health clinicians, working together with patients and families, in a systematic and cost-effective way to provide patient-centered care that may address mental health and substance abuse conditions, health behaviors including their contribution to chronic medical illnesses, life stressors, and crises, stress-related physical symptoms, and ineffective patterns of healthcare utilizations [9]. The practice of behavioral health in an integrated model addresses not only behavioral symptoms but also multiple psychological and behavioral factors that are associated with acute or chronic illness [13].

The practice of an integrated model of behavioral health can help address some of the inequities in mental health by reducing some of the social determinants and barriers to care experienced by marginalized populations, which include access to care such as finding practitioners, transportation costs, scheduling, and time. Integrating behavioral health with comprehensive primary healthcare can help increase the quality of care as well as reduce costs, leading to better health outcomes and ultimately a decrease in disparities [10–12].

The core principles of the IBH model are applicable across all age groups [9].

Inequities in Pediatric Mental Healthcare

Mental health conditions like anxiety and depression are increasingly a concern in the United States; an estimated one in every six children in the United States is affected by a mental health condition [14]. Untreated mental health conditions are a cause of serious morbidity *and contribute to decreased educational attainment, and in some cases can lead to suicide which is the second leading cause of death in adolescents aged 12–18* years old [15].

Despite this statistic, only half of children and adolescents with a mental health condition receive treatment from a mental health provider [14]; clearly, a gap of unmet mental healthcare exists in this patient population. In 2021, the American Academy of Pediatrics, American Academy of Child and Adolescent Psychiatry, and Children's Hospital Association declared a national emergency in children's mental health, recognizing a need for special attention to the issue considering its magnification by the COVID-19 pandemic [16]. This report noted an increase in emergency department visits for mental health concerns by 24% for children aged 5–11 and 31% for children 12–17 years, with an increase in 31% of suspected suicide attempts among girls 12–17 years in early 2021 [16]. These health concerns during the pandemic, coupled with an increase in grief from the loss of a parent, caregiver, and family members, add to the continued rise in the need for mental healthcare for children and adolescents.

While children and adolescents as a demographic collectively experience an unmet gap in their mental healthcare, some populations are at greater risk for worse mental health than their peers. These groups include the following:

1. *Black and Latinx Children and Adolescents*

Black and Latinx children and adolescents access mental healthcare at half the rate of their white counterparts, contributing to the profound mental healthcare access disparity that exists within these historically marginalized groups [17]. A rising concern for higher suicide rates in Black boys aged 5–11 and adolescent Black girls aged 12–17 has raised the alarm for the need for increased preventive measures such as earlier screenings as well as referrals [18]. Social determinants, which include higher poverty rates and uneven geographic distribution of resources, along with structural racism and discrimination, contribute to the inequities in access and disparities impacting outcomes for mental and behavioral health and have long-term impacts. Three notable disparities in mental and behavioral health for racial and ethnic minorities include diagnosis and treatment for externalizing behavior disorders, autism spectrum disorder (ASD), and suicide. These differences are marked by less likelihood of receiving outpatient treatment and less likelihood of being screened, diagnosed, and referred to a specialist [17]. Externalizing behavioral disorders in Black and Latinx children are more likely to be referred to emergency departments for aggression and agitation [17, 34].

Diagnosis of ASD among non-Hispanic Black children has been reported to be at a higher rate than among White children since 2018 [18]. Despite this statistic, the average reported delay in ASD screening from the time of parents' first concern can be as long as 3 years. This delay significantly contributes to higher rates of intellectual disability (44% versus 22%) and increased comorbidities among children from marginalized groups compared to non-Hispanic White children, primarily due to limited access to early, evidence-based services [19].

There are multiple factors that contribute to decreased and/or lack of access to mental and behavioral health services for racial and ethnic minorities. The range includes structural and perceptual. Structural barriers include insurance barriers, as well as community-level shortages of mental behavioral health providers, and barriers such as time, distance, and financial resources. On an individual level, competing demands for work and other responsibilities including parental perceptual awareness of and beliefs that mental and behavioral health are a significant problem that requires or needs any outside intervention can contribute to inequities. Importantly, stigma that families may have regarding mental behavioral concerns negatively impacts seeking preventive care as well as any previous history of adverse experiences with the healthcare system [47, 48]. Understanding the impact of these factors is an essential component in screening and planning for care.

2. *Sexual and Gender Minorities*

Youth who identify as a sexual and gender minority group, such as lesbian, gay, bisexual, transgender, queer, or questioning (LGBTQ), face multiple challenges that function as barriers to accessing mental and behavioral health services [44]. These barriers include fear of invalidation with gender identity (misgendering) and discrimination by providers and feeling the providers may be lacking in education for their specific health needs [22–24].

Adolescents seeking gender-affirming hormone therapy experience increased depression, anxiety, and difficulties relating to peers in part due to a lack of access to clinical infrastructure specifically tailored toward this group of patients [25].

Barriers to accessing care also include structural obstacles, such as lack of insurance coverage for gender-affirming care and insurance denials, which impact the majority of transgender youth. Additionally, recent political influences and laws in some states have further restricted access, even in cases where the benefits of these services meet rigorous criteria [25–27].

Youth and adolescents who belong to a sexual minority group are reported to have higher rates of experiencing biased-based bullying as well as family rejection, which puts them at higher risk for adverse mental behavior health outcomes. Adverse health outcomes, such as attempted suicide, have a higher rate in these youth compared to heterosexual peers [28]. It has been reported that compared to heterosexual cisgender peers, the odds of attempting suicide are more than three times higher for homosexual children (odds ratio [OR] 3.71, 95% CI 3.15, 4.37), more than fourfold higher for bisexual children (OR 4.87, 95% CI 4.76, 4.98), and over five times higher for transgender children (OR 5.87, 95% CI 3.51, 9.82) [28]. In 2019, 46.8% of high school students who identified as lesbian, gay, or bisexual reported having seriously considered suicide, and 23.4% reported having attempted suicide [28, 29].

Even with advances in public awareness, youth who identify as LGBTQ still face increased disparities from multiple sources, which include inequitable laws and policies and societal discrimination. Pediatricians are often the primary healthcare providers for transgender and gender-diverse (TGD) youth seeking advice and care. However, many may not have received adequate formal training to effectively meet the specific healthcare needs of this population [20].

It must also be made clear that mental illness in these youth is multi-factorial, including internal conflict between one's appearance and identity, coupled with limited availability of mental health providers and services with expertise in caring for youth, discrimination, stigma, and social rejection [20]. In addition, TGD youth experience increased homelessness, physical violence, and rejection from home as well as communities and are more susceptible to substance use and high-risk sexual behaviors, which can contribute to higher adverse MBH health outcomes [20–22].

3. *Children and Youth in Rural Communities*

Children and adolescents who live outside of major metropolitan and surrounding areas are particularly underserved in access to needed mental and behavioral health services [42, 43]. Rural communities although in the same state and counties have different cultures and populations than urban areas. Many of these differences impact overall health outcomes including mental health. The median income tends to be lower in rural areas, with fewer job opportunities. Employment is more often agrarian in nature, with higher self-employment rates that provide limited access to health insurance [38]. In addition, the completion of higher education rate is lower, with lesser high school graduation rates compared to urban areas [37].

Most youth with mental health conditions still do not receive needed interventions, largely because of the insufficient numbers of child mental health specialists and their concentration in urban/suburban areas and academic hubs [30, 31, 42]. It was noted by McDermott et al. that 60% of rural counties are designated as having a shortage of mental health practitioners [35]. Rural schools are less likely than urban schools to require that school counselors, social workers, and psychologists be certified or credentialed by state agencies or licensing boards and less likely to require school mental health workers to earn continuing education credits [36]. In addition, historical policy decisions for de-institutionalism, which led to the closure of large psychiatric institutions and a shift toward community-based care, left a higher toll and burden on many rural areas that were left without adequate community resources to support the need for mental health services adding to existing disparities.

Mental health providers that are local may also have inadequate access to evidence-based interventions [44]. Lack of access to insurance, low Medicaid utilization, and insufficient funding contribute to inequities in mental healthcare, as well as challenges in the sustainability and stability of the mental healthcare workforce [45, 46].

Disparities in both access to and quality of care for children and adolescents are particularly notable, especially due to the shortage of child and adolescent psychiatrists as well as mental and behavioral health specialists [42, 43]. While this shortage is a nationwide issue, it is especially pronounced in rural America, where psychiatric care is often provided by a fragmented network of family physicians, school counselors, mental healthcare workers, and child protective services caseworkers [41].

Geographic home location is also important, as suicide rates for adolescents and young adults are higher in rural communities compared to urban counterparts, a difference that has increased over time [32]. The age-adjusted rural suicide rate among people aged 15 and older is 35% higher [39]. Stigma in seeking care for mental health adds to the disparities in suicide as well as depression and anxiety disorders. Stigma is thought to be one of the main causes of delaying psychiatric care among the rural population [40]. Additionally, in smaller communities where people are more likely to know one another, concerns about a lack of anonymity often outweigh fears of confidentiality breaches [31, 38].

4. *Incarcerated Juveniles*

It is estimated that 66% of incarcerated juvenile males and 75% of incarcerated juvenile females meet the criteria of at least one mental health disorder, presenting a need for improved delivery of mental healthcare to this patient population [33]. Clearly, there is much work to be done to ensure an equitable delivery of mental healthcare for children and adolescents in the United States.

In summary, a comprehensive approach is essential to address the factors contributing to mental and behavioral health disparities, particularly among children and youth. Developing and implementing best-practice models that integrate behavioral health within the primary pediatric medical home is crucial. For example, the continuum of service might be split up into pre-diagnosis and diagnosis (prevention, screening, initial diagnosis); management of diagnosis (quality of treatment received, quantity of treatment received); and evaluation of management (outcomes). Since each stage of this continuum can be influenced by interventions at multiple levels, efforts to improve equitable access to children's mental health care must involve a collaborative approach. This includes engagement from clinicians, health systems, schools, community stakeholders, and legislators at the state and national levels.

Pediatric Patient-Centered Medical Home and Integration of Behavioral Health

Access to care is often a considerable barrier, as multiple factors—such as scheduling frequent appointments, traveling to those appointments, taking time off from school or work, and coordinating between providers—can make it difficult to obtain equitable healthcare. The pediatric patient-centered medical home (P-PCMH) functions as a whole-child approach to healthcare, existing as the intersection of multiple facets of care [49]. With a P-PCMH model, children and adolescents can receive comprehensive care at their pediatric primary care office with an improvement in coordination among the numerous other services involved in the delivery of care; the collective mission is to deliver more equitable, coordinated, patient-centered care.

Integrating behavioral healthcare into the P-PCMH model in theory mitigates the barriers to care often experienced by patients with the intent to deliver high-quality mental healthcare that is well-coordinated with the work of the existing pediatric primary care provider.

Catering to a unique patient population, pediatricians play an important role in framing the trajectory of children and adolescent health at a critical time in life. Many health behaviors with profound morbidity and mortality in early adulthood (such as obesity, depression, anxiety, and substance use disorders) are often established in childhood or adolescence [50, 51]. Due to expanded insurance coverage, most children and adolescents in the United States have access to a primary care physician or PCMH.

Integration of behavioral healthcare into the P-PCMH takes existing mental healthcare delivered by primary care providers (PCPs) and increases the use of evidence-based medication algorithms and evidence-based psychotherapy, collectively improving the treatment of the mental health conditions that can often persist into adulthood unaddressed if ineffectively managed in childhood [49]. Primary care in the United States has become a critical access point for patients to receive adequate mental healthcare; integrating mental healthcare into the PCMH can support primary care providers by increasing their comfort with managing these long-term conditions [52]. Not only does the integration of behavioral healthcare improve provider comfort in the treatment phase, but it also allows for earlier detection of mental health problems as it becomes a core component of these practices, making it less likely to be missed or misdiagnosed. There are numerous benefits that come from the integration of behavioral health into PCMHs that have already been seen in such practices in the United States [53]. One improvement in care seen from such a model is that PCPs can feel more comfortable that their patients are getting timely access to the mental healthcare they need. Patients saw improvement in common mental health conditions such as anxiety and depression, evident in reduced scores on the GAD-7 and PHQ-9. Integrated behavioral health is an effective approach to the diagnosis and treatment of pediatric mental health conditions.

IBH Models: Advantages and Challenges

Integrated behavioral health (IBH) features licensed mental health providers embedded within primary care offices, working closely with primary care providers to address the mental health needs of children and adolescents [53]. There are various models that can be used to meet the needs of the population being served and the primary practice. In general, integrated behavioral health (IBH) is an effective method in addressing the under-met mental health needs seen in the pediatric population [54]. IBH is a cost-effective and systematic approach to providing patient-centered care for the defined population. The care may address mental health and substance abuse conditions, health behaviors (including their contribution to chronic medical illnesses), life stressors and crises, stress-related physical symptoms, and ineffective patterns of healthcare utilization [55].

IBH helps reduce mental and behavioral health inequities, by providing increased access to care within the same practice or location, increasing the probability of follow-up and coordination of care with the primary care provider, and decreasing the stigma of receiving behavioral care as well as reducing costs [50, 55, 57, 58].

There are several different frameworks and two main models for IBH. Models are the approaches and frameworks that refer to the overarching conceptual structure that organizes how practices implement integrated care. Integrating behavioral health into primary care requires planning for what is the best fit for the practice and the needs and characteristics of the patient population. Integrating behavioral health into the primary care practice is not a small quality improvement project but a transformative undertaking for the entire practice.

The two main comprehensive models of IBH care are the following:

1. *Collaborative Care Model*

The Collaborative Care Model involves a team-based approach that includes consultation with a psychiatrist, proactive outreach and population management by a behavioral healthcare manager, and a measurement-guided care plan.

2. *Primary Care Behavioral Health Model*

The Primary Care Behavioral Health model incorporates a behavioral health clinician into the primary care team who works as a generalist in providing accessible services for behavioral health problems and bio-psychosocially influenced health conditions.

Other models of behavioral health integration include integration into specialty care settings and settings and integration of primary care into a behavioral health clinic.

Primary care practices often implement integrated care with a hybrid approach to these models, or with incorporation of some but not all of these components. Some examples include hiring an integrated behavioral health professional who provides generalist counseling services and also establishing a contract for telepsychiatry or partnering with a psychiatrist outside of their current resources but choosing to improve their coordination with outside behavioral health services with their care manager initiating outreach for high priority behavioral health conditions. The approach may also vary depending on local workforce availability and resources, including financial for the practice [53, 56, 57].

Challenges to implementation also include a chronic history of under-funding of both primary care and behavioral health services; despite the addition of some newer billing codes for integrated behavioral health, criticism lies in the insufficient coverage of the spectrum of IBH healthcare and incentive for volume versus quality [58].

Newer types of frameworks for implementation of IBH include:

1. *Comprehensive Health Integration (CHI)* [59]

The CHI framework includes eight evidence-based "Domains of Integration" and associated sub-domains that are an adaptation and expansion of the previously published General Health Integration (GHI) Framework for Behavioral Health organizations [59]. In CHI, each of the domains has been updated to be applicable to both Primary Healthcare (PH) and Behavioral Healthcare (BH) settings and to both adult and child populations. There are measurable standards with the framework that help document progress in each of the domains. These are organized by defining three "Integration Constructs" with performance metrics that provide an opportunity to demonstrate value.

The CHI framework can function as a measurement tool for assessing the level of integration within healthcare practices, programs, and provider organizations. It enables these entities to evaluate and demonstrate their progress in delivering integrated services to the populations they serve. Additionally, it provides a structured way to communicate this progress to payers and population managers.

The purpose of the CHI framework is to provide a comprehensive and practical guide for bidirectional integration—both the integration of PH into BH settings and behavioral health into primary healthcare settings. This framework is designed to be flexible and adaptable, making it applicable to child and adult populations, small and large healthcare providers, rural and urban settings, and organizations with varying levels of resources [59].

The processes identified in each domain are all related specifically to addressing PH and BH issues in an integrated manner. The eight broad domains are as follows:

1. Screening, Referral, and Follow-Up
2. Prevention and Treatment of Common Conditions
3. Continuing Care Management
4. Self-Management Support
5. Multidisciplinary Teamwork
6. Systematic Measurement and Quality Improvement
7. Linkage with Community/Social Services for SDOH
8. Financial Sustainability

2. *The Building Blocks of Behavioral Health Integration Framework* [55]

The Building Blocks of Behavioral Health Integration Framework is designed to align expectations across payers, providers, and patients. The framework can be used in alternative payment models supporting flexible approaches to implement BHI so that payers know how additional support is being used, providers are able to choose their approach based on patient needs and local resources, and there are standardized care delivery expectations for patients [55].

The key components of the framework include the following:

1. Foundational Care Delivery Expectations: Leadership in the practice for identifying patients who could benefit from the services and providing and linking them to care with follow-up and measurements in place.

2. Advanced Coordination and Care Management: Shared information and expectations between primary and behavioral health providers and linkages with social services and specialists as needed.
3. Integrated Behavioral Health Professional (IBHP): An integrated behavioral health professional works as part of the primary care practice.
4. Psychiatry: A psychiatrist supports complex diagnostic evaluation and therapy.
5. Advanced Care of Substance Use Disorders (ACSUD): Primary care provider provides treatment for Substance Use Disorders, such as tobacco, alcohol, and opioid use. Counseling is provided in the practice for these disorders.

These components are data-driven to support quality improvement, emphasize team-based care, and promote patient and family engagement while ensuring access to necessary resources.

Summary: Closing the Gap

Integrating behavioral health practice into the P-PCMH allows for an opportunity to broaden the scope of practice; this practice model presents an opportunity for behavioral health clinicians to more effectively follow developmental concerns, mental health consultations, and psychopharmacologic changes in order to optimally manage any number of behavioral health conditions [60]. In a span of 3 years, 10 of the 11 integrated practice models started in California continued to operate at the end of the study period, showing that these practices have a need in the broader community and can be an effective option for managing mental health conditions [53]. While integrated models are effective, disparities remain even despite their initiation, leaving room for improvement in the way that they are implemented and the practice design [61]. Rural and urban areas have historically been geographic categories that experience health disparities for a number of reasons; for example, these areas are often under-resourced, making the integration of behavioral health into the PCMH more challenging with fewer resources available to support patients [62]. Although designation as a federally qualified health center (FQHC) can help bring recognition to practices and health systems that are underserved, these safety net organizations report barriers to delivering behavioral healthcare, particularly for patients that are uninsured [63]. Integrating behavioral healthcare into the PCMH in these areas will be one step in improving access to mental healthcare for patients in these areas, but more steps are needed to close the gap on this disparity of care [63]. On the provider level, increasing the capacity of providers and staff to address barriers to care (identification of social determinants of health with appropriate action, integrating mental healthcare into pediatric graduate medical education) can help improve patient engagement in mental healthcare. Focus on clinical infrastructure, such as establishing relationships between pediatricians and mental health providers and adoption of routine screening for pediatric social-emotional concerns, can ensure that problems are identified and appropriately treated when present. On the care team level, increasing the use of paraprofessionals and advocating for policy change to support integrated practices can take steps to ensure the mental health of communities as a whole is addressed. Properly addressing pediatric mental health conditions is important and needed. While improvements to the delivery of mental healthcare for this population are necessary to optimize child and adolescent health, integrated behavioral health practices offer a practical way to broaden the scope of the P-PCMH while mitigating barriers to care that prevent children and adolescents from receiving the mental healthcare, they both need and deserve.

Future Directions

There is no one comprehensive model for IBH and the spread of integrated behavioral health and primary care outside of research and demonstration projects has been limited and sustaining successful programs has been challenging due to many of the factors listed in this chapter. There is increased interest in better understanding more about integration strategies and their implementation.

The newer frameworks Comprehensive Health Integration (CHI) and the Building Blocks of Behavioral Health Framework offer a way to standardization for integration and improved research on effectiveness, which can help with evidence of best practice and offer foundations for providers and practices.

References

1. Montoya-Williams D, Peña MM, Fuentes-Afflick E. In pursuit of health equity in pediatrics. J Pediatr X. (Internet). 2020 (cited 2023 Jan 2);5:100045. https://doi.org/10.1016/j.ympdx.2020.100045. Epub 2020 Aug 21. PMID: 33733084; PMCID: PMC7963264. Available from: https://pubmed.ncbi.nlm.nih.gov/33733084/.
2. Braveman P, Arkin E, Orleans T, Proctor D, Acker J, Plough A. What is health equity? Behav Sci Policy. (Internet). 2018 (cited 2022 Dec 29);4:1–14. Available from: https://behavioralpolicy.org/wp-content/uploads/2018/12/What-is-Health-Equity.pdf.
3. National Academies of Sciences, Engineering, and Medicine, Health and Medicine Division, Board on Population Health and Public Health Practice, Committee on Community-Based Solutions to Promote Health Equity in the United States. Communities in action: pathways to health equity. Washington, DC: National Academies Press.
4. Braveman P. Defining health equity. J Natl Med Assoc. (Internet). 2022 (cited 2022 Dec 29);114(6):593–600. https://doi.org/10.1016/j.jnma.2022.08.004. Epub 2022 Sep 24. PMID: 36167751. Available from: https://pubmed.ncbi.nlm.nih.gov/36167751/.
5. The American Academy of Pediatrics Policy statement on health equity and children's rights. Pediatrics. (Internet). 2010 (cited 2023 Jan 2);1259(4):838–49. Available from: https://publications.aap.org/pediatrics/article/125/4/838/73134/Health-Equity-and-Children-s-Rights?autologincheck=redirected.
6. Braveman P, Barclay C. Health disparities beginning in childhood: a life-course perspective. Pediatrics. (Internet). 2009 (cited 2023 Jan 3);124(Suppl 3):S163–75. Available from: https://pubmed.ncbi.nlm.nih.gov/19861467/.

7. Braveman PA. Swimming against the tide: challenges in pursuing health equity today. Acad Med. (Internet). 2019 (cited 2023 Jan 2);94:170–1. Available from: https://pubmed.ncbi.nlm.nih.gov/30431455/. [PubMed: 30431455].
8. Montoya-Williams D, Peña MM, Fuentes-Afflick E. In pursuit of health equity in pediatrics. J Pediatr X. (Internet). 2020 (cited 2023 Jan 2);5:100045. Available from: https://pubmed.ncbi.nlm.nih.gov/33733084/.
9. AHRQ: effective health care program: strategies for integrating behavioral health and primary care. (Internet) (cited 2024 Oct 25). https://effectivehealthcare.ahrq.gov/products/strategies-integrating-behavioral-health/protocol.
10. Katon W, Lin E, Von Korff M, et al. Collaborative care for patients with depression and chronic illnesses. N Engl J Med. 2010;363(27):2611–20. https://doi.org/10.1056/NEJMoa1003955. PMID: 21190455.
11. Solberg L, Crain A, Jaeckels N, et al. The DIAMOND initiative: implementing collaborative care for depression in 75 primary care clinics. Implement Sci. 2013;8:135. https://doi.org/10.1186/1748-5908-8-135. PMID: 24238225.
12. Unützer J, Katon W, Callahan C, et al. Collaborative care management of late-life depression in the primary care setting: a randomized controlled trial. JAMA. 2002;288(22):2836–45. https://doi.org/10.1001/jama.288.22.2836. PMID: 12472325.
13. Soares N, Apple RW, Kanungo S. The role of integrated behavioral health in caring for patients with metabolic disorders. Ann Transl Med. 2018;6(24):478.
14. Whitney DG, Peterson MD. US national and state-level prevalence of mental health disorders and disparities of mental health care use in children. JAMA Pediatr. 2019;173(4):389–91. https://doi.org/10.1001/jamapediatrics.2018.5399.
15. CDC: National Center for Health Statistics Adolescent Health: (internet access: Oct 2024). https://www.cdc.gov/nchs/fastats/adolescent-health.htm.
16. AAP, AACAP, CHA declare national emergency in children's mental health. AAP News. American Academy of Pediatrics. Accessed 20 July 2024. https://publications.aap.org/aapnews/news/17718/AAP-AACAP-CHA-declare-national-emergency-in.
17. Alegria M, Vallas M, Pumariega AJ. Racial and ethnic disparities in pediatric mental health. Child Adolesc Psychiatr Clin N Am. 2010;19(4):759–74. https://doi.org/10.1016/j.chc.2010.07.001.
18. Ring the alarm: the crisis of black youth suicide in America: Emergency Taskforce on Black Youth Suicide and Mental Health. https://theactionalliance.org/sites/default/files/ring_the_alarm-_the_crisis_of_black_youth_suicide_in_america_copy.pdf.
19. Maenner MJ, Shaw KA, Bakian AV, et al. Prevalence and characteristics of autism spectrum disorder among children aged 8 years — autism and developmental disabilities monitoring network, 11 sites, United States, 2018. MMWR Surveill Summ. 2021;70(11):1–16. https://doi.org/10.15585/MMWR.SS7011A1.
20. Rafferty J, Committee on Psychosocial Aspects of Child and Family Health, Committee on Adolescence, Section on Lesbian, Gay, Bisexual, and Transgender Health and Wellness. Ensuring comprehensive care and support for transgender and gender-diverse children and adolescents. Pediatrics. 2018;142(4):e20182162. https://doi.org/10.1542/peds.2018-2162. Epub 2018 Sep 17. Erratum in: Pediatrics. 2023 Oct 1;152(4):e2023063756. doi: 10.1542/peds.2023-063756. PMID: 30224363.
21. Tordoff DM, Wanta JW, Collin A, Stepney C, Inwards-Breland DJ, Ahrens K. Mental health outcomes in transgender and nonbinary youths receiving gender-affirming care. JAMA Netw Open. 2022;5(2):e220978. https://doi.org/10.1001/jamanetworkopen.2022.0978. Erratum in: JAMA Netw Open. 2022 Jul 1;5(7):e2229031. doi: 10.1001/jamanetworkopen.2022.29031. PMID: 35212746; PMCID: PMC8881768.
22. Chong LSH, Kerklaan J, Clarke S, Kohn M, Baumgart A, Guha C, Tunnicliffe DJ, Hanson CS, Craig JC, Tong A. Experiences and perspectives of transgender youths in accessing health care: a systematic review. JAMA Pediatr. 2021;175(11):1159–73.

23. Edwards A, Hung R, Levin JB, Forthun L, Sajatovic M, McVoy M. Health disparities among rural individuals with mental health conditions: a systematic literature review. Rural Ment Health. 2023;47(3):163–78. https://doi.org/10.1037/rmh0000228. Epub 2023 May 11. PMID: 37638091; PMCID: PMC10449379 in Accessing Health Care: A Systematic Review. JAMA Pediatr. 2021 Nov 1;175(11):1159–1173. https://doi.org/10.1001/jamapediatrics.2021.2061. PMID: 34279538.
24. Hoffmann JA, Alegría M, Alvarez K, et al. Disparities in pediatric mental and behavioral health conditions. Pediatrics. 2022;150(4):e2022058227. https://doi.org/10.1542/peds.2022-058227.
25. House H, Gaines S, Hawkins LA. Sexual and gender minority adolescents: meeting the needs of our LGBTQ patients and their families. Clin Pediatr Emerg Med. 2019;20(1):9–16. https://doi.org/10.1016/j.cpem.2019.02.004.
26. Kuper LE, Mathews S, Lau M. Baseline mental health and psychosocial functioning of transgender adolescents seeking gender-affirming hormone therapy. J Dev Behav Pediatr. 2019;40(8):589–96. https://doi.org/10.1097/DBP.0000000000000697.
27. Nahata L, Quinn GP, Caltabellotta NM, Tishelman AC. Mental health concerns and insurance denials among transgender adolescents. LGBT Health. 2017;4(3):188–93. https://doi.org/10.1089/lgbt.2016.0151.
28. Kremen J, Williams C, Barrera EP, et al. Addressing legislation that restricts access to care for transgender youth. Pediatrics. 2021;147(5). https://doi.org/10.1542/peds.2021-049940.
29. Di Giacomo E, Krausz M, Colmegna F, Aspesi F, Clerici M. Estimating the risk of attempted suicide among sexual minority youths. JAMA Pediatr. 2018;172(12):1145–52. https://doi.org/10.1001/jamapediatrics.2018.2731. [PubMed: 30304350].
30. Myers K, Comer JS. The case for telemental health for improving the accessibility and quality of children's mental health services. J Child Adolesc Psychopharmacol. 2016;26(3):186–91. https://liblynxgateway.com/wmed?url=https://www.proquest.com/scholarly-journals/case-telemental-health-improving-accessibility/docview/2113648650/se-2. https://doi.org/10.1089/cap.2015.0055.
31. Brooks D, Jani S. Rural and frontier communities. Child Adolesc Psychiatr Clin N Am. 2024;33(4):729–39. https://doi.org/10.1016/j.chc.2024.06.002. Epub 2024 Jul 20. PMID: 39277322.
32. Fontanella CA, Hiance-Steelesmith DL, Phillips GS, et al. Widening rural-urban disparities in youth suicides, United States, 1996–2010. JAMA Pediatr. 2015;169(5):466–73. https://doi.org/10.1001/jamapediatrics.2014.3561.
33. Vinson SY, Coffey TT, Jackson N, McMickens CL, McGregor B, Leifman S. Two systems, one population: achieving equity in mental healthcare for criminal justice and marginalized populations. Psychiatr Clin North Am. 2020;43(3):525–38. https://doi.org/10.1016/j.psc.2020.05.006.
34. Marrast L, Himmelstein DU, Woolhandler S. Racial and ethnic disparities in mental health care for children and young adults: a national study. Int J Health Serv. 2016;46(4):810–24. https://doi.org/10.1177/0020731416662736.
35. Mcdermott M, Drescher C, Smitherman T, et al. Prevalence and sociodemographic correlates of lifetime substance abuse among a rural and diverse sample of adolescents. Subst Abus. 2013;34(4):371–80.
36. O'Malley M, Wendt SJ, Pate C. A view from the top: superintendents' perceptions of mental health supports in rural school districts. Educ Adm Q. 2018;54(5):781–821.
37. Merchant JA, Coussens C, Gilbert D; The Institute of Medicine Roundtable on Environmental Health Sciences, Research, and Medicine. The Social Environment in Rural America. Rebuilding the unity of health and the environment in Rural America. Washington, DC: National Academies Press; 2006.
38. Murry VMB, Heflinger CA, Suiter SV, Brody GH. Examining perceptions about mental health care and help-seeking among rural African American families of adolescents. J Youth Adolesc. 2011;40(9):1118–31.

39. Nestadt P, Triplett P, Fowler D, et al. Urban-rural differences in suicide in the state of Maryland: the role of firearms. Am J Public Health. 2017;107:1548–53.
40. Eberhardt MS, Pamuk ER. The importance of place of residence: examining health in rural and nonrural areas. Am J Public Health. 2004;94:1682–6.
41. Reiss F. Socioeconomic inequalities and mental health problems in children and adolescents: a systematic review. Soc Sci Med. 2013;90:24–31.
42. Thomas CR, Holzer CE 3rd. The continuing shortage of child and adolescent psychiatrists. J Am Acad Child Adolesc Psychiatry. 2006;45:1023–31.
43. https://www.apa.org/pubs/reports/2011-report.pdf. Accessed 26 Nov 2024.
44. Comer JS, Barlow DH. The occasional case against broad dissemination and implementation: retaining a role for specialty care in the delivery of psychological treatments. Am Psychol. 2013;69:1–18.
45. Glisson C, Schoenwald SK, Kelleher K, Landwerk J, Hoagwood K, Mayberg S, Green P. Therapist turnover and new program sustainability in mental health clinics as a function of organizational culture, climate, and service structure. Admin Pol Ment Health. 2008;35:124–33.
46. Stirman SW, Kimberly K, Cook N, Calloway A, Castro F, Charns M. The sustainability of new programs and innovations: a review of the empirical literature and recommendations. Implement Sci. 2012;14:7–17.
47. Mojtabai R, Olfson M. National trends in mental health care for US adolescents. JAMA Psychiatry. 2020;77(7):703–14. https://doi.org/10.1001/JAMAPSYCHIATRY.2020.0279. [PubMed: 32211824].
48. Cook BL, Hou SSY, Lee-Tauler SY, Progovac AM, Samson F, Sanchez MJ. A review of mental health and mental health care disparities research: 2011–2014. Med Care Res Rev. 2019;76(6):683–710. https://doi.org/10.1177/1077558718780592. [PubMed: 29877136].
49. Shahidullah JD, Hostutler CA, Coker TR, Allmon Dixson A, Okoroji C, Mautone JA. Child health equity and primary care. Am Psychol. 2023;78(2):93–106. https://doi.org/10.1037/amp0001064.
50. Asarnow JR, Miranda J. Improving care for depression and suicide risk in adolescents: innovative strategies for bringing treatments to community settings. Annu Rev Clin Psychol. 2014;10:275–303. https://doi.org/10.1146/annurev-clinpsy-032813-153742schw.
51. Kolko DJ, Perrin E. The integration of behavioral health interventions in children's health care: services, science, and suggestions. J Clin Child Adolesc Psychol. 2014;43(2):216–28. https://doi.org/10.1080/15374416.2013.862804.
52. Acri MC, Bornheimer LA, O'Brien K, et al. A model of integrated health care in a poverty-impacted community in New York City: importance of early detection and addressing potential barriers to intervention implementation. Soc Work Health Care. 2016;55(4):314–27. https://doi.org/10.1080/00981389.2015.1137256.
53. Schweitzer J, Bird A, Bowers H, et al. Developing an innovative pediatric integrated mental health care program: interdisciplinary team successes and challenges. Front Psych. 2023;14:1252037. https://doi.org/10.3389/fpsyt.2023.1252037. Published 2023 Nov 16.
54. Remoue Gonzales S, Higgs J. Perspectives on integrated behavioral health in pediatric care with immigrant children and adolescents in a Federally Qualified Health Center in Texas. Clin Child Psychol Psychiatry. 2020;25(3):625–35. https://doi.org/10.1177/1359104520914724.
55. Gold SB, Gilchrist E, Kirchner S, Razeen B, Green LA, Perry Dickinson W. The building blocks of behavioral health integration. The Eugene S. Farley, Jr. Health Policy Center & the Practice Innovation Program at the University of Colorado Anschutz Medical Campus; 2022.
56. Fledderman N, DeLeon J, Patel DR. Integrated behavioral health: definitions and contexts. Pediatr Clin N Am. 2021;68(3):511–8. https://doi.org/10.1016/j.pcl.2021.02.007. PMID: 34044980.
57. Polaha J, Williams SL, Heflinger CA, Studts CR. The perceived stigma of mental health services among rural parents of children with psychosocial concerns. J Pediatr Psychol. 2015;40(10):1095–104.

58. Balasubramanian BA, Cohen DJ, Jetelina KK, et al. Outcomes of integrated behavioral health with primary care. J Am Board Fam Med. 2017;1(30):130–9. Miller BF, Ross KM, Davis MM, Melek SP, Kathol R, Gordon P. Payment reform in the patient-centered medical home: enabling and sustaining integrated behavioral health care. Am Psychol. 2017;72(1):55–68.
59. Chung H, Smali E, Narasimhan V, Talley R, Goldman ML, Ingoglia C, Woodlock D, Pincus HA. Advancing integration of general health in behavioral health settings: a continuum-based framework. National Council for Mental Wellbeing; 2020. https://www.thenationalcouncil.org/resources/advancing-integration-of-general-health-in-behavioral-health-settings-acontinuum-based-framework/.
60. Talmi A, Muther EF, Margolis K, Buchholz M, Asherin R, Bunik M. The scope of behavioral health integration in a pediatric primary care setting. J Pediatr Psychol. 2016;41(10):1120–32. https://doi.org/10.1093/jpepsy/jsw065.
61. Chakawa A, Crawford TP, Belzer LT, Yeh HW. Disparities in accessing specialty behavioral health services during the COVID-19 pandemic and why we need pediatric integrated primary care. Front Psych. 2024;15:1356979. https://doi.org/10.3389/fpsyt.2024.1356979. Published 2024 May 10.
62. Wielen LM, Gilchrist EC, Nowels MA, Petterson SM, Rust G, Miller BF. Not near enough: racial and ethnic disparities in access to nearby behavioral health care and primary care. J Health Care Poor Underserved. 2015;26(3):1032–47. https://doi.org/10.1353/hpu.2015.0083.
63. Rust G, Daniels E, Satcher D, Bacon J, Strothers H, Bornemann T. Ability of community health centers to obtain mental health services for uninsured patients. JAMA. 2005;293(5):554–6. https://doi.org/10.1001/jama.293.5.554-c.

Chapter 9
Special Populations Including Transgender and Questioning Youth

Donald E. Greydanus and Dilip R. Patel

Introduction

A foundational factor in the successful survival of *Homo sapiens* over the past millennia is the emergence of the complex phenomenon of human sexuality that has been amazingly analyzed by science, religion, and politics. In the twenty-first century, the byzantine features of this topic have emerged into a controversial web of debate and research [1, 2]. As our children emerge from infancy to prepare for adulthood, they may need guidance from their healthcare providers regarding concerns that may arise over their inevitable progression in their understanding and acceptance of human sexuality [3, 4]. Table 9.1 outlines the basic topics of this chapter's concepts.

Traditional aspects of human sexuality focus on three intrinsic features: biological sex, core gender identity, and gender role behavior. Further evaluation of this arena leads to the *LGBTQIA+* classification referring to persons described as lesbian, gay, bisexual, transgender, questioning (queer), intersexed, agender, asexual, pansexual, genderqueer, and others. This discussion considers definitions of these terms and then presents potential behavioral complications seen in our pediatric patients who may be on a life journey to become part of this fascinating *LGBTQIA+* group. Emphasis is on the potential transgender child or adolescent and that integrated behavioral health can be of help to these persons as well as the clinicians caring for them. This review starts with key definitions in this arena and includes some historical reflections as well.

D. E. Greydanus (✉) · D. R. Patel
Department of Pediatric and Adolescent Medicine, Western Michigan University Homer Stryker M.D. School of Medicine, Kalamazoo, MI, USA
e-mail: donald.greydanus@wmed.edu

R. W. Apple et al. (eds.), *Using Integrated Behavioral Health in Pediatric Practice*, https://doi.org/10.1007/978-3-031-85784-3_9

Table 9.1 Outline of chapter

1. Abstract
2. Introduction
3. Definitions of Human Sexuality Concepts
4. Transgender Teen and Young Adult
(a) *Prevalence: Homosexuality and Transgenderism*
(b) *Issues of Nomenclature and Diagnostic Considerations*
(c) *Behavioral and Mental Health Problems*
5. Conclusions

Definitions

In the nineteenth- to twenty-first-century studies of the growth of human beings from birth to adulthood, various classic stages have been identified that include the psychosexual development of Sigmund Freud (1856–1939), cognitive development of Jean Piaget (1896–1980), psychosocial development of Eric Erikson (1902–1994), moral development of Lawrence Kohlberg (1927–1987), and others (Table 9.2 [5–13],). From this and other research, definitions and descriptions have emerged regarding the enigma as well as the purpose of human sexuality as part of the overall presence of human development [14].

Classic analysis of human sexuality has focused on three themes: *biological sex, core gender identity*, and *gender role behavior* [15]. Such perusals over the history of humanity have debated the normalcy versus pathology of these challenging concepts with many fields entering this complex as well as changing debate that include the interplay of science, religion, and politics [1, 2, 14–19].

Biological Sex

The concept of *biological sex* is identified in a biological system based on the XX/XY sex chromosomes found in human beings and other mammals. It notes that a person's biological sex XX or XY is established at conception though research reveals that sex hormones in the postnatal period can also have effects on the growing fetus [15]. In this sex-determination system, the influence of biological factors leads to sexual distinctions of this person. Classic theory concludes that androgen steroid hormones present between the 6th and 12th fetal week induce the XY fetus to be a "normal" male from a biological and, to some measure, behavioral extent.

In this system, it is concluded that a "normal" female (XX) arises due to the existence of female hormones combined with the absence of a critical threshold of androgens in the fetus. This system is complex and still not well understood and seen, for example, in the identification of apparently limited circumstances or cases characterized by the absence of critical sex hormone levels (i.e., deficient or

Table 9.2 Classic stages of human development from nineteenth- to twenty-first-century research

Name of the development	Specific stages and ages in development
Psychosexual development of Sigmund Freud (Austrian neurologist; psychoanalysis founder)	1. Oral Stage: Birth to 18 months 2. Anal Stage: 18 months to 3 years 3. Phallic Stage: 3–6 years of age (Oedipus/Electra Complex) 4. Latency Stage: 6–12 years of age 5. Genital Stage: Ages of adolescence (12+)
Cognitive development of Jean Piaget (Swiss psychologist)	1. Sensorimotor Stage (0–2 years) 2. Preoperational Stage (2–7 years) 3. Concrete Operational Stage (7–11 years) 4. Formal Operational Stage (11 years plus)
Psychosocial development of Eric Erikson (German-born American psychoanalyst)	1. Basic trust vs. Mistrust Stage (Infancy) 2. Autonomy vs. Shame & Doubt Stage (Toddler years) 3. Initiative vs. Guilt Stage (Early Childhood) 4. Industry vs. Inferiority Stage (School Aged/Middle Childhood) 5. Identity vs. Role Confusion Stage (Adolescent Years) 6. Intimacy vs. Isolation Stage (Emerging Adulthood) 7. Generativity vs. Stagnation Stage (Middle Adult years) 8. Integrity vs. Despair Stage (Older Adult Years)
Moral development of American psychologist Lawrence Kohlberg (three levels: pre-conventional, conventional, and post-conventional; each level has 2 sub-stages)	1. Level 1: Pre-conventional (a) Stage 1: Punishment and obedience (b) Stage 2: Instrumental purpose orientation 2. Level 2: Conventional (a) Stage 3: Good Boy/Nice Girl (b) Stage 4: Law and Order 3. Level 3: Post-conventional or Principled (a) Stage 5: Social Contract (b) Stage 6: Universal Ethical Principles (not everyone reaches this highest level or moral development)

excessive) with resultant alteration of what is considered to be a "normal" female or male. The perplexing paradox of this biological sex system is also identified by the unusual presence of a chromosomal aberration inducing an intersex individual that has a prevalence of 0.18% and indicates various mixtures of male as well as female characteristics [20, 21].

The oft-perceived enigmatic nature of the biological sex system includes other perplexities leading to such conditions as the Klinefelter syndrome, Turner syndrome, and congenital adrenal hyperplasia (late-onset adrenal hyperplasia). *Klinefelter syndrome* is found in males and most cases are due to a 47,XXY karyotype because of sex chromosome aneuploidy; less frequent causes are from higher-grade aneuploidies such as 48,XXXY or 48,XXYY, an aberrant X chromosome such as 47,iXq,Y, and even a mosaicism such as 47,XXY/46,XY [22]. *Turner syndrome* is identified in females because of the absence of the second sex chromosome (45,X) or portions thereof [23, 24]. If there is an excess of androgens due to abnormal adrenal gland steroidogenesis, *congenital adrenal hyperplasia* (CAH) results—most commonly due to 21-hydroxylase deficiency and less commonly due to others such as 11β-hydroxylase and 3β-hydroxysteroid dehydrogenase deficiency [25]. CAH can occur in males or females with varying presentations based on the precise state of enzyme deficiency that occurs.

Core Gender Identity/Gender Role Behavior

As complex and controversial as the concept of biological sex can be, perhaps concepts of *core gender identity* and *gender role behavior* may be even more contentious and enigmatic for society and researchers in the twenty-first century. Theories of child development generally conclude that children typically self-identify themselves as "male" or "female" by 3 years of age; also, they usually establish non-sexual gender role behavior at this age, for example, little girls playing with dolls and wearing dresses in contrast to little boys who usually would not be involved in such behavior.

The self-concepts of "femininity" versus "masculinity" are seen in young childhood and reinforced or challenged by personal feelings and societal/familial inputs as childhood emerges into adolescence and adulthood. Views of childhood development usually conclude that having a heterosexual or homosexual orientation may develop in childhood (i.e., 6–8 years of age) but exploration of a physical sexual behavior with orgasm is identified in the adolescent years with further variations or adaptions arising during the adult years. Despite contemporary religious–political concerns in this regard, observations and research in the twentieth and twenty-first centuries reveal that human sexuality is fluid, is more complex than known effects of sex hormones, and includes variations as found in the *LGBTQIA+* classification referring to persons described as lesbian, gay, bisexual, transgender, questioning (queer), intersexed, agender, asexual, pansexual, genderqueer, and others (see Table 9.3) [1–4, 13, 15–19, 26–31].

As research and controversy continue in such changing arenas, more traditional terms are challenged and potentially rejected by some in society. For example, the concept of *heteronormativity* involves acceptance of heterosexuality as being normal and homosexuality as being abnormal. Such a concept is challenged by those supporting the fluidity of gender theories with the acceptance of various views on human sexuality [30, 31]. This may lead to confusion on the part of some children, adolescents, and young adults dealing with emerging concepts of human sexuality and the potential development of mental health concerns or disorders.

Thus, it is critical that persons in the healthcare profession provide guidance for these pediatric persons in this regard which can include the use of integrated

Table 9.3 Definitions of various terms in human sexuality

Asexuality (hypo-sexuality)
This refers to an adolescent or adult who reports no interest in nor drive regarding sexual eroticism; hypo-sexuality refers to a *limited* interest or drive in sexual eroticism.
Biological Sex
See Text.
Bisexuality
This describes an adolescent or adult who reports erotic desire toward both males and females but not always in equal measures.
Cisgender(Cis)
This refers to a person who reports a gender identity that is equivalent to the one given at birth: a male remains a male and a female remains a female. This person does not report being provided the "wrong" sex identification.
Core Gender Identity
See text.
Cross-Dressing Behavior
This refers to the behavior of pubertal adolescents or adults who derive non-erotic pleasure from dressing in clothes opposite to their biological sex. It can be seen in various persons, including those who are heterosexual or homosexual, and may occur for a variety of reasons (i.e., entertainment, culture, others). Those persons who derive erotic pleasure from such pleasure that leads to serious distress in their lives or prevents normal (ordinary) day-to-day living may have a psychiatric disorder called transvestic disorder or transvestic fetishism.
Gender Dysphoria
This term refers to the consequential or weighty discomfort (anguish) stimulated in persons who find that the sex given to them by parents/healthcare team at birth is not consistent with what their feelings or emotions tell them they are.
Genderqueer [29]
This term is illustrative of the 21st concept of the fluidity of human sexuality and refers to adults who may have changing concepts of genders that include feeling they are neither male nor female at one time and/or perhaps one or the other at other times. Terms used may be genderqueer or non-binary genders.
Gender Role Identity
See text.
Gender Role Behavior
See text.
Genetic Sex
This is a term in the sexuality literature that identifies the sex of a person based on the chromosomes that are present such as XY, XX, XO, XXY, XYY, and others. See text.
Heterosexuality
This is a term in the human sexuality literature describing a pubertal adolescent or adult reporting significant eroticism toward the opposite sex (i.e., females for males, males for females) and little if at all toward the same sex. Such eroticism involves a person's sexual desire, speculations, and encounters. In various religious and political agendas, it is considered the normal state of erotic wishes and behavior.

(continued)

Table 9.3 (continued)

Homosexuality
This is a term in the human sexuality literature describing a pubertal adolescent or adult reporting significant eroticism toward the same sex (i.e., females for females, males for males) and little if at all toward the opposite sex. Such eroticism involves a person's sexual desire, speculations, and encounters. In various religious and political agendas, it is considered an abnormal state of erotic wishes and behavior. Homosexual males are called gay persons and homosexual females are called lesbian persons.
LGBTQ
This term refers to adolescent or adult persons who describe themselves as lesbian, gay, bisexual, transgendered, or questioning (i.e., not sure what sexual orientation one is and perhaps seeking clarification)
LGBTQIA+
This is an expanded term that indicates and illustrates the expanding features of the fluidity of sexuality: lesbian, gay, bisexual, transgender, questioning (queer) intersexed, agender, asexual, pansexual, genderqueer, and others
Pansexuality (Omnisexuality)
This term describes pubertal adolescents or adults who feel their sexual or emotional attraction to others is not subject to nor contingent on the specific gender or sex of others. This is illustrative of the twenty-first-century concept of the fluidity of human sexuality.
Transsexualism (Transgender)
This term refers to pubertal adolescents or adults who conclude their assigned anatomic sex or gender identity is inconsistent with their feelings; thus, the assigned female identifies as being a male while the assigned male self-identifies as a female. In a culture that is against such a concept due to religious and/or political agendas, this can lead to considerable behavioral consequences for these persons. See text.

behavioral health in pediatric practice [32]. Potential problems and management issues in the lives of transgender persons are now discussed as an example of such persons who are dealing with fluidity in human sexuality; indeed, some may find frightening confusion in their transition from childhood to adolescence and adulthood while dealing with living in current society as potential or established transgender persons [1–3, 15, 33].

Transgender Teen and Young Adult

Prevalence (Homosexuality and Transgenderism)

Despite timeless theological and bureaucratic exhortations that the normal state of human sexuality involves XY males and XX females who are heterosexual, researchers and non-heterosexual persons have provided information in the twentieth and twenty-first centuries that human sexuality is a fluid and fascinating process of *Homo sapiens* that extends beyond heterosexuality [1, 18, 19]. Pioneering publications occurred in the mid-twentieth century involving surveys of 5000 adult males and 6000 adult females in the 1930s and 1940s; this monumental work was led by

American sexologist and biologist (zoologist) Alfred Charles Kinsey (1894–1956) with his colleagues including Wardell B. Pomeroy (American sexologist and psychologist; 1913–2001), Clyde Martin (American sexologist; 1918–2014) and Paul Henry Gebbard (American anthropologist and sexologist; 1917–2015) [34, 35].

In their often disputed works, they concluded that exclusive homosexuality (i.e., sexual fantasy and sexual behavior) is found in 4% of adult males and 2% of adult females [34, 35]. Their research led to the now classic Kinsey 7-point scale of sexual orientation in which 0 is exclusively heterosexual in sexual behavior as well as fantasy and a 6 is exclusively homosexual in sexual behavior and fantasy [34, 35]. Though the percentages of adults who range from 0 to 6 are often debated by some, the concept is identified that a wide variety of normal human sexuality is found apart from exclusive heterosexuality [1, 15, 36, 37].

As children and adolescents mature, they develop more understanding of their sexual identities, which can involve a variety of sexual fantasies and experimentations. American adolescent medicine specialist Gary Remafedi published a 1992 study that surveyed 34,706 Minnesota students from grades 7 to 12; his research revealed that 88.2% felt they were principally heterosexual while 10.7% were not sure of their sexual orientation and 1.1% identified as being bisexual or essentially homosexual [38]. The inevitable journey of children and adolescents toward an adult understanding and acceptance of their actual sexual orientation and identity can be confusing, challenging, and conflictual—especially if they arrive at conclusions at odds with the dictums of family and society. The confusion that this may engender may lead to some to question who they are in terms of a sexual being.

American sociologist Richard R. Troiden has presented a four-stage model of gay identity development as noted in Table 9.4 [39, 40]. In *Stage One*, an individual engages in variable homosexual experiences as a child and/or teenager as there is learning acquired in the negative perspective generally found in society regarding a gay lifestyle. *Stage Two* reflects the conflicts this person has in struggling to understand that the anti-homosexual societal attitude applies to him or her and eventually *Stage Three* may arise in which the person recognizes that s/he is gay, seeks some involvement in gay culture, and seriously reflects on the concept that they can live as a homosexual person.

In *Stage Four*, there is acceptance (affirmation or integration) of being a homosexual person in which one's eroticism (i.e., sexual desire, speculations, and encounters) is toward the same sex (female to female or male to male). Some persons can be halted at any stage while others may eventually arrive in their journey of life in Stage Four over years or perhaps a lifetime. Other models are being developed by researchers in the study of acquiring a homosexual lifestyle in humans [41].

Table 9.4 Troiden's stages of gay identity development [39, 40]

1. Stage One: Sensitization
2. Stage Two: Dissociation and Signification
3. Stage Three: Coming Out
4. Stage Four: Acceptance

In the potentially labyrinthine peregrination for the acquisition of an adult sexual orientation, some persons come to the realization or questioning state that they have been labeled by family and/or society with the wrong sex category. As listed in Table 9.3, these human beings may acquire the label of being transgender persons [15, 33]. The acknowledgment of transgender human beings has taken many millennia of human history due to the conflict of such a concept presented to general human society. Plutarch (46 to 119 AD) was a Greek philosopher, historian, and priest at the Temple of Apollo in Delphi (Greece) who wrote about an intersex deity called "the great mother" and other Greek legends detailed the lives of ancient Amazons including Amazon females who were male-like in many ways including their clothes and fighting skills [42, 43].

In the twentieth century, after millennia of myths and theological turmoil, researchers began to provide some detailed data on the subject of transgenderism. For example, Harry Benjamin (1885–1986) was a German–American endocrinologist and a sexologist who provided information on the reality of what was called transsexualism in the middle of the twentieth century [44, 45]. The term, transgenderism, replaced the term transsexualism over time for many, and Harry Benjamin was honored for his research in various ways including the initiation of the Harry Benjamin International Gender Dysphoria Association in 1979, which itself transitioned into the World Professional Association for Transgender Health (WPATH) [33].

Another influential twentieth-century researcher in this arena was New Zealand American sexologist and psychologist John William Money (1921–2006), who stimulated the study of transsexualism that included the development of its medical management; this included modus operandi involving appropriate psychological, medical, and surgical stratagem that initiated sex reassignment surgery in 1966 [33, 46–48].

As we are in the middle of the third decade of the twenty-first century, studies have shown society the existence of transgender persons and some children as well as adolescents will declare themselves in this group during their adolescence and/or adulthood after a potentially turbulent journey of human sexuality self-realization and experimentation. Some will have variable periods of questioning who they are and may benefit from appropriate healthcare providers and mental health professionals working with them. Some may develop other conclusions after being in a questioning state for variable periods of time in their *LGBTQIA+* journey.

Studies continue to search for the prevalence of transgenderism in current society. Some research on adults suggests that 0.4–0.6% are transgender and some conclude that 0.7% of 13–17-year-olds are transgender youth [33, 49, 50]. WPATH has concluded that transgender female (male to female) prevalence is about 1 in 12,000 and transgender male (female to male) prevalence is about 1 in 30,000; up to 1.3% of middle school pupils identify themselves as transgender [33]. Thus, the studies endure and healthcare professionals must provide empathic, comprehensive care to these individuals. In this regard, it is important to understand what problems these persons may be at risk for and how to help them.

Issues of Nomenclature and Diagnostic Considerations

Healthcare provided to a child or adolescent with potential transgenderism and/or confusion about their sexual identity should be non-judgmental, sensitive, and comprehensive and integrate behavioral health principles. This pediatric person faces a myriad of sometimes overwhelming challenges complicating their journey to healthy adulthood. In a thorough evaluation of their pediatric patients, clinicians may learn that this patient expresses views consistent with questioning their sexual identity or consistent with possible transgenderism. This child or adolescent may be exposed to disturbing and frightening information from family and other elements of society including social media.

It is important for the clinician to understand that this pediatric patient (child or adolescent) may develop a myriad of behavioral and mental health problems as well as disorders. The clinician can work with integrated behavioral health professionals to provide an immediate evaluation while developing an expeditious plan of action to help their patient and family. This is also the case for the child and adolescent who deal with seeking to acquire other non-heterosexual identities (i.e., homosexual, bisexual, others) as noted in Table 9.3 [51].

The clinician typically utilizes a diagnosis of gender dysphoria when evaluating patients having anguish over realizations or feelings that the sex label provided to them at birth is not consistent with what they feel from emotions within themselves. Such labels can be upsetting to these patients who may be provided other perceived labels of negativity from miscellaneous theological and societal groups (including family and peers). The clinician can consult with the 2013 DSM-5 book from the American Psychiatric Association for guidance in the diagnosis of gender dysphoria (GD) that recommends two categories of GD, both requiring specific criteria lasting at least 6 months in which there is GD in children versus GD in adolescents and adults [52].

Differences in diagnosis are found in these two groups including, for example, the need for the presence of at least six of eight listed criteria for children versus at least two of six listed criteria for GD in adolescents and adults [52]. In both criteria, the diagnosis includes considerable distress within the person because of the identified discordance and it should be specified if the GD is found with congenital adrenal hyperplasia, androgen insensitivity syndrome, or other sex development disorders [52]. In the criteria of GD in adolescents and adults, it is necessary to note if the person with this diagnosis has shifted into a post-transition state involving living in the selected gender and receiving (or preparing to receive) appropriate hormonal and/or surgical management.

The 2013 DSM-5 evolved into its 2022 text revision compendium (DSM-5 TR) that continued with its detailed discussion of gender dysphoria [53]. Nomenclature continues to evolve and in the DSM-5 TR these phrases are used: individual assigned male at birth or individual assigned female at birth (versus natal male/natal female), experienced gender (versus desired gender), and gender-affirming treatment regimen (versus cross-sex treatment regimen) [52–54]. Also, some clinicians around the

Table 9.5 Differential diagnosis of gender dysphoria [52]

1. Nonconformity to gender roles
2. Transvestic disorder
3. Body dysmorphic disorder
4. Psychosis (schizophrenia, others)
5. Others (i.e., conditions not meeting DSM-5 GD diagnosis)

world prefer to utilize concepts from the World Health Organization International Classification of Diseases (ICD) regarding gender identity-related diagnoses; the 1994 ICD 10 was replaced with the ICD 11, which was implemented in 2022; it is a reliable clinical tool for healthcare professionals with excellent reliability and clinical utility compared to the DSM 5 as well as DSM 5 TR [55].

A sine qua non axiom for the trained clinician is to consider the differential diagnosis of conditions one assesses and manages [56]. When evaluating a potential diagnosis of gender dysphoria, the DSM-5 suggests several possibilities as listed in Table 9.5 [33, 52, 53, 57–59]. The clinician and healthcare team evaluating this person must be well-trained in this arena and thoroughly understand GD as well as its differential diagnoses while remaining nonjudgmental and sensitive in interactions with this patient [33, 60]. If overtime, a diagnosis of transgenderism is made, referral to a team specializing in the management of these persons is recommended so that appropriate as well as timely management goals can be established with regard to psychological support, hormonal treatment (i.e., gender-affirming treatment management), and/or appropriate gender reassignment surgery [33, 60, 61].

Behavioral and Mental Health Problems

The increased risk of behavioral and mental health problems in those in various places on a journey toward a lifestyle of transgenderism is not surprising, considering the negative milieu in which these persons and others in the *LGBTQIA+* population exist; see Table 9.6 [33, 51]. A few are discussed now, and this emphasizes the need for behavioral services including counseling that should be available to these persons and the potential benefit of integrated behavioral services in pediatric practice, as recommended in this chapter as well as the book [32].

Bullying

In a study of 14- to 19-year-olds (1177) from this group (i.e., transgender, genderqueer, cisgender sexual minority), poly-victimization (i.e., 5 or more experiences with victimization) was reported in 39.3% [62]. In this group of poly-victimization, the most common form of victimization was school-based bullying, which was reported at 69.2% that included physical, verbal, or relational bullying [62]. This

Table 9.6 Increased risk for potential behavioral/mental health issues of transgender persons [33, 51]

1. Anxiety and anxiety disorders
2. Autism spectrum disorder (ASD)
3. Bullying (cyber-bullying)
4. Depression and depression disorders
5. Eating disorders
6. Suicidality and overt suicide
7. Others

study of victimization included cyberbullying, sexual victimization, child maltreatment, physical assault, and others [62]. Thus, clinicians dealing with transgender patients should inquire regarding the potential for various forms of bullying, especially in the school milieu [62, 63].

Suicidality

Research has revealed that being a member of the *LGBTQIA+* community is a risk factor for suicidality and completed suicides that include children, adolescents, and young adults [33, 64, 65]. In a study of 120,617 adolescents aged 11–19 years, almost 14% revealed a history of a suicide attempt with the highest report noted in female to male adolescents at 50.8% [66]. In this same study, the suicide attempt rate was 41.8% among those identifying as neither female nor male (explicitly), 29.9% for the male to female adolescents, 27.9% for those listed as questioning, 17.6% among female adolescents, and 9.8% with male adolescents [66].

In another report of 4464 adolescents, suicidal ideation was reported in 49.29% of transgender youth, 41.31% of gender expansive youth, 19.08% of female adolescents, and 10.82% of male adolescents; gender expansive youth were described as those questioning the typical conclusions in society regarding gender roles/norms and identities [67]. Risk factors for suicidality in this group included such issues as depression, victimization by peers (including cyber-bullying), dating violence, substance abuse, feeling unsafe at school, limited social support, and others [67, 68]. Our LGBTQIA+ youth potentially pay a high personal price because of the stigmatization, prejudice, and discrimination they may encounter in society.

Conclusions

Sexual orientation is a fluid process, and in the fascinating journey of acquisition of an orientation accepted by a person, sometimes the conclusion is that a transgender person is found in adolescence or adulthood. Some have a journey in which they question who they are and may eventually arrive in the LGBTQIA+ community. It is important that clinicians caring for these children and adolescents obtain a careful evaluation of their young patients, including asking about their sexual orientation. If they are in the LGBTQIA+ arena, many possible problems await them partially due to the theological, political, and social conflicts this may confront them. Negative issues that await these young patients include bullying (cyberbullying), anxiety, depression, suicidality, and other behavioral problems as well as disorders [33, 68]. It is critical that the caring clinician identify these issues and arrange for expeditious mental health evaluation as well as management. Having an integrated behavioral health approach in the office is an important and recommended step in this direction [32].

References

1. Ventriglio A, Bhugra D. Sexuality in the 21st century: sexual fluidity. East Asian Arch Psychiatr. 2019;29(1):30–4.
2. Logie CH, Perez-Brumer A, Parker R. The contested global politics of pleasure and danger: sexuality, gender, health and human rights. Glob Public Health. 2021;16(5):651–63. https://doi.org/10.1080/17441692.2021.1893373.
3. Fonseca H, Greydanus DE. Sexuality in the child, teen, and young adult: concepts for the clinician. Prim Care. 2007;34(2):275–92; abstract vii. https://doi.org/10.1016/j.pop.2007.04.015.
4. Rosenthal SI, Blythe MJ. Adolescent sexuality. Adolesc Med State Art Rev. 2007;18:425–587.
5. Pancost SL, Holowicki AN, Belachew BS. Normal child and adolescent psychological development. In: Greydanus DE, Patel DR, Nazeer A, Apple RW, Merrick J, editors. Behavioral pediatrics. Introduction. 5th ed. New York: Nova Science Publishers, ch 2.; 2022. p. 21–43.
6. Freud S. Three essays on the theory of sexuality, vol. 7. London: Hogarth Press; 1953. p. 125–243.
7. Shulman ME. What use is Freud? J Am Psychoanal Assoc. 2021;69(6):1093–113. https://doi.org/10.1177/00030651211059546.
8. Green A. Has sexuality anything to do with psychoanalysis? Int J Psychoanal. 1995;76(Pt 5):871–83.
9. Scott HK, Cogburn M. Piaget. 2023 Jan 9. In: StatPearls [Internet]. Treasure Island (FL): StatPearls Publishing; 2024.
10. Flavell JH. Psychoanalysis and developmental psychology. Introduction (Jean Piaget). Int J Psychiatry. 1967;3(2):75–81.
11. Voyat G. Jean Piaget: 1896–1980. Am J Psychol. 1981;94(4):645–8.
12. Kohlberg L, Elfenbein D. The development of moral judgments concerning capital punishment. Am J Orthopsychiatry. 1975;45(4):614–40.
13. Sachdeva S, Singh P, Medin D. Culture and the quest for universal principles in moral reasoning. Int J Psychol. 2011;46(3):161–76.
14. Benagiano G, Mori M. The origins of human sexuality: procreation or recreation? Reprod Biomed Online. 2009;18(Suppl 1):50–9.
15. Greydanus DE, Dickson CA, Omar HA, Vu CT. Pediatric and adolescent sexuality: an overview. In: Omar HA, Greydanus DE, Patel DR, Merrick J, editors. Pediatric and adolescent sexuality and gynecology. Principles for the primary care clinician. 2nd ed. New York: Nova Science Publishers, ch 1.; 2021. p. 3–62.
16. DuBois LZ, Shattuck-Heidorn H. Challenging the binary: gender/sex and the bio-logics of normalcy. Am J Hum Biol. 2021;33(5):e23623. https://doi.org/10.1002/ajhb.23623.
17. Weiss E. No bones about it: sex is binary. Arch Sex Behav. 2024. https://doi.org/10.1007/s10508-024-02851-3.

18. Kellogg Spadt S, Rosenbaum TY, Dweck A, Millheiser L, Pillai-Friedman S, Krychman M. Sexual health and religion: a primer for the sexual health clinician (CME). J Sex Med. 2014;11(7):1607–18; quiz 1619. https://doi.org/10.1111/jsm.12593.
19. Gruskin S, Yadav V, Castellanos-Usigli A, Khizanishvili G, Kismödi E. Sexual health, sexual rights and sexual pleasure: meaningfully engaging the perfect triangle. Sex Reprod Health Matters. 2019;27(1):1593787. https://doi.org/10.1080/26410397.2019.1593787.
20. Sax L. How common is intersex? A response to Anne Fausto-Sterling. J Sex Res. 2002;39(3):174–8. https://doi.org/10.1080/00224490209552139.
21. Lee PA, Mazur T, Houk CP. DSD/intersex: historical context and current perspectives. J Pediatr Endocrinol Metab. 2023;36(3):234–41. https://doi.org/10.1515/jpem-2022-0582.
22. Bonomi M, Rochira V, Pasquali D, Balercia G, Jannini EA, Ferlin A, Klinefelter ItaliaN Group (KING). Klinefelter syndrome (KS): genetics, clinical phenotype and hypogonadism. J Endocrinol Investig. 2017;40(2):123–34. https://doi.org/10.1007/s40618-016-0541-6.
23. Gravholt CH, Viuff M, Just J, Sandahl K, Brun S, van der Velden J, et al. The changing face of Turner syndrome. Endocr Rev. 2023;44(1):33–69. https://doi.org/10.1210/endrev/bnac016.
24. Steiner M, Saenger P. Turner syndrome: an update. Adv Pediatr Infect Dis. 2022;69(1):177–202. https://doi.org/10.1016/j.yapd.2022.03.004.
25. Fraga NR, Minaeian N, Kim MS. Congenital adrenal hyperplasia. Pediatr Rev. 2024;45(2):74–84. https://doi.org/10.1542/pir.2022-005617.
26. Garnets LD. Sexual orientations in perspective. Cultur Divers Ethnic Minor Psychol. 2002;8(2):115–29. https://doi.org/10.1037/1099-9809.8.2.115.
27. Hines M. Sex hormones and human destiny. J Neuroendocrinol. 2009;21(4):437–8. https://doi.org/10.1111/j.1365-2826.2008.01788.x.
28. Mahler L, Mundle G. A need for orientation: the WMA statement on natural variations of human sexuality. Int Rev Psychiatry. 2015;27(5):460–2. https://doi.org/10.3109/09540261.2015.1086321.
29. Richards C, Bouman WP, Seal L, Barker MJ, Nieder TO, T'Sjoen G. Non-binary or genderqueer genders. Int Rev Psychiatry. 2016;28(1):95–102. https://doi.org/10.3109/09540261.2015.1106446.
30. Pollitt AM, Mernitz SE, Russell ST, Curran MA, Toomey RB. Heteronormativity in the lives of lesbian, gay, bisexual, and queer young people. J Homosex. 2021;68(3):522–44. https://doi.org/10.1080/00918369.2019.1656032. Epub 2019 Aug 22.
31. Anderson J, Maugeri J. Correlates of attitudes toward bisexuality: a systematic review and meta-analysis. J Homosex. 2024;71(1):259–92. https://doi.org/10.1080/00918369.2022.2112524.
32. Malik S, Joychan S, Goslee J, DeBianco M, Addesso L, Hashemi N, Nazeer A. Integrated mental health in primary care offices. In: Greydanus DE, Patel DR, Nazeer A, Apple RW, Merrick J, editors. Behavioral pediatrics. Introduction. 5th ed. New York: Nova Science Publishers, Chapter 1.; 2022. p. 3–19.
33. Agana MG, Greydanus DE, Indyk JA, Calles JL Jr, Kushner J, Leibowitz S, et al. Caring for the transgender adolescent and young adult: current concepts of an evolving process in the 21st century. Dis Mon. 2019;65(9):303–56. https://doi.org/10.1016/j.disamonth.2019.07.004.
34. Kinsey A, Pomeroy W, Martin C. Sexual behavior in the human male. Philadelphia: WB Saunders; 1948.
35. Kinsey A, Pomeroy W, Martin C, Gebbard P. Sexual behavior in the human female. Philadelphia: WB Saunders; 1953.
36. Bell A, Weinberg M. Homosexuality: a study of diversity among men and women. New York: Simon Schuster; 1978.
37. McConaghy N, Armstrong B, Birrell P, Buhrich N. The incidence of bisexual feelings and opposite sex behavior in medical students. J Nerv Ment Dis. 1979;167(11):685–8.
38. Remafedi G, Resnick M, Blum R, Harris L. Demography of sexual orientation in adolescents. Pediatrics. 1992;89(4 Pt 2):714–21.

39. Troiden RT. Becoming homosexual: a model of gay identity acquisition. Psychiatry. 1979;42:362–73.
40. Troiden R. Homosexual identity development. J Adolesc Health Care. 1989;9(2):105–13.
41. Jaspal R. Social psychological aspects of gay identity development. Curr Opin Psychol. 2022;48:101469. https://doi.org/10.1016/j.copsyc.2022.101469.
42. McInerney J. Plutarch's manly women. In: Rosen RM, Sluiter I, editors. Andreia: studies in manliness and courage in classical Athens. Mnemosyne, Bibliotheca Classica Batava, Supplementum, vol. 238. Leiden/Boston: Brill; 2003. p. 319–44.
43. Penrose WD Jr. Introduction: the appeal of the Amazons. J Lesbian Stud. 2024;28(2):205–32. https://doi.org/10.1080/10894160.2024.2319942.
44. Benjamin H. Clinical aspects of transsexualism in the male and female. Am J Psychother. 1964;18:458–69.
45. Benjamin H. Sexual problems at the consultation hour of the general practitioner. Landarzt. 1966;42(20):885–90.
46. Bullough VL. The contributions of John Money: a personal view. J Sex Res. 2003;40(3):230–6.
47. Green R. John Money, Ph.D. (July 8, 1921–July 7, 2006): a personal obituary. Arch Sex Behav. 2006;35(6):629–32.
48. Ehrhardt A. John Money, Ph.D. J Sex Res. 2007;44(3):223–4.
49. Shumer DE, Nokoff NJ, Spack NP. Advances in the care of transgender children and adolescents. Adv Pediatr Infect Dis. 2016;63(1):79–102.
50. Flores AR, Herman JL, Gates GT, Brown TN. Age of Individuals who identify as transgender in the Unites States. Los Angeles: Williams Institute; 2017. https://williamsinstitute.law.ucla.edu/wpcontent/uploads/TransAgeReport.pdf.
51. Feinstein BA, van der Star A, Dorrell KD, Blashill AJ. Sexual orientation and mental health in a US cohort of children: a longitudinal mediation study. J Child Psychol Psychiatry. 2024;65(2):188–98. https://doi.org/10.1111/jcpp.13873.
52. American Psychiatric Association. Diagnostic and statistical manual of mental disorders. 5th ed. Washington, DC: American Psychiatric Association; 2013. p. 451–9.
53. American Psychiatric Association. Diagnostic and statistical manual of mental disorders. 5th ed., Text revision. Washington, DC: American Psychiatric Association; 2022.
54. First MB, Yousif LH, Clarke DE, Wang PS, Gogtay N, Appelbaum PS. DSM-5-TR: overview of what's new and what's changed. World Psychiatry. 2022;21(2):218–9. https://doi.org/10.1002/wps.20989.
55. de Vries ALC, Beek TF, Dhondt K, de Vet HCW, Cohen-Kettenis PT, Steensma TD, Kreukels BPC. Reliability and clinical utility of gender identity-related diagnoses: comparisons between the ICD-11, ICD-10, DSM-IV, and DSM-5. LGBT Health. 2021;8(2):133–42. https://doi.org/10.1089/lgbt.2020.0272.
56. Feinberg AN, Reddy VN. Development of a differential diagnosis from the history and physical examination. In: Greydanus DE, Feinberg AN, Patel DR, Homnick DN, editors. The pediatric diagnostic examination. New York: McGraw Hill Companies, Inc. ch 4.; 2008. p. 59–68.
57. Marino JL, Lin A, Davies C, Kang M, Bista S, Skinner SR. Childhood and adolescence gender role nonconformity and gender and sexuality diversity in young adulthood. JAMA Pediatr. 2023;177(11):1176–86. https://doi.org/10.1001/jamapediatrics.2023.3873.
58. Fisher KA, Marwaha R. Paraphilia. 2023 Mar 6. In: StatPearls [Internet]. Treasure Island (FL): StatPearls Publishing; 2024.
59. Jassi A, Krebs G. Body dysmorphic disorder. Psychiatr Clin North Am. 2023;46(1):197–209. https://doi.org/10.1016/j.psc.2022.10.005.
60. Micangeli G, Profeta G, Colloridi F, Pirro F, Tarani F, Ferraguti G, Spaziani M, Isidori AM, Menghi M, Fiore M, Tarani L. The role of the pediatrician in the management of the child and adolescent with gender dysphoria. Ital J Pediatr. 2023;49(1):71. https://doi.org/10.1186/s13052-023-01466-z.

61. Roden RC, Billman M, Francesco A, Mullin R, Tassi C, Wozolek B, et al. Treatment goals of adolescents and young adults for gender dysphoria. Pediatrics. 2024;153(1):e2023062202. https://doi.org/10.1542/peds.2023-062202.
62. Sterzing PR, Ratliff GA, Gartner RE, McGeough BL, Johnson KC. Social ecological correlates of polyvictimization among a national sample of transgender, genderqueer and cisgender sexual minority adolescents. Child Abuse Negl. 2017;67(1):1–12.
63. Gower LA, Rider GN, McMorris BJ, Eisenberg ME. Bullying victimization among LGBTQ youth: critical issues and future directions. Curr Sex Health Rep. 2018:1–9. https://doi.org/10.1007/s11930-018-0169-y.
64. Silenzio VM, Pena JB, Duberstein PR, Cerel J, Knox KL. Sexual orientation and risk factors for suicidal ideation and suicide attempts among adolescents and young adults. Am J Public Health. 2007;97(11):2017–9. https://doi.org/10.2105/AJPH.2006.095943.
65. Lovero KL, Dos Santos PF, Come AX, Wainberg ML, Oquendo MA. Suicide in global mental health. Curr Psychiatry Rep. 2023;25(6):255–62. https://doi.org/10.1007/s11920-023-01423-x.
66. Toomey RB, Syvertsen AK, Shramko M. Transgender adolescent suicide behavior. Pediatrics. 2018;142(4):e20174218. https://doi.org/10.1542/peds.2017-4218.
67. Garthe RC, Blackburn AM, Kaur A, Sarol JN Jr, Goffnett J, Rieger A, et al. Suicidal ideation among transgender and gender expansive youth: mechanisms of risk. Transgend Health. 2022;7(5):416–22. https://doi.org/10.1089/trgh.2021.0055.
68. Greydanus DE, Nazeer A, Qayyum Z, Patel DR, Rausch R, Hoang LN, et al. Pediatric suicide: review of a preventable tragedy. Dis Mon. 2024:101725. https://doi.org/10.1016/j.disamonth.2024.101725.

Chapter 10
The Role and Importance of Integrated Behavioral Health for Pediatric Patients with Disabilities

Tierra Jolly, Sreevidya Kurra, and Cheryl A. Dickson

Introduction

This chapter will cover the basic tenets of Integrated Behavioral Health Services and their application to pediatric patients with disabilities. It will go over the principles and benefits of IBH, application to pediatric care, specific interventions and assessment tools, definition of pediatric disabilities, and a deeper dive into mental health in disabled children. The purpose of this chapter is to highlight the benefits of IBH in holistic treatment and management of pediatric disabilities.

IBH is defined, according to the Lexicon for Behavioral Health and Primary Care Integration, as the care that results from a practice of primary care and behavioral health clinicians, working together with patients and families, using a systematic and cost-effective approach to provide patient-centered care for a defined population. This care may address mental health and substance abuse conditions, health behaviors, life stressors and crises, stress-related physical symptoms, and ineffective patterns of health utilization [1]. The integrated model of care differs from traditional mental health clinics in regards to assessment, treatment, and collaboration within the healthcare team [2]. Service delivery is also briefer than traditional clinics in regards to number and length of sessions [2].

United States national estimates suggest that nearly 12.6 million children have special health care needs and 1.2 million children have a medical complexity that requires extensive health care services [3]. The National Survey of Children's Health from 2019 to 2020 found the prevalence of children with special health care

T. Jolly · S. Kurra (✉)
Western Michigan University Homer Stryker MD School of Medicine, Kalamazoo, MI, USA
e-mail: sree.kurra@wmed.edu

C. A. Dickson
Pediatrics and Adolescent Medicine, Western Michigan University, Homer Stryker M.D. School of Medicine, Kalamazoo, MI, USA

R. W. Apple et al. (eds.), *Using Integrated Behavioral Health in Pediatric Practice*, https://doi.org/10.1007/978-3-031-85784-3_10

needs to be 14.1 million. Special health care needs were also more common among non-Hispanic Black children and children living in poverty [4]. Among the disabled youth, individuals exhibit psychiatric and behavioral co-morbidity at rates two to three times greater than the general population. About 30–35% of people with intellectual and developmental disabilities experience a psychiatric disorder [2]. The high rates of depression, anxiety, and other comorbid psychiatric conditions in patients with disabilities impact overall health, well-being, pain, and quality of life [2]. Access to integrated behavioral health services reduces barriers to care, increases service utilization, and enhances treatment outcomes. Having all providers in the same location also addresses poor communication [2]. For these reasons, it is paramount that integrated behavioral and medical care services be offered to pediatric patients with disabilities and their families. Throughout the rest of this chapter, we will offer several different models and specific IBH interventions.

Understanding IBH: Principles and Benefits

The IBH model differs from primary care in many ways. At its essence, each member of the team brings with them a unique set of competencies and must acknowledge and respect the expertise of different disciplines. This requires a clear understanding of one's role on the team and effective communication between team members. It also requires administrative and professional staff to work together in a coordinated manner [1]. By doing so, the healthcare team is able to have a holistic approach to each patient.

Some of the specific barriers to care noted within the pediatric disability population include fragmented medical care, transportation, quality of life, and financial challenges/insurance-related barriers [4]. By providing care to these patients through an IBH model, we can focus on improved access to care, better health outcomes, and increased patient and family satisfaction. The IBH model also reduces healthcare costs in the long-term by addressing mental health needs early on and preventing escalation of symptoms which may need more intensive interventions [1].

IBH Models and Their Application in Pediatric Care

Coordinated

The key characteristic of this model is effective interdisciplinary communication between the pediatrician and behavioral health consultant. Pediatricians can consult with a behavioral health specialist via telephone regarding appropriate intervention and treatment. There can also be involvement of care coordinators who serve as the intermediary between the physicians and mental health providers. This model is cost effective since behavioral health consultants do not have to be located at the practice setting or be hired full time [1].

These services can be helpful for rural practices and for addressing the needs of underserved patients, due to the lack of on-site coordination. The intervention is brief and immediate. Coordinated services can increase access to care by connecting earlier with specialized providers who are better trained to triage and provide advice for behavioral concerns [5].

Colocated

The primary care provider and behavioral health provider are located in the same practice setting; however, they function independent of one another. There is not necessarily a collaboration between the two entities—each provider has separate treatment plans. Being located in the same setting has its advantages in that they are able to consult when necessary and are easily accessible. They also share the same electronic medical record, increasing access to information [1].

Previous studies looking at a co-located model have suggested that the location of services in the primary care setting may impact attendance and service use [5]. Specifically, within our population where transportation is a barrier to care, having our integrated health services team under one roof will address key social determinants of health. Disadvantages of this model include disjointed care plans between the PCP and behavioral health provider.

Fully Integrated/Collaborative

In a fully integrated model, the behavioral health consultant is available and consulted during all scheduled pediatric office visits. There is a unified treatment plan that involves both the pediatric care and behavioral management plans. Many integrated health models involve a method of universal behavioral health screening of patients presenting to the PCP [5]. Some programs additionally work with families and teachers to support effective collaboration [5]. The fully integrated health model does not serve to replace more extensive regular behavioral care evaluation and management. Rather, it serves to complement delivery of behavioral health in a primary care setting [1].

Benefits of this model include increased access to treatment and less need for outside referrals [5]. This would serve as the best model for pediatric patients with disabilities because of increased attention to the individualized patient. It also addresses the health disparities within the population, specifically fragmented medical care. Studies have shown that care for this population should include a family-centered approach where coordinated care through a single provider should engage in shared decision making with patients and families to define goals and solve problems [4]. Some of the disadvantages of this model may be resource availability and funding.

Hybrid

The specific needs of the medical practice and the patient population it serves are the key determinants of the most preferred IBH model. Each model alone may not best serve the population, in which case a hybrid approach may be implemented [1].

Primary Care Behavioral Health (PCBH)

The main goal of the PCBH model is to enhance the primary care team's ability to manage and treat behavioral health problems and biopsychosocial influenced health conditions. The model incorporates the behavioral health consultant into the primary care team to extend and support the team. Specially, the BHC serves as a generalist, is easily accessible, is team-based, works with a high volume of patients, serves as an educator, and is a routine part of care. The BHC starts by using a focused visit to assist with specific symptoms or functional improvement. Patients are followed up by the PCP and BHC. Once symptoms begin to improve, the PCP assumes sole oversight but can re-engage the BHC at any time [6].

While fully integrated programs focus on the individual patient and improving their outcome, the PBCH model aims to improve care of the entire practice population. It aims to improve overall population health by increased access to the PCP and increased PCP comfortability in working with biopsychosocial issues. This model also serves to provide brief, low-intensity interventions to large numbers of patients [1].

Defining Disability

In this chapter, we embrace the World Health Organization's International Classification of Functioning, Disability, and Health (ICF) and acknowledge its role in shaping our conception of "disability." The ICF provides a standard language and framework to describe an individual's health that de-emphasizes the cause of an individual's disability; instead, it focuses on the impact of that disability on an individual's body functions and structure, activities and participation, within the unique environmental and personal context in which they live [7]. Ayoub et al. used this ICF framework to further develop their own four categories of disability:

- Physical disabilities: These can be permanent, like cerebral palsy or spina bifida, or temporary, like a broken bone or concussion.
- Chronic conditions requiring accommodations: This category includes physical (i.e., asthma, diabetes) and mental health conditions (i.e., anxiety, depression) that require ongoing management and may necessitate accommodations in various settings.

- Sensory disabilities and conditions, like hearing and/or vision impairments.
- Cognitive, educational, neurodevelopmental, and social (CENS) disabilities: This category encompasses a wide range of diagnoses, including autism spectrum disorder (ASD), attention-deficit hyperactivity disorder (ADHD), and conditions associated with intellectual disability, like trisomy 21, Fragile X syndrome, and fetal alcohol syndrome [3].

We have opted to use these broad parameters for disability in the service of both inclusivity and logistical necessity; the literature we review uses a dizzying array of terms to describe the population at hand: special health care needs, disability, special needs, intellectual developmental disability, learning disability, impairment, limitation. Throughout this chapter, whenever possible, we will offer examples for each of these four disability categories.

Prevalence and Impact of Mental Health Conditions in Disabled Children

Research consistently shows that children with disabilities experience mental health conditions at significantly higher rates than typically developing children [8–12]. This pattern is observed across various types of disabilities and in diverse geographical settings. However, the exact prevalence rates vary depending on the specific disability, the methodology used in the study, and the source of the data [11]. Additionally, identifying mental health conditions in children with disabilities can be difficult for providers [10].The nature of a child's disability can make it difficult for them to communicate their feelings and experiences. Physicians may also mistakenly attribute symptoms of a patient's mental health symptoms to their disability diagnosis. This leads to under-diagnosis of discrete psychiatric conditions; this is especially the case with patients who have more than one disability diagnosis [10].

Clinical samples find that almost half of children with physical disabilities meet criteria for a diagnosis of a mental health disorder [8]. This percentage is found to be lower in general population studies; here, 20–30% of children with physical disabilities are affected [13]. Even higher rates are found among children with cognitive, educational, neurodevelopmental, and social disabilities (CENS), approximately 40% of whom have a diagnosable mental health condition [9] (Table 10.1).

Overall, children with cerebral palsy (CP) are 2.7–7.1 times more likely than their non-CP peers to have depression, anxiety, and behavior/conduct problems [14]. Research on children with intellectual disability has identified a slightly higher prevalence of anxiety, depression, oppositional defiant disorder, and conduct disorder compared to children without intellectual disability [10]. Notably, the presence of one psychiatric disorder significantly increases the risk of other disorders. A study reported that 58% of children with a new diagnosis of a physical disability or chronic condition requiring accommodations (including asthma, diabetes, epilepsy, food allergy, and juvenile idiopathic arthritis) had multiple mental health disorders

Table 10.1 Prevalence and association of physical conditions and mental disorders by gender and age group

	Prevalence, %						Gender (Reference: Female)[a]		Age Group (Reference: >18 years)[a]			
		Gender		Age Group					<13 years		13–18 years	
	Total ($N = 9014$)	Male ($n = 4349$)	Female ($n = 4665$)	<13 years ($n = 3585$)	13–18 years ($n = 3678$)	>18 years ($n = 1751$)	aOR	(95% CI)	aOR	(95% CI)	aOR	(95% CI)
Medical specialty/systems[b]												
Allergy/immunologic												
Severe allergies	0.9	1	0.9	0.9	1.1	0.6	1.11	(0.72–1.72)	1.34	(0.67–2.67)	1.63	(0.83–3.20)
Asthma/respiratory	1.2	1.2	1.1	1.2	1.1	1.1	1.12	(0.76–1.66)	0.99	(0.58–1.69)	0.96	(0.56–1.65)
Autoimmune/inflammatory	8.9	7.9	9.8	7.3	9.9	9.9	0.77	(0.67–0.90)	0.7	(0.57–0.85)	0.96	(0.79–1.17)
Cardiologic	3.5	3.4	3.5	3.3	3.2	4.5	0.97	(0.77–1.21)	0.71	(0.53–0.96)	0.69	(0.52–0.93)
Endocrine/metabolic	6.1	5.4	6.8	4.8	7.7	5.6	0.76	(0.64–0.90)	0.84	(0.65–1.09)	1.38	(1.09–1.76)
Eye/ear/nose/throat	3.3	3.1	3.4	3.4	3.4	2.8	0.89	(0.70–1.12)	1.21	(0.86–1.70)	1.19	(0.85–1.67)
Gastroenterologic	6.9	7.6	6.2	5.4	7.5	8.6	1.24	(1.05–1.46)	0.55	(0.44–0.70)	0.81	(0.66–1.00)
Hematologic	3.9	4.3	3.6	3.5	4.2	4.3	1.26	(1.02–1.56)	0.79	(0.59–1.06)	0.97	(0.73–1.29)
Nephrology/urologic	2.6	2.1	3.1	2.2	2.7	3.1	0.67	(0.51–0.87)	0.73	(0.51–1.04)	0.86	(0.61–1.20)
Neurologic												
Birth anomalies	15	15.5	14.5	16.9	14.4	12.1	1.03	(0.92–1.16)	1.43	(1.21–1.70)	1.19	(1.00–1.42)
CNS	19.6	20.5	18.8	16	19.2	27.7	1.15	(1.04–1.28)	0.47	(0.41–0.55)	0.6	(0.53–0.69)
Developmental	18	21.4	14.8	19.8	18	14	1.53	(1.38–1.71)	1.47	(1.25–1.73)	1.33	(1.13–1.56)
Oncologic	3.1	3.2	3	2.6	2.9	4.6	1.07	(0.84–1.36)	0.55	(0.41–0.75)	0.6	(0.45–0.81)
Orthopedic	7.9	7	8.8	6.7	9.1	7.9	0.76	(0.65–0.89)	0.84	(0.68–1.05)	1.15	(0.94–1.42)

Mental disorders[c]												
Anxiety disorders	11.7	8.8	14.4	10.5	12.7	11.8	0.58	(0.51–0.67)	0.96	(0.80–1.15)	1.14	(0.96–1.36)
ADHD	17.6	22.5	12.9	23.2	17.5	6.2	1.88	(1.68–2.11)	4.38	(3.55–5.41)	3.18	(2.57–3.93)
Behavior disorders	18.2	20.9	15.7	15.5	22.9	13.8	1.51	(1.35–1.69)	1.19	(1.01–1.41)	2.01	(1.71–2.35)
Mood disorders	12.4	9.2	15.5	5.1	15.7	20.4	0.6	(0.52–0.68)	0.22	(0.19–0.27)	0.75	(0.65–0.87)
Subclinical psychosis symptoms	21.4	22.5	20.3	18.5	25	19.5	1.2	(1.08–1.33)	0.96	(0.83–1.12)	1.44	(1.25–1.66)
Children's Global Assessment Scale score ≤70	23.3	24.7	22	19.4	25.2	27.5	1.23	(1.12–1.36)	0.65	(0.57–0.74)	0.92	(0.81–1.05)

Merikangas et al. [13]

[a]OR based on logistic regression models controlling for gender, age, race/ethnicity, and maternal education

[b]Physical conditions based on electronic medical chart review and parent informant report (or proband report for youth aged ≥18 years)

[c]Diagnostic and Statistical Manual of Mental Disorders, Fourth Edition indices of mental disorders: diagnosis algorithms considered endorsement of screen question, symptom count, duration, distress, and impairment. Anxiety disorders = agoraphobia, generalized anxiety disorder, panic disorder, separation anxiety disorder; Behavior disorders = oppositional defiant disorder, conduct disorder; Mood disorders = major depressive disorder and mania; psychosis symptoms were based on subpsychotic positive symptoms (PRIME-Screen Revised), subthreshold negative/disorganized symptoms (6 SIPS ratings), and/or positive psychosis screen

at initial assessment, although this number decreased to 42% after 6 months [8]. There also appears to be a direct association between the severity of a child's functional impairment and the presence of a mental health disorder [13].

Statistics are equally appalling when disabled children reach adulthood. According to the U.S. Department of Health and Human Services, one in three adults with disabilities reports frequent mental distress—defined as 14 or more self-reported mentally unhealthy days in the past 30 days—which is associated with mental health disorders. They are also more likely to experience other factors associated with a higher occurrence of mental health disorders, like underemployment, poverty, and limited health care access [15]. This distress can lead to serious consequences: in the UK, disabled adults were four times more likely to report a suicide attempt in the last 12 months compared to non-disabled adults [16].

The relationship between disability and mental health is complex and bidirectional. Children who have disabilities are often exposed to social stigmatization, discrimination, and exclusion, which may cause feelings of loneliness, low self-esteem, and difficulties in forming relationships [17]. These experiences make them more vulnerable to mental health issues, like depression and anxiety [11]. Disabilities are often accompanied by a variety of practical challenges and functional limitations that can negatively impact mental well-being. For example, restricted mobility may impede participation in activities, leading to social isolation and frustration [14, 17]. In addition, the chronic pain that can accompany disabilities is, in itself, a risk factor for depression [14]. CENS can impact social development and increase the risk of mental health challenges. Difficulties with communication and social interaction can lead to frustration, anxiety, and difficulty forming meaningful connections with peers [9, 12, 14].

Not only can disability increase the risk of developing mental health conditions, but pre-existing mental health conditions can exacerbate the challenges associated with disability even more difficult to manage [16]. Depression can negatively impact motivation and alter pain perception, making it harder to manage physical symptoms or engage in physical or occupational therapies. Comorbid mental health conditions can also interfere with treatment adherence, potentially leading to increased disability [18]. Finally, the stigma associated with mental illness can make it harder to seek support and participate in social activities, further limiting opportunities for social connection and potentially worsening mental health [11, 16]. Multimorbidity—the co-occurrence of mental health conditions and physical disabilities—can have a compounding effect on an individual's overall quality of life [8, 18].

Individuals with disabilities clearly have a critical need for IBH, which employs a variety of holistic care models to address both their physical and mental health needs [12]. Early identification and intervention for mental health conditions are essential to minimize those conditions' impact on disability and improve overall well-being. As a result, both the American Association of Pediatrics and the American Academy of Child and Adolescent Psychiatry recommend the screening and assessment of children's mental health through the child's medical home [19]. As most initial disability diagnoses are made by primary care providers, pediatricians are uniquely prepared to initiate both mental health care and disability care for children with disabilities and have the opportunity to engage with patients and their families in a familiar setting, without stigma [12, 19].

However, this opportunity stands in stark contrast to the unfortunate reality: for children with disabilities, mental health services remain extremely hard to access within a system riddled with significant barriers to care. First, there is limited availability of specialized mental health providers for children with disabilities. Of the existing pediatric mental health programs, many have admission criteria or other hurdles to access care; the need for a formal referral from a primary care provider, the exclusion of some disabling conditions, long wait lists, limited insurance coverage, and an uneven distribution between providers in urban and rural areas all result in the mental health concerns of disabled children remaining significantly under met [10–12, 19, 20]. Second, pediatricians believe that they should be the providers responsible for identifying mental health and behavioral disorders in their patients. Despite this, many claim a lack of training or experience required to assess, diagnose, or treat mental health conditions in children with disabilities [19]. Results from a series of interviews with autistic adults and community health clinicians demonstrated that most of the barriers to care they experienced involved clinicians' limited knowledge, lack of experience, poor competence, and low confidence working with autistic patients [21]. In a survey of parents of children with ASD, 42% reported their child's health care provider did not understand the impact autism had on all aspects of their life and care [22]. Next, like many parents, they found that their pediatrician's office was not designed to accommodate the sensory and physical needs of children with disabilities. Instead, there were loud noises, bright lights, long wait times, and a general lack of accessible equipment that overwhelm many disabled children. This leaves them agitated and unable to participate in their care or be properly evaluated by healthcare providers [3, 12, 22]. Differences in communication styles also create a barrier to accessing mental health care for patients who are nonverbal or use augmented assistive communication devices [10, 12, 22, 23].

Finally, the fragmented nature of healthcare systems presents tremendous challenges for children with disabilities who require services across multiple sectors. Families are left to navigate complex systems on their own, and a lack of communication and coordination between providers results in missed opportunities for early intervention and truly holistic care [11, 18, 21]. It is absolutely essential to note here that children with hearing impairment were less likely to have access to a medical home, community services, or adequate health insurance compared to other children with disabilities; children with sensory disabilities were also more likely to report a poor quality of life compared to children with other disabilities [3]. For children with any disability, these access issues are compounded by their exclusion from research trials and a significant gap in research focused specifically on their mental health needs. Unsurprisingly this has led to a lack of evidence-based interventions for this patient population [3, 9–11].

Specific IBH Interventions and Assessment Tools

University of Rochester Complex Care Center (CCC) Model of Integrated Behavioral Health

Holderle et al. [2] discuss a novel model of integrated behavioral health. In this model, they target a high needs patient population of adults (19+) with complex pediatric-onset conditions such as cystic fibrosis, intellectual and developmental disabilities, and sickle-cell disease. The goal of the model is to utilize a population-health approach for meeting patient behavioral healthcare needs.

Initially the team includes a full-time licensed social worker, but later expands to two part-time licensed psychologists and a consulting psychiatrist. Benefits of having a psychiatrist on board include avoiding referrals to an outside clinic for appointments, which may require long wait times. Patients with disabilities are given the Glasgow Depression Scale for People with Learning Disability, the GAD-7, the Drug Abuse Screening Test, and AUDIT alcohol consumption questions. Patients who are identified as needing behavioral health treatment are referred to a member of the IBH team for an initial evaluation. Other services provided by this model include caregiver support groups, telemedicine appointments, and inpatient visitation and consultation.

After implementation, the authors received positive formal feedback from patients stating they felt comfortable and appreciated the ability to coordinate appointments with multiple providers in the same day. Some of the challenges they faced included longer appointments (>60 min) for patients with disabilities to meet their care needs and lack of outpatient providers/service agencies to help with transitioning into adulthood. There were also barriers during hospitalization due to lack of familiarity with developmental disabilities and communication issues. The study also mentions the need for a social worker due to many patients living in group homes, which complicates implementation of environmental or behavioral interventions.

The Behavioral Health Stratified Treatment (B.E.S.T.) Program

Berg et al. [24] talk about the B.E.S.T program, which is an integrated behavioral health program for youth (ages 13–20) with intellectual and/or developmental disabilities. Key components of the program include classifying risk for depression and anxiety, tiered mental health interventions, and data sharing between care coordinators and B.E.S.T. staff. Tier assignment for intervention is based on PHQ-A, GAD-7, and MINI-KID questionnaires. Youth may be reassigned to a different tier based on a 6-month re-assessment.

The B.E.S.T program presents a unique case of integrated behavioral health. They talk about the importance of preventive mental health interventions during the key developmental period of adolescence rather than treatment after onset of clinical depression or anxiety. They also discuss the benefits of a telehealth platform and online module format to deliver this care, including low cost and easier accessibility for patients with socioeconomic and geographic barriers.

Barriers to Implementing IBH and Strategies to Overcome Them

Mental health care is an essential component of the overall medical care provided to children with disabilities [12]. However, major barriers hinder the effective delivery of IBH models. The primary challenges include limited provider training and expertise, fragmented healthcare systems, and the persistent stigma surrounding both disability and mental illness. These barriers often overlap, creating a complex environment that hinders comprehensive care delivery.

Educating Providers

A significant barrier to implementing IBH is the lack of training and experience among healthcare providers. This knowledge gap can lead to missed diagnoses, inadequate treatment, and difficulty recognizing the special mental health needs of children with disabilities [16, 18, 21, 25]. Educating healthcare providers about these specific needs is paramount.

One potential solution is integrating technology into training programs to increase provider knowledge [3, 10, 11, 21]. Tele-education networks can offer easily accessible coursework and training, especially to practicing providers in underserved communities [26]. For instance, Project ECHO Autism STAT uses video conferencing to link frontline primary care providers with autism experts, who mentor and teach best practices through case-based learning [27]. In this way, the program trains primary care providers to accurately diagnose and treat ASD, increasing the capacity of community-based providers to better serve children with ASD. ECHO Autism STAT also allows children to be evaluated and diagnosed in their home communities, reducing the need for long distance travel to access specialized care. This model has the potential to reduce diagnostic delays and improve access to early intervention services [20, 27]. Additionally, telerehabilitation for children with CENs and their families is at least as effective in improving outcomes, and frequently more so, than traditional face-to-face methods [18].

Another solution is the strategic inclusion of disability education in medical education. Developed to address training gaps in pediatric residency programs, the Special Care Optimization for Patients and Education (SCOPE) program emphasizes home visits and expands curricula that typically lack exposure to the family-centered medical home model and other important aspects in coordinating care for a child with a disability [3, 28, 29]. Families participating in SCOPE report high satisfaction levels with the program; residents are seen as understanding the impact of the child's condition on family life and responsive to family concerns [28, 29]. SCOPE is a promising model that provides hands-on experience, practical tools, and mentorship support to equip future pediatricians with the knowledge, skills, and attitudes needed to provide high-quality, family-centered care to children with disabilities.

Fragmented Systems

Beyond limited physician training, the fragmented nature of healthcare systems is also a barrier to IBH implementation for children with disabilities. This fragmentation forces families to navigate complex systems on their own, makes it challenging for primary care providers and specialists to coordinate care, and causes delays in diagnosis and treatment. Researchers have specifically noted the disconnect between community mental health and disability care providers, which leads to communication breakdowns and barriers to access for people with disabilities [21]. This lack of integration highlights a critical need for better coordination between providers and systems to ensure seamless, comprehensive care.

Strategies for addressing this fragmentation include the development of standardized referral pathways, shared care plans, and regular communication between providers [12]. Integrated models of care, rather than siloed services, can help streamline access to comprehensive care [25]. Collaborative care models, like those proposed by Cates and Soares, involve embedding behavioral health specialists within a primary care setting [19]. Co-location can facilitate early identification and intervention of mental health concerns, reduce stigma related to seeking mental health care, and encourage communication between primary care providers and behavioral health specialists [16]. It also offers opportunities to share electronic health records, create standardized referral pathways, and implement of collaborative care plans [12].

Project Austin, an initiative launched at Children's Nebraska, is an outstanding example of improved care coordination. This program provides continuity of care for children with disabilities as they transition from a hospital setting with specialized care to their home and community [30]. Project Austin does this through a multifaceted approach that centers on the creation of individualized Emergency Medical Plans (EMPs); these detail a child's medical history, treatment needs, and specific procedures allowed in an emergency [31]. The program is transitioning to a QR code system, allowing first responders to instantly access the child's EMP in an emergency setting [31]. Additionally, Project Austin also provides training to emergency personnel, so they are well-equipped to manage the unique needs of children with medical complexity [31]. With its system based on shared information, clear communication, and specialized training, Project Austin integrates hospital-based care and community-based emergency services, for more timely interventions and better outcomes for children with disabilities. Notably, Children's Nebraska cites a 55% reduction in organizational costs after implementing the program [30].

Reducing Stigma

Stigma associated with both disability and mental illness is another significant barrier to seeking and receiving appropriate mental health care [11, 17]. This fear of judgment can deter families from disclosing their child's mental health needs, leading to delayed interventions and worsening conditions. Pediatric providers must foster inclusive healthcare environments that encourage families to seek help [3, 25].

Reducing stigma must begin with disability training for healthcare staff. Offering flexible appointment scheduling, making facilities accessible, and engaging families as partners in care are also essential steps toward creating truly welcoming environments [3, 12, 18]. The Quick Tips Card (QTC) is a tool that empowers parents of children with ASD to communicate their child's unique needs to medical personnel. The QTC is completed by parents and shared with physicians before an appointment begins. It offers a standardized, proactive approach for parents to communicate individualized information with the care team, like communication styles, sensory preferences, and calming strategies. This lets providers individualize their approach to an appointment according to the child's needs, in order to reduce challenging behaviors and improve visit outcomes [22].

Technology can also be used to foster communication and reduce shame related to chronic conditions. BostonBreathes is a web-based platform for children with asthma, that allows patients to track their symptoms, access educational resources, and engage in two-way communication with their healthcare team. This platform illustrates how technology can be used for more than provider education; it is also a powerful tool for streamlining communication between stakeholders and empower patients to participate as part of their own care team [3, 32].

Future Directions and Conclusion

There is enormous potential of integrated behavioral health (IBH) models to improve access to mental health services, particularly within primary care settings. Bultas et al. [22] argue for reducing barriers to care for children with autism within office-based healthcare settings. Soares et al. [23] advocate for the role of IBH in addressing the complex needs of patients with metabolic disorders, who often experience co-occurring mental health conditions. Research by Sterling et al. [23, 33] demonstrates positive long-term outcomes of implementing a SBIRT (Screening, Brief Intervention, and Referral to Treatment) model for depression and substance use among adolescents in primary care settings. This all suggests that early identification and intervention within IBH models can lead to reduced need for specialized mental health services and improved overall well-being.

There is an urgent need to address the mental health disparities faced by children with disabilities. By dismantling barriers to access and promoting a holistic approach to care, we can improve their well-being and ensure they receive the support they deserve. Recommendations include continuing to identify areas for future research and policy development to improve the integration of IBH into pediatric healthcare for children with disabilities as well as advocating for increased funding, workforce development, and implementation of evidence-based practices.

References

1. Fledderman N, DeLeon J, Patel DR. Integrated behavioral health: definitions and contexts. Pediatr Clin N Am. 2021;68(3):511–8. https://doi.org/10.1016/j.pcl.2021.02.007.
2. Holderle KE, Poleshuck E, Rosenberg T, Pulcino T. Integrated behavioral health in primary care for adults with complex childhood onset medical and developmental diagnoses. J Clin Psychol Med Settings. 2022;29(3):586–95. https://doi.org/10.1007/s10880-021-09798-w.
3. Ayoub MC, Rava J, Lewis Hunter A, Kuo AA. Facilitators and barriers to care for patients with disabilities in primary pediatrics. Pediatr Ann. 2022;51(6):e243–53. https://doi.org/10.3928/19382359-20220407-07.
4. Flasch EA. Health equity and children with medical complexity/children and youth with special health care needs: a scoping review. J Pediatr Health Care. 2024;38(2):210–8. https://doi.org/10.1016/j.pedhc.2023.07.007.
5. Njoroge WF, Hostutler CA, Schwartz BS, Mautone JA. Integrated behavioral health in pediatric primary care. Curr Psychiatry Rep. 2016;18(12):106. https://doi.org/10.1007/s11920-016-0745-7.
6. Reiter JT, Dobmeyer AC, Hunter CL. The primary care behavioral health (PCBH) model: an overview and operational definition. J Clin Psychol Med Settings. 2018;25(2):109–26. https://doi.org/10.1007/s10880-017-9531-x.
7. World Health Organization. Towards a Common Language for Functioning, Disability and Health ICF towards a Common Language for Functioning, Disability and Health: ICF the International Classification of Functioning, Disability and Health. 2002. https://cdn.who.int/media/docs/default-source/classification/icf/icfbeginnersguide.pdf.
8. Butler A, Van Lieshout RJ, Lipman EL, et al. Mental disorder in children with physical conditions: a pilot study. BMJ Open. 2018;8(1):e019011. https://doi.org/10.1136/bmjopen-2017-019011.
9. Glasson EJ, Buckley N, Chen W, et al. Systematic review and meta-analysis: mental health in children with neurogenetic disorders associated with intellectual disability. J Am Acad Child Adolesc Psychiatry. 2020;59(9). https://doi.org/10.1016/j.jaac.2020.01.006.
10. Totsika V, Liew A, Absoud M, Adnams C, Emerson E. Mental health problems in children with intellectual disability. Lancet Child Adolesc Health. 2022;6(6):432–44. https://doi.org/10.1016/s2352-4642(22)00067-0.
11. Lal S, Tremblay S, Starcevic D, Mauger-Lavigne M, Anaby D. Mental health problems among adolescents and young adults with childhood-onset physical disabilities: a scoping review. Front Rehabil Sci. 2022;3:904586. https://doi.org/10.3389/fresc.2022.904586.
12. Heslon K, Hanson JH, Ogourtsova T. Mental health in children with disabilities and their families: red flags, services' impact, facilitators, barriers, and proposed solutions. Front Rehabil Sci. 2024;5:1347412. https://doi.org/10.3389/fresc.2024.1347412. Published 2024 Feb 12.

13. Merikangas KR, Calkins ME, Burstein M, et al. Comorbidity of physical and mental disorders in the neurodevelopmental genomics cohort study. Pediatrics. 2015;135(4):e927–38. https://doi.org/10.1542/peds.2014-1444.
14. Whitney DG, Warschausky SA, Peterson MD. Mental health disorders and physical risk factors in children with cerebral palsy: a cross-sectional study. Dev Med Child Neurol. 2018;61(5):579–85. https://doi.org/10.1111/dmcn.14083.
15. Cree RA, Okoro CA, Zack MM, Carbone E. Frequent mental distress among adults, by disability status, disability type, and selected characteristics — United States, 2018. MMWR Morb Mortal Wkly Rep. 2020;69(36):1238–43. https://doi.org/10.15585/mmwr.mm6936a2.
16. Meltzer H, Brugha T, Dennis MS, et al. The influence of disability on suicidal behaviour. Alternatives. 2012;6(1):1–12. https://doi.org/10.1016/j.alter.2011.11.004.
17. Maxey M, Beckert TE. Adolescents with disabilities. Adolesc Res Rev. 2016;2(2):59–75. https://doi.org/10.1007/s40894-016-0043-y.
18. Scott KM, Von Korff M, Alonso J, et al. Mental–physical co-morbidity and its relationship with disability: results from the World Mental Health Surveys. Psychol Med. 2008;39(1):33–43. https://doi.org/10.1017/s0033291708003188.
19. Cates K, Soares N. Need for integrated behavior health model in primary care. Pediatr Clin N Am. 2021;68(3):533–40. https://doi.org/10.1016/j.pcl.2021.02.009.
20. Sohl K, Mazurek MO, Brown R. ECHO Autism: using technology and mentorship to bridge gaps, increase access to care, and bring best practice autism care to primary care. Clin Pediatr. 2017;56(6):509–11. https://doi.org/10.1177/0009922817691825.
21. Maddox BB, Crabbe S, Beidas RS, et al. "I wouldn't know where to start": perspectives from clinicians, agency leaders, and autistic adults on improving community mental health services for autistic adults. Autism. 2019;24(4):136236131988222. https://doi.org/10.1177/1362361319882227.
22. Bultas MW, McMillin SE, Zand DH. Reducing barriers to care in the office-based health care setting for children with autism. J Pediatr Health Care. 2016;30(1):5–14. https://doi.org/10.1016/j.pedhc.2015.08.007. Epub 2015 Oct 9. PMID: 26455786.
23. Soares N, Apple RW, Kanungo S. The role of integrated behavioral health in caring for patients with metabolic disorders. Ann Transl Med. 2018;6(24):478. https://doi.org/10.21037/atm.2018.10.62. PMID: 30740409; PMCID: PMC6331357.
24. Berg KL, Mihaila I, Feinstein RT, Shiu CS, Gussin H, Acharya K, Gladstone TRG, Bernard L, Best M, Renz E, Abdallah G, Weldy S, Herrman D, Lynch E, Gerges M, Perez P, Buchholz KR, Msall M, Aaron S, Mutti M, et al. BEhavioral Health Stratified Treatment (B.E.S.T.) to optimize transition to adulthood for youth with intellectual and/or developmental disabilities. Contemp Clin Trials. 2024;136:107374. https://doi.org/10.1016/j.cct.2023.107374.
25. Suen CG, Campbell K, Stoddard G, Carbone PS. Patient-centered outcomes in an interdisciplinary clinic for complex children with autism. J Dev Behav Pediatr. 2020;42(3):182–90. https://doi.org/10.1097/dbp.0000000000000877.
26. Sockalingam S, Kirvan A, Pereira C, et al. The role of tele-education in advancing mental health quality of care: a content analysis of project ECHO recommendations. Telemed J E Health. 2021;27(8):939–46. https://doi.org/10.1089/tmj.2021.0122.
27. Sohl K, Levinstein L, James A, et al. ECHO (Extension for Community Healthcare Outcomes) Autism STAT: a diagnostic accuracy study of community-based primary care diagnosis of autism spectrum disorder. J Dev Behav Pediatr. 2023;44(3):e177–84. https://doi.org/10.1097/dbp.0000000000001172.
28. Bogetz JF, Gabhart JM, Rassbach CE, et al. Outcomes of a randomized controlled educational intervention to train pediatric residents on caring for children with special health care needs. Clin Pediatr (Phila). 2015;54(7):659–66. https://doi.org/10.1177/0009922814564050.
29. Bogetz J, Gabhart J, Rassbach C, et al. Special care optimization for patients and education (SCOPE): training pediatric residents about children with special health care needs. MedEdPORTAL Publ. Published online. 2013. https://doi.org/10.15766/mep_2374-8265.9627.

30. Home – Project Austin. Project Austin. Published September 25, 2024. Accessed 21 Oct 2024. https://www.projectaustin.org/.
31. Project Austin. Children's Nebraska. https://www.childrensnebraska.org/hospital-experience/support-services/project-austin/.
32. Wiecha JM, Adams WG, Rybin D, Rizzodepaoli M, Keller J, Clay JM. Evaluation of a web-based asthma self-management system: a randomised controlled pilot trial. BMC Pulm Med. 2015;15:17. https://doi.org/10.1186/s12890-015-0007-1. Published 2015 Feb 25.
33. Sterling S, Parthasarathy S, Jones A, Weisner C, Metz V, Hartman L, Saba K, Kline-Simon AH. Young Adult Substance Use and Healthcare Use Associated With Screening, Brief Intervention and Referral to Treatment in Pediatric Primary Care. J Adolesc Health. 2022;71(4S):S15–S23. https://doi.org/10.1016/j.jadohealth.2021.11.033. PMID: 36122965.

Chapter 11
Integrated Behavioral Health Challenges for Ethnic Minority Populations

Summer Chahin, Juanita Moses, and Cheryl A. Dickson

Introduction

Mental Health Crisis

Youth in the United States are currently facing a mental health crisis [1]. This trend has been seen across all age groups, especially during the Covid pandemic era [1]. Research has found that in 2023, 20% of adults experienced some symptoms of anxiety and/or depression [2, 3]. Additionally, from 2020 to 2023, approximately 10% of Americans reported experiencing at least some symptoms of depression [3–6].

In terms of the youth in the USA, rates of mental health challenges were increasing even prior to the pandemic, especially youth who were at least 12 years old or older [4]. Research has found that approximately 15% of suicides occur in the 10- to 24-year-old range, which is the second leading cause of death in this age group [4]. This is also over a 50% increase since the year 2000 [4–6]. Research has also shown that from 2010 to 2020, high school students have reported feelings of hopelessness and sadness, with a nearly 40% increase in these feelings in this time span [7]. More recently, it was found that 40% of high school students reported feelings of hopelessness in 2023 [4–7].

S. Chahin (✉) · J. Moses
Western Michigan University Homer Stryker M.D. School of Medicine, Kalamazoo, MI, USA
e-mail: Summer.chahin@wmed.edu; Juanita.moses@wmed.edu

C. A. Dickson
Pediatrics and Adolescent Medicine, Western Michigan University, Homer Stryker M.D. School of Medicine, Kalamazoo, MI, USA
e-mail: Cherly.dickson@wmed.edu

R. W. Apple et al. (eds.), *Using Integrated Behavioral Health in Pediatric Practice*, https://doi.org/10.1007/978-3-031-85784-3_11

Mental health crises like this can significantly impact several areas of an individual's and society's functioning, including the family unit, school, the work force when caregivers need to leave work to support the child, the economy, our neighborhoods, among many others. Additionally, beyond Covid, there are many factors impacting these changes in youth mental health over time including gun violence, the way youth interact with social media, social connectedness, neighborhood factors, health literacy and misinformation, well-being, safety, and success in school, exposure to interpersonal violence at home, and caregiver well-being and support. These are all important factors to consider when navigating how to support youth living with mental health conditions and how it may impact their day-to-day functioning.

Integrated Behavioral Health Services and Utilization Rates

Integrated Behavioral Health Care (IBH) is a service focused on a whole-person patient-centered approach in managing medical and behavioral health concerns in one location. This is a service delivered by both psychologists and medical providers following the main principles that physical, behavioral, and social health are all interconnected. One of the main benefits of IBH is that it can help lower healthcare utilization and lower healthcare costs. An additional benefit of integrating psychologists and other mental health providers into primary care and specialty clinics is that an individual or family can receive all of their healthcare needs in one place which leads to individuals being more likely to follow up and receive necessary cares.

The added benefit of integrating psychological and behavioral health services into primary care offices is valuable and an effective solution in finding ways to increase access to mental health services and a way to decrease barriers to access to these services. This is also an ideal solution to increasing health equity in medical care. Health equity has been a buzz word in healthcare in recent years and is defined as "...The state in which everyone has a fair and just opportunity to attain their highest level of health." [2, 3, 5–7] Indeed, those who have limited access to opportunities and resources are more likely to struggle with healthcare challenges in the long run. It's particularly important to focus on how to increase access to resources for marginalized communities (e.g., ethnic minorities, LGBTQIA+ communities, those experiencing homelessness, those living in rural areas, etc.) who are disproportionately impacted by the mental health crisis. However, this chapter will focus on IBH services for ethnic minorities, specifically.

Behavioral health needs cost Americans approximately 400 billion dollars in healthcare costs per year and are often found to be one of the top leading causes of disease burden in the USA [8, 9]. Researchers have found that implementing an IBH model in primary care can reduce emergency room visits by 6–7% [10]. In terms of utilizing IBH, researchers found a 143% increase in utilization of behavioral health and psychological care in integrated care models compared to a 12% increase in non-integrated models of healthcare.

In a different scoping review, researchers found 26 other studies that highlight the reduction of emergency room visits with the implementation of integrated behavioral health care in the hospital setting and in primary care [11]. Within this review, several researchers discovered that integrating behavioral health care into their hospital decreased the use of emergency rooms for behavioral health-related needs [12–16]. There were some researchers who found that the length of stay in the hospital decreased with the availability of integrated behavioral health [13].

As highlighted above, there are several benefits to implementation of and utilization of integrated behavioral health services. However, there remain many significant barriers for minority populations to access and utilize these services. The remainder of this chapter will focus on different ethnic minority groups, the mental health prevalence and mental health service utilization rates for each minority group, the unique challenges and barriers each minority group faces, unique cultural considerations for each minority group, and some potential strategies for overcoming barriers and increase utilization within each minority group.

Challenges in Utilizing Integrated Behavioral Health Services for Ethnic Minorities

African American/Black

African Americans are defined as "a person whose origins are in any of the Black racial groups of Africa." [15] The term "Black" "is broader and more inclusive than African American. Use of the capitalized Black recognizes that language has evolved and, especially in the United States, the term reflects a shared identity and culture beyond skin color." [15]

According to the United States Census Bureau [5], 13.9% of the population of the United States is African American/Black [17]. Additionally, approximately 13.2% of the childhood population is African American/Black [17]. According to [5], approximately 9% of non-Hispanic African American/Black who are 5 years or older and living in the United States speak a language other than English at home, and approximately 3% speak English less than "very well." [17]

Research has found that the African American/Black population makes up approximately 20% of the group living with mental health concerns [18]. Unfortunately, Black adolescents have been found to be an especially disadvantaged group who are often misdiagnosed [18, 19]. Research has found that access to mental health services is especially challenging for this group due to the high rates of overdiagnosis of some mental health disorders such as schizophrenia or conduct disorder and underdiagnosis of other mental health disorders such as mood or anxiety disorders [19].

Suicide has become an exceptionally challenging issue within the African American/Black population, but especially within the adolescent and young adult age range. Researchers have recently found that suicide was the third leading cause of death among the 10- to 24-year-old African American/Black group [17]. Additionally, in 2020, the rate of suicide was 4x higher in male adolescents who are Black compared to their female counterparts [17]. Further, Black females were approximately 60% more likely to have a suicide attempt compared to their white female counterparts [17].

According to SAMHSA (2024), 15% of Black individuals aged 18 or older received any mental health treatment in the past 12 months compared to 27% of white individuals [6]. Further, 7% of Black individuals received medication treatment for mental health concerns in the last 12 months compared to 21% of white individuals [6]. Additionally, 56% Black individuals 18 or older with an episode of major depression received treatment for depression compared to 69% of white individuals [6].

Historically, there have been many barriers and issues in accessing healthcare and mental healthcare services for this population. Barriers to access and utilization of mental health services among Black communities are deeply rooted in both historical and contemporary factors, many of which perpetuate a cycle of trauma, mistrust, and limited access to care. One of the most significant historical events that continues to shape mental health outcomes for Black individuals is slavery. The forced displacement, dehumanization, and violence experienced by enslaved Africans have had enduring psychological effects that reverberate through generations.

This historical trauma has contributed to heightened vulnerability to mental health struggles such as depression, anxiety, and post-traumatic stress disorder (PTSD) in the Black population.

The impact of trauma is further exacerbated by contemporary issues such as police violence and the systemic racism that underpins it. Black individuals in the USA face the constant threat of police violence, whether by witnessing it firsthand, hearing about it in their communities, or seeing it broadcasted on social media. The murder of George Floyd in 2020, which was filmed and widely shared, marked a significant moment that amplified the trauma many Black people already carried from years of police brutality.

In addition to the psychological impact of trauma, Black individuals often face structural and systemic barriers to accessing mental health services. A lack of adequate health insurance is one of the most significant obstacles [20]. In many cases, Black individuals are either uninsured or underinsured, making it difficult to afford necessary care [20]. Even when insurance is available, the scarcity of affordable mental health services in many Black communities remains a critical issue. Furthermore, the opposition to the expansion of Medicaid, particularly in southern states, has left many Black individuals without access to essential healthcare, including mental health services [21].

These structural barriers are compounded by a general mistrust in the healthcare system, rooted in its history of exploitation and mistreatment of Black people. The infamous Tuskegee Experiment, in which Black men with syphilis were denied treatment for decades, is just one example of the deep-rooted mistrust that many Black individuals have toward mental health professionals [22]. There are also several studies highlighting the challenges with mental health screeners and measurement tools that are often used and have been found to not be culturally appropriate [23, 24]. There is also a lack of appropriately trained or racially congruent providers, with only 4% of psychologists in the United States identifying as Black [25, 36].

When healthcare providers fail to recognize or address these unique stressors, or when there is a lack of culturally competent care, Black individuals may feel alienated or unheard, further discouraging them from seeking support. The compounded effects of historical trauma, ongoing violence, systemic barriers, and a lack of trust in the healthcare system have created a complex and persistent challenge for Black communities in accessing and utilizing mental health services.

There are a few strategies individuals and organizations can implement to reduce barriers to engagement in mental health services for this population. For example, it is always important to start with critical self-reflection within individual providers and maintain curiosity and cultural sensitivity. At the organizational level, it is important to implement comprehensive analyses related to racial equity and organizational processes. It is also pertinent to recognize the unique mental health challenges faced by this specific population and how the needs of Black individuals, youth, and family are different from other ethnic groups. Providers and organizations should also focus on de-stigmatizing mental health, treatment, and the barrier stigma creates in accessing care.

Further, there should be increased attention on education to major stakeholders including government officials and non-profits that can support individuals and families in paying medical costs or finding affordable healthcare coverage. Further, as mentioned before, there is a significant lack of Black mental health providers and culturally competent providers. Providers and organizations should hold cultural sensitivity training, work on recognizing biases they hold and listen to and respect the beliefs, histories, perspectives that minority individuals bring and advocate for minority colleagues as well. Organizations should also consider partnering with key community stakeholders that hold significance for the Black community such as church leaders.

Hispanic/Latino American

The Hispanic/Latino American population in the USA is very diverse, encompassing people from many different nations and races. The term "Hispanic" refers to language and includes people with ancestry from a country whose primary language is Spanish. "Latino" and its similar variations refer to geography, specifically people with origins from any country in Latin America, which includes Mexico, Central and South America, and the Caribbean.

In the 2020 U.S. Census, this was the second largest racial or ethnic group (after the non-Hispanic white population), making up 18.7% of the total population, and 25.7% of the pediatric population under [18, 26]. The five largest subgroups by origin in descending order are Mexican, Puerto Rican, Salvadoran, Dominican and Cuban [25]. Nearly three in four speak English at least "very well," though just over two in three reports speaking a language other than English at home [25, 26].

Describing immigration by generation is a way to categorize people based on their country of birth and the country of birth of their parents and grandparents.

First-generation immigrants were born outside the USA, but if they migrate when they are children, they may be referred to as 1.5-generation immigrants. Second-generation immigrants were born in the USA but have at least one foreign-born parent. Third-generation immigrants have two US born parents and at least one foreign-born grandparent.

According to a recent report based on data from 2021, about one in three of all US Hispanics were foreign-born ("first-generation") immigrants [25]. Overall, just over four out of five Hispanics are US citizens, and nearly four out of five of the Hispanic/Latino population have lived in the USA for over 10 years [25]. It is estimated that nearly 25% of the total US foreign-born population of any race is undocumented and include those who either enter without permission from the US government or enter with a legal visa that is no longer valid [27]. Of this group, nearly 75% are Hispanic or Latino [27].

The diversity in immigrant experience has a variable effect on mental health. Many members of the Hispanic/Latino American population have lived in the USA for multiple generations, are well-established, and have similar rates of mental illness and access to health care as their white counterparts. However, undocumented immigrants crossing the border may have exposure to physical, verbal, psychological, and/or sexual violence as part of their journey, and upon arrival in the USA may have trouble with housing, employment, and access to healthcare. A review of undocumented immigrant adults showed common mental health concerns experienced included depression, anxiety, PTSD, and substance use [28]. Research has shown that factors such as immigrant generation (i.e., first-generation, second-generation), age of immigration, and duration as an immigrant in the receiving nation have important implications for the relationship between immigrant status and mental disorders [29].

A study published in 2010 showed unique migration stressors (i.e., involuntary migration, exposure to traumatic events during migration, and discrimination) in first-generation immigrant Latino youth increased the risk of both depressive symptoms and anxiety. However, time in the USA and support from family and teachers reduced these risks [30].

There has been a recent increase in anti-immigrant sentiment in political rhetoric and mass media, and many Latino immigrants have been labeled as foreigners, stereotyped as criminals, and accused of abusing access to government services [27]. This has led to increased discrimination experienced by many Hispanic/Latino Americans, regardless of immigration status. A recent study showed immigration-related discrimination is associated with elevated depression and anxiety regardless of one's own and parental immigration status [31].

A recent narrative revealed more than 20% of Hispanic/Latino American adults report having a mental illness. However compared to the 52% of white patients who received mental healthcare in 2021, only 36% of Hispanics and Latinos received care [32]. Hispanic/Latino American youth consistently report the highest rates of feeling sad or hopelessness in the past year when compared to their non-Latino white and black counterparts [33]. Just over 20% of Hispanic/Latino American adolescents seriously considered suicide in 2021, which was similar to the non-Hispanic white population, though the death rate from suicide was slightly lower [26]. Hispanics/Latino American children were half as likely to receive mental health treatment compared to non-Hispanic whites [34]. This population may experience several barriers to access of mental health services that contribute to this. Further, Hispanics/Latino Americans have the highest uninsured rate of any racial or ethnic group in the United States. According to 2022 ACS estimates, 16.8% of Hispanics/Latinos (of any race) had no health insurance coverage compared to 5.3% of non-Hispanic whites [26].

Although much of this population speak English well, approximately 25% may have difficulty with a language barrier. Interpreting services may not always be readily available, and even when they are, patients may choose to decline services for various reasons, including privacy, fear, time, or simply a desire to minimize extra attention to themselves. Several studies have found that bilingual patients are evaluated differently when interviewed in English as opposed to Spanish and that Hispanics are more frequently undertreated [25]. Regardless of language proficiency, the patient may be more comfortable communicating mental health concerns in their native language. Providers can advocate for scheduling extra time if possible, ensuring patients are aware of privacy rules and encouraging patient use of interpreting services as needed.

There may be a lack of knowledge and/or awareness about mental health problems and available services, including difficulty recognizing mental illness and identifying psychiatric symptoms when the presenting concern is a somatic symptom [34, 35]. Providers need to be aware of this and screening tools can be utilized to aid with accurate diagnosis.

According to 2021 data from the American Psychological Association, Latinos make up a mere 8% of the psychology workforce [36]. Lack of culturally tailored services and culturally competent mental health professionals can affect effective mental health care for this population. Advocating for educational pipelines for diverse candidates will ultimately improve culturally appropriate care. Providers also need to be aware of their personal biases and take opportunities to educate themselves on cultural differences.

Although the Hispanic/Latino American population is very diverse, there are some common characteristics that are shared by many in this group. These include attitudes toward family, traditional gender roles, and religion. *Familismo* is a cultural value that emphasizes the importance of family and is a core part of Hispanic and Latino culture. It includes a strong sense of loyalty to family, belief in familial honor, commitment and dedication to family, and seeking advice and support from family. A 2010 study showed high levels of *familismo* were protective against negative mental health outcomes [37].

Traditional gender role norms are known as *machismo* and *marianismo,* and describe a set of values, attitudes, and beliefs about masculinity and femininity, respectively. *Machismo* traditionally encompasses positive and negative aspects of masculinity, including bravery, honor, dominance, aggression, sexism, sexual prowess, and reserved emotions, among others. *Marianismo* emphasizes the role of women as family- and home-centered; it encourages passivity, self-sacrifice, and chastity. *Machismo* and *marianismo* are intertwined, co-existing constructs that describe socially acceptable norms and beliefs that support men and women in traditional gender roles emphasizing a patriarchal power structure. A study in 2016 supports that some aspects of these multidimensional constructs may be associated with negative cognitive-emotional factors such as depression, anxiety, anger, and cynical hostility [38]. An understanding of this potential aspect of culture is important for healthcare providers working with this population.

Religion may be important to Hispanic/Latino American families, as 3 out of 4 identify as Christian, with approximately 50% identifying as Catholic. In 2018, a study showed religious fundamentalism was associated with more negative attitudes toward people with mental illness, which can increase stigma and decrease the likelihood of seeking mental health care [35]. Providers can help equalize mental health and physical health concerns and help educate patients on their interconnectedness and the importance of addressing both.

Undocumented immigrants are less likely to seek health care for multiple reasons, including lack of insurance and limited financial means, fear of detection by immigration officials, and fear of being turned away or mistreated by health care providers [27]. Community health centers currently provide the most care for the undocumented [27]. They are positioned to provide culturally appropriate care but are often overstretched and not adequately reimbursed for their work. Providers can advocate for supporting these centers through either local insurance programs or additional funding.

Integrated behavioral health is uniquely positioned to assist in improving access to mental health care in the Hispanic/Latino American population. For reasons previously discussed, this population may be less likely to pursue assessment and treatment for mental health concerns. However, integrating this into the primary care setting has already shown to be helpful. In 2024, researchers showed US children were just over twice as likely to receive mental health treatment if their primary place of care was a primary care office, and they had a well child exam in the last year [34].

Asian American

Asian Americans are also a very diverse group. They have origins in over 20 countries and have unique histories, cultures, languages, religions, history of immigration, and other characteristics [39, 40]. The 2020 US Census Bureau uses a definition of Asian as a person having origins in any of the original peoples of the Far East, Southeast Asia, or the Indian subcontinent including, for example, Cambodia, China, India, Japan, Korea, Malaysia, Pakistan, the Philippine Islands, Thailand, and Vietnam [26].

This group accounts for about 6% of the US population, with the five largest subgroups of Asian Americans in descending order being Indian, Chinese, Filipino, Vietnamese, and Korean American [17, 26]. Historically, Asian Americans were often statistically grouped together with Pacific Islanders (AAPI). In 1997, these groups were separated into two separate categories, and in 2024 they continued to revise and further define these populations for more accurate reporting [26]. However, traditionally these groups may still be combined in studies and discussions.

The number of immigrants from Asian countries in the United States grew considerably with the passage of the 1965 Immigration and Nationality Act [41]. Asian Americans are now the fastest growing racial minority in the USA, and it is predicted that by 2060, 1 in 10 American youths will be of Asian origin [42]. Nearly 6 in 10 of Asian Americans were born in another country, in contrast to 14% of the total American population [39]. Nearly 70% report speaking English "very well," though nearly 3 in 4 may speak a language other than English at home [26]. As noted previously, this is a diverse population, and statistics on mental health may vary by subgroup, however due to some cultural similarities, data is often extrapolated to encompass the Asian American population.

In 2020, a study showed AAPI youth may be under diagnosed for conditions like depression and ADHD and relatively over diagnosed for anxiety and adjustment disorders [43]. In a study of adolescent Asian Americans (11–18yo), nearly half reported baseline depression or suicidality [44]. Suicide was the leading cause of death in Asian American young adults (15–24yo), though the overall suicide rate was less than half compared to non-Hispanic whites [2, 26]. In general, this group has a lower rate of substance use disorder compared to the general US population [45]. Mental illness is often stigmatized in Asian cultures, leading to underreporting and somatic presentations of mental health issues [46–48].

Previous studies show Asian Americans are less likely than Caucasians to seek mental health treatment [49]. For the adult population, recent data show Asian Americans were 50% less likely to receive mental health care [6, 26]. Having a parent with a mental health diagnosis increases the likelihood of a child receiving treatment, highlighting the importance of addressing parental mental health [34].

Barriers to accessing mental health services are numerous and may include stigma associated with mental health disorders, the model minority stereotype, language differences, availability of appropriate staff, and lack of adequate insurance coverage [45, 49]. Mental illness may be considered a weakness and may be seen as a source of burden and/or shame in this population. First-generation immigrants may be more likely to lack understanding about mental health, which can lead to denial or neglect of these issues [45]. In order to minimize stigma and shame and preserve self-esteem, some Asian American family members may discourage treatment of their children for fear of a breach in confidentiality and fear of destroying a family reputation.

Asian Americans are often perceived to achieve a higher degree of socioeconomic success in comparison to the average population. In 2019, over half of Asian adults had a bachelor's degree, compared to one-third of both total immigrant and US born adults. However, education levels vary widely based on the Asian country of origin [41]. This contributes to the "myth of the model minority," which is based on stereotypes. This myth characterizes Asian Americans as a polite, law-abiding group who have achieved a higher level of success than the general population through some combination of innate talent and immigrant striving [50]. Asian American children may be expected to have higher academic achievement and innate musical abilities. This can lead to pressure to try to meet the expectations of society and oftentimes family, which can lead to undue stress and challenges with mental health.

The 2000 College Health Assessment Survey showed that Asian American college students were 1.6 times more likely than white students to seriously consider attempting suicide in the previous year [51]. The myth erases the differences among individuals, ignores the diversity of Asian American cultures, and is harmful to the struggle for racial justice [50]. It also perpetuates the "foreignness" of Asian Americans, leading to the common question familiar to many in this population, "So where are you *really* from?" Combined with the stigma often associated with mental illness, it may discourage this population from seeking care.

Language barriers can also lead to lack of addressing mental health and/or misinterpretation of responses to relevant questions. Screening questionnaires are often not available in multiple Asian languages. If interpreting services are not readily available, children sometimes serve as interpreters, which is not ideal.

Shortage of mental health providers can lead to long wait times for patients to access care. If available providers lack cultural awareness, this can discourage patients from seeking care and may interfere with accurate diagnosis [34]. Racial concordance would be ideal, but the need for these mental health providers exceeds the availability in this realm [43]. According to the American Psychological Association, in 2016, just 4% of active psychologists were Asian.

In 2022, rates of lack of health insurance were similar between Asian Americans and non-Hispanic whites at about 5% [26]. Though most have some form of health insurance, the cost of mental health services can be prohibitive depending on the type of insurance coverage [45]. For example, with high-deductible private insurance plans, families may have to pay for the majority of care out of pocket, and the cost can discourage families from complying with treatment recommendations.

With relatively recent immigration for many subgroups in the Asian American population, there is a role for the discussion of acculturation and enculturation. In general, acculturation is the process of adapting to a new culture, and enculturation is the process of learning one's native culture. Asian American youth may face stress trying to navigate these two processes, leading to family conflicts, identity confusion, and poor mental health [46, 47, 51]. Parents may not approve of how their child is adopting US cultural practices, but youth may not have adequate knowledge of, or even desire to pursue knowledge of their native culture. Hansen's law states "what the son wishes to forget, the grandson wishes to remember," referring to the tendency for second-generation immigrants to distance themselves from their ethnic heritage, while their grandchildren later seek to rediscover it.

Asian American youth may experience discrimination based on their appearance, religion, culture, and perception of foreignness [46]. Both microaggressions and macroaggressions may be noted. Microaggressions are defined as "brief and commonplace daily verbal, behavioral, and environmental indignities, whether intentional or unintentional, that communicate hostile, derogatory, or negative racial slights and insults to the target person or group." [52]

Macroaggressions refer to the systemic and institutionalized forms of bias and oppression that impact the lives of entire groups of minoritized people. The experience of this racism can lead to severe mental health issues such as anxiety and depression [42]. With the recent Covid-19 pandemic, Asian American youth and young adults reported increased experiences of anti-Asian harassment and violence. The majority reported an increase in their depressive symptoms, and many felt less safe and even avoided public spaces due to fear of being targeted [53].

Many Asian cultures are collectivistic, which means that people are seen as part of a group rather than as individuals. In contrast, the USA is a Western society that is considered an individualized society, where people are seen as independent and autonomous, and social behavior is dictated by the preferences of individuals. This dichotomy can play a significant role in cultural barriers in mental health care. For example, a Western clinician may feel the individual is too enmeshed with their family and see it as unhealthy and recommend setting more boundaries. However, the Asian American patient may feel it is normal for them, and not be interested in changing the family dynamic, but instead may be willing to endure or persist for the sake of the group.

In a collectivist society, effective treatment involves a multipronged approach. This may include individual, group, family, and community interventions, along with medication management [46, 53]. Culturally adapted cognitive behavioral therapy (CBT) and attachment-based family therapy (ABFT) are highlighted as effective methods [46]. Engaging families through cultural and religious gatherings can help destigmatize mental health issues and promote resilience. Providers must navigate the different value systems of the parent–child dyad without ostracizing either generation to deliver effective care [46].

As mentioned previously, integrated behavioral health is an excellent option for this population, as US children were just over twice as likely to receive mental health treatment if their primary place of care was a primary care office [34]. It is important for providers to examine their own biases, educate themselves about cultural variations, and work to empower minority youth [42]. Future efforts should focus on culturally tailored interventions and sustainable partnerships between clinical and community organizations to bridge gaps in care [34].

Arab American/Middle Eastern North African

According to the Census Bureau, the definition of Middle Eastern North African is, "...geographically based and includes Arabic-speaking groups, such as Egyptian and Jordanian, and non-Arabic speaking groups, such as Iranian and Israeli. It also includes ethnic and transnational groups from the region, such as Assyrian and Kurdish." [54] Further, Arab American is defined as a group of immigrants and descendants of immigrants who come from the Arabic world [55]. Over 3.5 million individuals identified as MENA in the 2020 census which accounts for 1.5% of the "White alone or in combination" category and over 2.5 million individuals identified as MENA only [54]. Approximately 47% of the MENA population in the United States is comprised of individuals from Lebanon, Iran, and Egypt (Table 11.1) [17].

Mental health related topics continue to be taboo and stigmatized within the Arab world. However, according to researchers, there is a significant prevalence of mental health concerns within the Middle East with estimates of up to 34% of the population experiencing at least one mental health related concern [56]. Approximately 30% of this population were found to be depression and anxiety, with the highest impact being on women, those who are impacted by conflict, violence, and displacement, and those who are from vulnerable populations [56].

Recent research has also found that mental health concerns increased 14% over a 30-year range with the highest increases in Bulimia and Schizophrenia and biggest decreases in developmental intellectual disabilities such as ADHD, conduct disorder, and autism spectrum disorders [56]. Data on the mental health of the Arab American population is scarce because, until recently, this community was not identified as a separate ethnic group which has made it challenging to receive appropriate medical and psychological needs that are specific to this group. There is more literature on adult utilization rates, but it is even more scarce for pediatric and adolescent groups.

The traditions among the MENA community are strong, even with Arab Americans living within the United States. The Arab American population is one of the groups with the lowest rates of utilization of mental health services. There are also several barriers to accessing mental health care for this group within the United States. Researchers have found that adolescent and youth population from Arab American communities also have low rates of mental health care utilization.

Research highlights several barriers to this including: desires to avoid damage to personal and familial reputation, challenges with communicating mental health needs to caregivers, gender roles and norms within the MENA community and expectations around mental health, and the quality and appropriateness of available services for the culture and traditions. There are also low rates of mental health care utilization in adults from MENA communities and instead the community turns to

Table 11.1 Breakdown of age and sex group in the United States MENA Community [17]

Middle Eastern North African identifying	Age group	% in each age group
	Under 18 years old	26%
	18 to 44 years	42%
	45 to 64 years	22%
	65 years and older	11%
	Sex group	
	Female	49%
	Male	51%

elder family members and religious leaders for support when mental health concerns arise [57].

Indeed, individuals from the Arab diaspora experience mental health challenges and these challenges can be exacerbated after migration to the United States. There is a strong sense of cultural pride for those who are a part of the MENA community. Culturally, there is a value placed on "purity" and maintaining a "good familial reputation." Due to these values, those from MENA communities may suffer in silence due to the value placed on maintaining a certain image, especially as a woman.

There is also a strong tradition in the MENA and Arab American communities surrounding marriage, as this is the most important thing a woman can do, even more important than education. There are also cultural beliefs that allowing a woman or girl to receive mental health treatment would negatively impact any chance they have of getting married and attempt to marry off their daughters before any damage can be made to the daughter or families reputation. Additional beliefs within the community include that mental health related information appearing in an individual's medical record could impact their future employability [58]. There are others who have beliefs that receiving mental health care services could impact the individual's ability for future child-rearing and parenting [58].

The topic of mental health concerns in this community is still surrounded by significant shame and stigma. These matters are also required to stay within a family unit and are not spoken of outside of the home. There are several examples highlighting these values and how it maintains the stigma around mental health in this culture. For example, if children are yelled at or scolded, it's because they deserved it: if a child or adolescent shows symptoms of depression, then they are deemed as lazy, or if a child or adolescent states a boundary or asks for a need to be met, then they are being disrespectful and ungrateful for what they are being given. The attitudes, traditions, and misinformation related to mental health migrate with families as they come to the United States and further maintain the stigma and barriers associated with seeking out mental health supports.

Further, there are several additional barriers that exist for the MENA community when it comes to finding or engaging in mental health care services. If an individual who is part of the MENA community attempts to initiate services, they are met with many challenges including potentially not being able to afford mental health services. There are some individuals, especially women, who do not have the additional autonomy to seek out services, particularly if they live with their family or husbands who may not allow them to receive those services or discuss family matters with strangers or outside of the home. There are others who also seek out services but then have a language barrier and do not speak English or have a language barrier and cannot find a provider who can conduct services in their required language or dialect, or understands the culture or religious beliefs and traditions that are specific to the MENA community.

There are several strategies to consider utilizing to engage members of the MENA community in mental health services and to support breaking down the existing barriers to engagement for the community. One major area includes educating families and individuals. Providers could consider tailoring education to fit the values and traditions of the culture but using specific verbiage over other words. For example, one may consider leaving out terms such as "mental health" and "therapy" from discussions on this topic and discussing these concerns in the context of stress, trauma, and other similar verbiage which tends to resonate better with members of the MENA community.

Another strategy which one may use in order to attempt to increase engagement is re-framing discussions of mental health for members of the MENA community. Providers could consider discussing the benefits of therapy. For example, providers could discuss mental health in the context of how therapy could improve school performance and grades which is a strong value in the Arab world. Providers could take this approach to get buy-in from families and individuals and then continue to converse about mental health concerns or diagnoses.

Along the same lines, providers could consider utilizing metaphors in conversations about mental health. Specifically, members of the MENA community value physical health and have stronger buy-in when discussing their physical health. Thus, providers could consider discussing mental health in the context of a metaphor related to one's physical health (e.g., mental health as a muscle, emotional first aid, burnout as exhaustion, mental health as an immune system, stress as a pressure cooker, mental health check-ups, anxiety as a stomachache, or depression as a broken bone).

Summary/Conclusion

Integrated behavioral health services remain the gold standard for primary care services as it is a team-based approach that includes a psychologist on the healthcare team and is a means to support the physician and patient [59]. Although IBH can provide increased access to mental health services, ethnic minorities continue to experience significant challenges due to barriers in access for needed mental health services.

These barriers are similar across the various ethnic minority sub-populations and include systemic issues such as lack of health insurance, transportation, discrimination and availability of mental health providers as well as cultural which include stigma related to need for mental health care, lack of trust of the system, and lack of cultural competence including language of providers. A key summary of specific factors to consider for each ethnic-minority group as reported in this chapter for providers to understand in assessment of mental health and design of an Integrated Behavioral Health model within their practice include are highlighted in the following:

African Americans (AA) youth have been found to be an especially disadvantaged group who are often misdiagnosed [19]. In addition, research shows AA youth are more often over diagnosed with some mental health disorders such as conduct disorders and schizophrenia while being underdiagnosed for other disorders such as anxiety and mood disorders [19]. The need for improved mental health services is crucial as suicide rates are highest in AA males and females [3]. Stigma as well as historical trauma are significant considerations for decreased access and utilization of mental health care services. Providers must consider these issues in designing and delivering mental health care for this population.

Uniquely, Hispanic and Latinx youth challenges with mental health care include factors such as immigrant generation (i.e., first-generation, second-generation), age of immigration, and duration as an immigrant in the receiving nation have important implications for the relationship between immigrant status and mental disorders [29]. Additional mental health problems for youth in this population are the stress from immigration-related discrimination which has been shown to increase depression and anxiety regardless of one's own and parental immigration. Providers should include an understanding of the political climate and immigration in assessing the mental health status and needs for this sub-population.

Asian American youth may experience discrimination based on their appearance, religion, culture, and perception of foreignness [46]. The impact of racism, which increased with COVID –19, added to severe mental health issues such as anxiety and depression [42]. Barriers to accessing mental health services are numerous and may include stigma associated with mental health disorders, the model minority stereotype, language differences, availability of appropriate staff, and lack of adequate insurance coverage [45–49]. Providers should consider the importance of family dynamics and cultural identity and stereotypes for designing mental health care services for this population.

Finally, Middle Eastern North African (MENA) community data is limited because, until recently, this community was not identified as a separate ethnic group which has made it challenging to receive appropriate medical and psychological needs that are specific to this group. Family traditions are strong, and the Arab American population is one of the groups with the lowest rates of utilization of mental health services. The topic of mental health concerns in this community is still surrounded by significant shame and stigma. These matters are also required to stay within a family unit and are not spoken of outside of the home. As suggested in this chapter, providers can consider re-framing discussions of mental health for members of the MENA community, focusing on the benefits for therapy for example with improved school performance.

In summary, in addition to the specific recommendations listed, there is a need to increase the availability of mental health providers. Suggestions include increasing the pipeline for training mental health providers, including programs to increase diversity and incorporating cultural sensitivity training as well as developing programs for practices to participate in a coordinated system to receive IBH services virtually across different counties. Finally, payment for IBH providers should be critically evaluated as there needs to be an increase in reimbursement for services.

References

1. CDC National Center for Health Statistics and U.S. Census Bureau. Household Pulse Survey (2020–2024). Anxiety and Depression; 2024.
2. Center for Disease Control and Prevention. 2024. Health disparities in suicide.
3. Center for Behavioral Health Statistics and Quality SA and MHSA. Substance Abuse and Mental Health Services Administration. 2023 Companion infographic report: results from the 2021, 2022, and 2023 National Surveys on Drug Use and Health (SAMHSA Publication No. PEP24-07-020); 2024.
4. Goodwin RD, Dierker LC, Wu M, Galea S, Hoven CW, Weinberger AH. Trends in U.S. depression prevalence from 2015 to 2020: the widening treatment gap. Am J Prev Med. 2022;63(5):726–33.
5. Center for Disease Control and Prevention. Youth risk behavior survey data summary & trends report: 2013–2023; 2024.
6. SAHMSA. SAMHSA, 2024. Results from the 2023 National Survey on Drug Use and Health: Mental Health Detailed Tables; 2024.
7. National Center for HIV/AIDS VHS and TPD of A and SHealth. Youth risk behavior survey data summary & trends report 2009–2019; 2020.
8. Kamal R, Cox C, Rousseau D. Costs and outcomes of mental health and substance use disorders in the US. JAMA. 2017;318(5):415.
9. Melek S, Norris D, Paulus J, Matthews K, Weaver A, Davenport S. Potential Economic Impact of Integrated Medical-Behavioral Healthcare: Updated Projections for 2017; 2017.
10. Thapa BB, Laws MB, Galárraga O. Evaluating the impact of integrated behavioral health intervention: evidence from Rhode Island. Medicine. 2021;100(34):e27066.
11. Mao W, Shalaby R, Agyapong VIO. Interventions to reduce repeat presentations to hospital emergency departments for mental health concerns: a scoping review of the literature. Healthcare. 2023;11(8):1161.
12. Celano CM, Healy B, Suarez L, Levy DE, Mastromauro C, Januzzi JL, et al. Cost-effectiveness of a collaborative care depression and anxiety treatment program in patients with acute cardiac illness. Value Health. 2016;19(2):185–91.
13. Beere D, Page IS, Diminic S, Harris M. A mixed methods evaluation of an integrated adult mental health service model. BMC Health Serv Res. 2019;19(1):691.
14. Breslau J, Leckman-Westin E, Han B, Pritam R, Guarasi D, Horvitz-Lennon M, et al. Impact of a mental health based primary care program on emergency department visits and inpatient stays. Gen Hosp Psychiatry. 2018;52:8–13.
15. National Institute of Health. U.S. Department of Health and Human Services. 2024. Race and National Origin: NIH Style Guide.
16. Chen D, Torstrick AM, Crupi R, Schwartz JE, Frankel I, Brondolo E. Reducing emergency department visits among older adults. J Integr Care. 2019;27(1):37–49.
17. U.S. Census Bureau. census.gov. 2023. U.S. Census Bureau Quick Facts selected: United States.
18. Pederson AB. Management of depression in black people: effects of cultural issues. Psychiatr Ann. 2023;53(3):122–5.
19. Opara I, Weissinger GM, Lardier DT, Lanier Y, Carter S, Brawner BM. Mental health burden among black adolescents: the need for better assessment, diagnosis and treatment engagement. Soc Work Ment Health. 2021;19(2):88–104.
20. Yearby R, Clark B, Figueroa JF. Structural racism in historical and modern US health care policy. Health Aff. 2022;41(2):187–94.
21. Grogan CM, Park S (Ethan). The racial divide in state Medicaid expansions. J Health Polit Policy Law. 2017;42(3):539–72.
22. Howell J. Understanding black distrust of medicine. 2021.
23. Allden K, Jones L, Weissbecker I, Wessells M, Bolton P, Betancourt TS, et al. Mental health and psychosocial support in crisis and conflict: report of the mental health working group. Prehosp Disaster Med. 2009;24(S2):s217–27.

24. Ali GC, Ryan G, de Silva MJ. Validated screening tools for common mental disorders in low and middle income countries: a systematic review. PLoS One. 2016;11(6):e0156939.
25. Moslimani M, Hugo Lopez M, Noe-Bustamante L. Pew Research Center. 2023. 11 facts about Hispanic origin groups in the U.S.
26. Office of Minority Health. U.S. Department of Health and Human Services Office of Minority Health. 2024 [cited 2024 Dec 16]. Asian American Health. Available from: https://minorityhealth.hhs.gov/asian-american-health
27. Ornelas IJ, Yamanis TJ, Ruiz RA. The health of undocumented Latinx immigrants: what we know and future directions. Annu Rev Public Health. 2020;41(1):289–308.
28. Garcini LM, Murray KE, Zhou A, Klonoff EA, Myers MG, Elder JP. Mental health of undocumented immigrant adults in the United States: a systematic review of methodology and findings. J Immigr Refug Stud. 2016;14(1):1–25.
29. Salas-Wright CP, Vaughn MG. A "refugee paradox" for substance use disorders? Drug Alcohol Depend. 2014;142:345–9.
30. Potochnick S. The academic adaptation of immigrant students with interrupted schooling. Am Educ Res J. 2018;55(4):859–92.
31. Rodriguez VE, Enriquez LE, Ro A, Ayón C. Immigration-related discrimination and mental health among Latino undocumented students and U.S. citizen students with undocumented parents: a mixed-methods investigation. J Health Soc Behav. 2023;64(4):593–609.
32. Morales Lugo N. Unidos US Blog. 2024. Rompiendo Barreras: Dismantling Barriers to Latino Mental Health Care.
33. Isasi CR, Rastogi D, Molina K. Health issues in Hispanic/Latino youth. J Latina/o Psychol. 2016;4(2):67–82.
34. Elliott TR, Choi KR, Elmore JG, Dudovitz R. Racial and ethnic disparities in receipt of pediatric mental health care. Acad Pediatr. 2024;24(6):987–94.
35. Adams KS, Tost JR, Whatley MA, Brown MC, Dochney BJ, Taylor JM, et al. Relationship of Christian beliefs to attitudes toward people with mental illness. Am J Psychother. 2018;71(3):104–9.
36. American Psychiatric Association. Mental Health Disparities: Hispanics and Latinos. 2017.
37. Ayón C, Marsiglia FF, Bermudez-Parsai M. Latino family mental health: exploring the role of discrimination and familismo. J Community Psychol. 2010;38(6):742–56.
38. Nuñez A, González P, Talavera GA, Sanchez-Johnsen L, Roesch SC, Davis SM, et al. Machismo, marianismo, and negative cognitive-emotional factors: findings from the Hispanic community health study/study of Latinos sociocultural ancillary study. J Latina/o Psychol. 2016;4(4):202–17.
39. Budiman A, Ruiz N. https://www.pewresearch.org/short-reads/2021/04/29/key-facts-about-asian-americans/. 2021. Key facts about Asian Americans, a diverse and growing population.
40. Hong GK, Garcia M, Soriano M. Responding to the challenge. In: Handbook of multicultural mental health. Elsevier; 2013. p. 591–607.
41. Hanna M, Batalova J. Migration policy institute. 2021. Immigrants from Asia in the United States.
42. Shaligram D, Chou S, Chandra RM, Song S, Chan V. Addressing discrimination against Asian American and Pacific islander youths: the mental health Provider's role. J Am Acad Child Adolesc Psychiatry. 2022;61(6):735–8. https://doi.org/10.1016/j.jaac.2021.11.021. Epub 2021 Nov 26. PMID: 34843926. J Am Acad Child Adolesc Psychiatry [Internet]. 2022 Jun 1;61(6):735–8. Available from: www.jaacap.org
43. Lee CS, Wong YJ. Racial/ethnic and gender differences in the antecedents of youth suicide. Cultur Divers Ethnic Minor Psychol. 2020;26(4):532–43.
44. Iyer P, Parmar D, Ganson KT, Tabler J, Soleimanpour S, Nagata JM. Investigating Asian American adolescents' resiliency factors and young adult mental health outcomes at 14-year follow-up: a nationally representative prospective cohort study. J Immigr Minor Health. 2023;25(1):75–85.

45. Tanqueco R, Patel S, Watts V. psychiatry.org. 2020 [cited 2024 Dec 15]. Mental Health Facts for Asian Americans/Pacific Islanders. Available from: https://www.psychiatry.org/getmedia/1b7f4da3-d5ca-43be-b5ee-8cead4c12668/Mental-Health-Facts-for-Asian-Americans-Pacific-Islanders.pdf
46. Sharma N, Shaligram D, Yoon GH. Engaging South Asian youth and families: a clinical review. Int J Soc Psychiatry. 2020;66(6):584–92.
47. Balis T, Postolache TT. Ethnic differences in adolescent suicide in the United States. Int J Child Health Human Dev. 2008;1(3):281–96.
48. Choi H, Stafford L, Meininger JC, Roberts RE, Smith DP. Psychometric properties of the DSM scale for depression (DSD) with Korean-American youths. Issues Ment Health Nurs. 2002;23(8):735–56.
49. Abright AR, Chung H. Depression in Asian American children. West J Med. 2002;176(4):244–8.
50. Blackburn SS. Learning for Justice. 2019. What is the model minority myth?
51. Lau AS, Jernewall NM, Zane N, Myers HF. Correlates of suicidal behaviors among Asian American outpatient youths. Cult Divers Ethn Minor Psychol. 2002;8(3):199–213.
52. Sue DW, Capodilupo CM, Torino GC, Bucceri JM, Holder AMB, Nadal KL, et al. Racial microaggressions in everyday life: implications for clinical practice. Am Psychol. 2007;62(4):271–86.
53. Huynh J, Chien J, Nguyen AT, Honda D, Cho EE, Xiong M, et al. The mental health of Asian American adolescents and young adults amid the rise of anti-Asian racism. Front Public Health. 2023;10:958517.
54. Marks R, Jacobs P, Coritz Alli. United States Census Bureau. 2023. Lebanese, Iranian and Egyptian Populations Represented Nearly Half of the MENA Population in 2020 Census.
55. Arab American Institue. 2024. The story of Arab Americans is the story of America.
56. Effatpanah M, Nakhostin-Ansari A, Gorgani F, Khotbehsara ST, Seifi S, Nasoori H, et al. Burden and epidemiology of mental disorders in the Middle East and North Africa from 1990 to 2019: findings from the global burden of disease study. Balkan Med J. 2024;41(2):121–9.
57. Zolezzi M, Alamri M, Shaar S, Rainkie D. Stigma associated with mental illness and its treatment in the Arab culture: a systematic review. Int J Soc Psychiatry. 2018;64(6):597–609.
58. Qushua N, Smith-Appelson J, Sarraf D, Stark L, Seff I. Seeking approval first: mental health care utilization and engagements among MENA adolescents in the United States. Child Youth Serv Rev. 2023;155:107262.
59. Schrager S. Integrating behavioral health into primary care. Fam Pract Manag. 2021;28(3):3–4.

Part III
Pediatric Subspecialties

Chapter 12
Pediatric Subspecialties: Gastroenterology Clinics

Rebecca Rausch, Lindsey P. Dopheide, and Nicholas R. Bovio

Introduction

Gastrointestinal (GI) diseases or disorders are associated with substantial costs and are responsible for millions of health care encounters annually in the United States [1]. Functional GI disorders are now referred to as disorders of the gut-brain interaction (DGBI) [2]. Specific to children and adolescents, DGBI are the highly prevalent GI disorders with estimates of 24.7% of infants and toddlers and 25% of children and adolescents meeting diagnostic criteria for a functional GI disorder [3]. These diagnoses dominate pediatric gastroenterology outpatient practice, accounting for more than 50% of initial visits [4]. Children with organic GI disease or functional GI disorders demonstrate lower health-related quality of life across multiple domains (physical, emotional, social, and school) when compared to healthy controls and those with a functional GI disorder demonstrate lower health-related quality of life than those with an organic GI diagnosis [5].

GI symptoms in DGBI may be related to visceral hypersensitivity, altered gut-microbiota, motility disturbance, altered immune/mucosal functioning, and dysregulation of central nervous system processing, or any combination of the above [6].

R. Rausch (✉)
Pediatric and Adolescent Medicine, Western Michigan University, Homer Stryker M.D. School of Medicine, Kalamazoo, MI, USA
e-mail: Rebecca.rausch@Wmed.edu

L. P. Dopheide
Western Michigan University, Kalamazoo, MI, USA
e-mail: lindsey.dopheide@wmich.edu

N. R. Bovio
Western Michigan University Homer Stryker M.D. School of Medicine, Kalamazoo, MI, USA
e-mail: nicholas.bovio@wmed.edu

R. W. Apple et al. (eds.), *Using Integrated Behavioral Health in Pediatric Practice*, https://doi.org/10.1007/978-3-031-85784-3_12

These diagnoses are best understood and treated from a biopsychosocial perspective [7]. The biopsychosocial framework includes environmental, psychological, and biological factors that contribute to not only the development, but also the maintenance of FGIDs [7]. With this said, it has been recommended that psychological therapies that focus on GI diagnoses, referred to as brain-gut behavior therapies (BGBT), be incorporated into integrated care of DGBIs [8]. However, there can be difficulties in connecting individuals to mental health treatment. There has been a growing interest in and call for multidisciplinary integrated care for DGBI [9]. This chapter aims to review BGBTs, evidence of psychological interventions for select pediatric GI diagnoses, and approaches to integration of psychology services into gastroenterology services, including the available research data on this integration.

Brain-Gut Behavior Therapies (BGBT)

The next section provides an overview of three different empirically supported brain-gut behavior therapies (BGBT): cognitive behavioral therapy, gut-directed hypnotherapy, and mindfulness-based interventions. The discussion of each therapy includes the aim of the treatment, the treatment components, and an overview of what the patient can expect from the treatment. Only some patients with GI symptoms recognize the significant impact of stress and mood on their symptoms—as such all three BGBTs discussed address the treatment of psychological stress in patients [8].

Cognitive Behavioral Therapy (CBT) Cognitive behavioral therapy (CBT) is one of the most studied BGBT and one of the most widely used interventions for disorders of the gut-brain interaction (DGBI) [10]. The focus of CBT in the treatment of DGBI is helping patients unlearn maladaptive coping skills that they rely on because of both the symptoms they experience, and the stress associated with experiencing those symptoms [8]. Hypervigilance about bodily sensations can cause anxiety, which in turn increases the likelihood of experiencing the feared somatic symptoms [11]. CBT practices are intended to interrupt that cycle by helping the patient recognize how their thoughts impact their feelings and behaviors [11]. According to Keefer and colleagues [8], CBT targets psychological stress, negative emotions, maladaptive cognitive processes, avoidance tendencies, psychological comorbidity, somatization, abuse, and early-life experiences.

CBT can target a variety of presenting and comorbid concerns experienced by patients with DGBI. These patients tend to overestimate the probability of a negative event occurring, focus on the negative aspects of the situation, have core beliefs associated with perfectionism, and have a rigid coping style [12]. The CBT classification encompasses an entire class of treatments based on various cognitive behavioral theoretical models, although all CBT models typically include similar components [10]. Some of the typical components include psychoeducation about CBT and the gut-brain axis, relaxation training (i.e., diaphragmatic breathing and progressive muscle relaxation), cognitive restructuring (adopting a more realistic view of their symptoms), coping skills training (replacing maladaptive learned strategies with those that are more productive), and exposure techniques (designed to engage patients in ways that help them overcome fear-based avoidance patterns) [10]. Typically, therapy lasts six to twelve sessions and includes homework assignments that patients complete as a means of practicing the various skills and techniques they are taught during treatment [10].

Although a full summary of the research highlighting the efficacy of CBT with DBGI is beyond the scope of the current work, Palsson and Ballou [10] highlighted the efficacy of CBT with disorders such as irritable bowel syndrome, functional dyspepsia, non-cardiac chest pain (sometimes associated with gastroesophageal reflux), and inflammatory bowel disease (including both Crohn's disease and ulcerative colitis). Research focused on telehealth CBT treatments for DGBI has increased given the demand for virtual services due to the Covid-19 pandemic [13]. As demand for psychotherapy-based treatments for DGBI increases, additional research is needed to ensure improved access, reduced cost, and empirical validation for various DGBI [10].

Gut-Directed Hypnotherapy The overall goal of gut-directed hypnotherapy is to create a state of relaxation to help patients gain better control of their gut functioning [14]. The belief is that increased openness to therapist suggestion occurs when patients are in a heightened state of awareness (i.e., hypnosis) [8]. While in the hypnotic state, the therapist can introduce techniques and provide suggestions for the patient to implement once they are no longer in the hypnotic state [10]. Patients are encouraged to shift their focus from their gut having control of them, to the mantra that they are in control of their gut [15]. Gut-directed hypnotherapy targets psychological stress, maladaptive cognitive processes, and somatization [8].

Typically, hypnotherapy is conducted individually during weekly sessions (sessions are typically 30 to 60 minutes and occur for 6 to 12 weeks) [16]. There is some support for gut-directed hypnotherapy provided via telehealth after treatment modalities had to rapidly shift because of the Covid-19 pandemic [16]. Since there are many myths and misconceptions surrounding clinical hypnotherapy, the first session often serves as an introduction to gut-directed hypnotherapy and includes education on the basic anatomy and physiology of the gut [15].

Gut-focused hypnotherapy relies heavily on visual imagery on the part of the patient, for example, a patient with functional bowel disorder who might refer to their gut as a river or a patient with abdominal pain might use a deflating balloon as a metaphor to reduce bloating [15]. The therapist also provides strategies for feelings of anxiousness and catastrophizing (i.e., catastrophizing is taking a small problem and turning it into something greater or assuming the worst outcome) [15]. Some researchers suggest that gut-directed hypnotherapy leads to changes in neuroplasticity of peripheral and central gut-brain pathways [15]. For more specific information about the protocol for gut-directed hypnotherapy, see the supplemental materials of Vasant and Whorwell [15]. Although most research using gut-directed hypnotherapy has focused on irritable bowel syndrome, there is evidence of the efficacy of hypnotherapy with functional dyspepsia, non-cardiac chest pain (sometimes associated with gastroesophageal reflux), and inflammatory bowel disease [10].

Mindfulness-Based Interventions Mindfulness interventions can help by teaching the patient to attend to the present moment and accept any experienced sensations without judgement [17]. Mindfulness-based interventions work by targeting psychological stress and negative emotions [8]. Mindfulness therapy trains patients to appreciate their daily lives and live in the moment by utilizing attention regulation and openness to their current experiences [18], despite the pain and symptoms they may be experiencing.

Mindfulness at its very basis includes two components: self-regulation of attention and attitude towards one's experience in the moment [19]. The intervention requires the patient to pay absolute attention to the present experience and allow themselves to fully accept their experiences with openness and curiosity [19]. These mindfulness techniques can be especially useful to patients with DGBI because of the increased stress they tend to experience [8]. A specific example of a mindfulness-based approach is mindfulness-based stress reduction (MBSR). MBSR is a manualized workshop that lasts eight weeks and aims to teach participants to practice mindfulness [20]. Although less researched than other BGBTs, mindfulness techniques can be taught by a variety of professionals and there is the potential for group-based or online distribution [8].

Evidence of Psychological or Behavioral Treatments

Functional Abdominal Pain Disorders Functional abdominal pain disorders (FAPDs) in pediatrics are defined by the Rome IV criteria to include irritable bowel syndrome (IBS), functional dyspepsia, abdominal migraine, and functional abdominal pain not otherwise specified [21]. Prevalence FAPDs in pediatric populations has been estimated to be 8.2% [22]. Compared to healthy peers, FAPDs are associated with decreased quality of life [23]. Psychosocial factors are associated with symptoms in FAPDs, for example within IBS; however, somatization and pain catastrophizing have been shown to mediate the relationship between anxiety/depression and symptom severity in children diagnosed with IBS [24]. These diagnoses can carry a high financial cost, with total annual costs per patient diagnosed with IBS or functional abdominal pain/FAPDS estimated to be €2512.31 based on a study conducted in the Netherlands [25] and the mean all-cause incremental spending of United States children diagnosed with IBS reported to be $6364.60 annually, compared to controls when adjusting for age and gender [26].

Three recent systematic reviews focused on psychological treatment for FAPDs have been published. Gordon et al. [27] conducted a systematic review and meta-analysis of randomized controlled trials that compared psychological interventions (including CBT, yoga, hypnotherapy, and guided imagery) and any control condition or no intervention for youth between the ages of 4 and 18 years old. Results revealed moderate certainty that when compared to no intervention, CBT was associated with higher treatment success in addition to lower pain frequency and pain intensity. In terms of results related to hypnotherapy compared to no intervention, there was low certainty that hypnotherapy resulted in higher treatment success. As such, CBT and hypnotherapy may be considered as treatments for FAPDs.

Chen et al. [28] examined the efficacy of CBT for both functional and recurrent abdominal pain disorders in children and adolescents, with a specific aim of examining longer term outcomes. Results indicated that at the post-treatment time point, CBT had significant effects in reduced pain intensity, depression, and solicitousness. At the three month follow-up period, pain intensity and total social cost were significantly decreased, while total health cost did not demonstrate significant change. At the 12 month follow-up point, pain intensity was decreased. Additionally, CBT treatment was associated with improvement in quality of life. These results help to highlight the sustained impact of CBT on reduced intensity of pain up to the 12 month follow-up point and authors suggested including CBT in management for youth with FAPDs.

A third systematic review and meta-analysis that focused on CBT for FAPDs was conducted by Ma et al. [29] and included 14 studies. Low to moderate quality evidence was found that when compared to control groups, participation in CBT was associated with the following outcomes: improvement in general functional impairment, abdominal pain symptoms, psychological states, and higher treatment success. While positive results were found at short-term follow-up points, discrepancies were reported for treatment effects at both mid- and long-term follow-up points, pointing to the need for longer-duration studies.

Inflammatory Bowel Disease Inflammatory bowel disease (IBD), which consists of ulcerative colitis and Crohn's disease, involves chronic patterns of inflammation of the gastrointestinal (GI) tract [30]. Comorbid symptoms of anxiety and depression can lead to worsened outcomes for IBD patients and once mood or anxiety symptoms are present, research shows that they are likely persistent [31]. This makes sense, given that inflammation can be exacerbated by the body's stress response (i.e., anxiety) [30]. Patients with IBD often experience anxiety associated with their GI symptoms, which can in turn increase the intensity of their GI symptoms [30]. Aliu and colleagues [30] argued that psychoeducation should be the first step in treating IBS-like symptoms of IBD as patients may not understand the relationship between the gut-brain axis and how interrelated their symptomology may be.

Seaton and colleagues [32] found that across 28 randomized control trials, psychological mood interventions significantly reduced levels of inflammation in adults with IBD. Not only can psychological interventions help reduce the comorbid mood disorders often seen with IBD, but psychological interventions also work to reduce inflammation caused by IBD [32]. Greater inflammation reduction occurred in patients with the most improvements in mood. This finding led Seaton and colleagues [32] to argue that the reason for the improvement in IBD symptoms is likely improved mood. Regardless of the exact mechanism of action targeted by psychological therapies, the integration of psychological interventions in IBD treatment can help improve patient outcomes and their general sense of wellbeing [32].

On the other hand, Riggott and colleague's [31] findings were inconclusive as to whether psychological intervention improved outcomes of IBD. However, the authors still indicated that there is support for introducing psychological interventions for the treatment of IBD. At the very least, they advocated for mental health screening for patients with IBD to determine the presence of comorbid mental health disorders. Future research is needed to determine whether improved mental health is the cause of the improved IBD symptoms or whether patients with improved mental health are more likely to manage their IBD symptoms more efficiently [32].

Functional Constipation Functional constipation has been shown to be one of the most prevalent functional GI disorders among both toddlers and children/adolescents [3]. Functional constipation is characterized by at least two of the following occurring at least once over the course of a week for at least one month: two for less bowel movements in the toilet peer week with a developmental age of four or greater, at least one instance of fecal incontinence per week, history of purposeful stool retention or retentive posturing, painful or harm bowel movements, large fecal mass in the rectum, or large diameter stools [21].

Functional constipation can have a significant impact on the lives of children and their families. Children with functional constipation have lower health related quality of life when compared to healthy reference samples [33]. Further, children with constipation report lower quality of life than children with IBD or gastroesophageal reflux disease [34]. Regardless of the presence of fecal incontinence, emotional and behavioral problems are more common in youth with functional constipation [35]. Specifically, the prevalence of behavior problems has been shown to be three to four times greater in children with functional constipation when compared to normative populations [36]. Psychosocial problems during early childhood have been shown to be risk factors for constipation and soiling in school age children [37].

Clinical guidelines on the evaluation and treatment of functional constipation in children and infants were published in 2014 by the North American Society for Pediatric Gastroenterology, Hepatology (NASPGHAN) and Nutrition and European Society for Paediatric Gastroenterology Hepatology and Nutrition (ESPGHAN) [38]. With consideration that only one study met inclusion criteria to be considered and, routine use of intensive, behavioral therapy (in addition to conventional treatment) was not recommended for treating childhood constipation (although quality of this evidence was considered low). Authors did recommend demystifying and providing guidance on toilet training when treating childhood constipation and noted that there may be benefit to referring to a mental health provider when children have constipation and behavioral concerns. Additionally, multidisciplinary treatment of childhood functional constipation was not recommended; however, there were no randomized controlled trials found that focused on this modality of treatment [38]. However, further research in this area has led to the idea that behavioral approaches show promise in the care of functional constipation or encopresis.

Hankinson et al. [39] evaluated the impact of both medical and behavioral treatments for chronic constipation in children. Within this multidisciplinary chronic constipation clinic, patients met with both a nurse practitioner and a behavioral psychologist. The initial visit included 30 minutes with the nurse practitioner and 30 minutes with the behavioral psychologist. During the meeting with the nurse practitioner, constipation was assessed, organic causes were evaluated, a diagnosis of functional constipation was made, and medication intervention was prescribed (colon disimpaction if needed and daily maintenance therapy). The visit with the behavioral psychologist focused on evaluation of participant history, compliance with medical regimen, toileting behaviors, and use of reinforcement approaches. Intervention was individualized based on presentation and symptoms, but included aspects of psychoeducation, behavioral methods for skill building and motivation, medication adherence, and pain management if needed. However, the primary emphasis was on developing a toilet sit schedule with relaxation strategies and use of reinforcement. Follow-up visits included problem solving recommended interventions and those who did not attend follow-up visits were contacted by phone to discuss symptoms and interventions. Authors reported that symptoms (frequency of bowel accidents, pain, use of diapers, and perception of constipation frequency) improved following treatment. Most saw improvement after a single visit. Authors did report that for those who initially presented with frequent bowel accidents, more extended treatment was necessary to achieve optimal outcomes.

Most recently, a 2023 study by Lamparyk et al. [40] reported results of a functional constipation shared medical appointment. This study focused on children between the ages of three years old and seven years old who had a diagnosis of functional constipation with or without encopresis. Exclusion criteria included children with a congenital abnormality that could not allow continence to be achieved through the mixture of behavioral and medical approaches alone or those with a significant psychological or developmental comorbidity that would not allow them to be successful with group participation. The group treatment approach was interdisciplinary, with the treatment team comprised of a pediatric psychologist, a pediatric gastroenterologist, a certified child-life specialist, and a licensed clinical counselor. The first visit included an individual session with the shared medical appointment team and focused on orienting to the biopsychosocial model, building rapport, medication adherence, and psychoeducation. The pediatric gastroenterologist also completed a medical examination and adjusted medications (possibly prescribing a clean-out if needed). The next three sessions were group based, with children and parents meeting separately. Sessions focused on a variety of aspects of education on constipation, medications, behavioral reinforcement strategies, and maintenance factors. The base of the treatment included soft and regular bowel movements and toilet sits that are relaxed and positive. Follow-up appointments were also offered, either with new, active cohorts working through the four session protocol or as a standalone follow-up group. Results indicated that parental treatment satisfaction was high and outcomes included either improvement or resolution of constipation in 83.7% of participants and improvement or resolution of encopresis in 64.7% of participants. These initial outcomes point towards the use of shared medical appointments with interdisciplinary care as a promising treatment approach for this population.

Rumination Syndrome Rumination syndrome (RS) is characterized by the repetitive regurgitation of recently swallowed food, which is subsequently re-swallowed or spit out [41]. Recognized as both a functional gastrointestinal disorder and a feeding and eating disorder according to the Rome IV criteria and DSM-5, RS primarily affects children but is prevalent across all age groups [41]. Despite its favorable prognosis, RS can lead to medical and psychosocial complications, such as esophageal injury and significant impairments in quality of life [41].

The pathophysiology of RS remains unclear, with hypotheses suggesting it may involve maladaptive behavioral responses to gastrointestinal stimuli or abnormal autonomic regulation [42]. Emerging behavioral and psychotherapy approaches are becoming more important in managing RS, especially since pharmacological treatments are limited. Diaphragmatic breathing (DB) is the most commonly utilized technique, which involves controlled breathing to counteract the retrograde flow of gastric contents [41]. DB can be paired with biofeedback or electromyography to enhance its effectiveness. Additional nonpharmacological treatments include cognitive-behavioral therapy, relaxation training, chewing gum, and hypnosis. Recent findings suggest that pediatric intensive outpatient programs incorporating behavioral therapies have been found to be as effective and less costly than inpatient management of rumination syndrome [43].

Management of RS should involve a multidisciplinary team consisting of gastroenterologists, psychologists, and dieticians. One study found that the development and distribution of rumination syndrome educational materials to gastroenterologists increased the rate at which patients were referred to behavioral therapy [44]. Given the efficacy of behavioral therapies, a collaborative approach is essential for effective management of the condition.

Functional Esophageal Disorders Functional esophageal disorders are disorders of the gut-brain axis characterized by esophageal symptoms that are not associated with underlying structural, inflammatory, or motility dysfunction [45]. This category of disorders includes but is not limited to functional chest pain, heartburn, reflux hypersensitivity, globus, and dysphagia [46]. The pathophysiology of functional esophageal disorders is related to esophageal visceral hypersensitivity and hypervigilance [46]. These processes lead to symptoms that cause significant distress and functional impairment. Traditional therapies for these disorders include neuromodulator agents including tricyclic antidepressants, selective serotonin reuptake inhibitors, gabapentin, and trazadone [46]. Recently, nonpharmacological brain-gut behavioral therapies (BGBTs) including cognitive behavioral therapy (CBT), gut-directed hypnotherapy, mindfulness-based interventions, and self-management programs have been gaining prominence in the treatment of functional esophageal disorders [46]. Recent evidence from a study by Hurtte et al. [47] found that global symptom burden and health-related quality of life were significantly improved in patients with functional esophageal disorders that underwent multimodal therapy compared to neuromodulator therapy alone [47]. In addition, assessment tools including the Northwestern Esophageal Quality of Life (NEQOL) and Esophageal Hypervigilance and Anxiety Scale (EHAS) have been developed to monitor the behavioral components of functional esophageal disorders [46]. Future clinical research directions include earlier implementation of BGBT in treatment algorithms, development of esophageal specific outcome measures, and investigating the overlap between functional and organic esophageal disorders.

Outcomes Associated with Integrated Care

Time and time again, research shows that integrated care leads to better patient outcomes than gastroenterological care alone [9]. The various benefits include reduction of both psychological and GI symptoms, decreased time on behalf of medical providers, and the potential for additional educational opportunities for both patients and medical providers.

Bray et al. [48] used a matched cohort model to compare the efficacy of an integrated multidisciplinary treatment approach (compared to a standard treatment approach) in the management of functional gastrointestinal disorders (FGIDs) in adults. They found that not only did the patients who received the multidisciplinary care have reduced levels of anxiety and depression, but also experienced reduced levels of gastrointestinal symptoms [48]. In a randomized controlled study, Basnayake and colleagues [49] found that adult patients who received care in a multidisciplinary clinic reported superior symptom improvement, increased psychological well-being, and increased quality of life than those who received care from a standard gastroenterologist. Additionally, the families of pediatric patients with chronic abdominal pain who participated in a multidisciplinary abdominal pain clinic reported higher levels of satisfaction with the services received compared to the families of pediatric patients seen in a traditional GI clinic [50].

Although various studies have reported mixed results regarding patient utilization of services following integrated care, many studies indicate various reductions in health care utilization for patients who receive multidisciplinary care. Basnayake and colleagues [49] reported that adult patients seen in a multidisciplinary clinic were less likely to see their primary care provider during the 12 months following treatment and were less likely to have endoscopies and blood tests performed outside the multidisciplinary care setting. Kinsinger and colleagues [51] found that adult patients who engaged in integrated psychological treatment received fewer GI-related medical procedures, although they found no significant difference in physician office visits for those involved in integrated care. However, although psychological interventions required the patient to put in more work initially, there is less of a time investment overall and significantly less time required from medical providers [51]. In a comparison of pre- and post-integration outcomes, Winnick and colleagues [52] found that pediatric patients who participated in a billed visit with a psychologist had a significant decrease in the total days seen by their medical providers. Additionally, Chu et al. [53] saw a decrease in emergency department visits for children who were seen by a multidisciplinary team that included a pediatric gastroenterologist, a pain medicine physician, and a pain psychologist.

Finally, integration of psychological treatment into medical practices typically leads to more opportunities for educating physicians about the brain-gut interaction. Turner and colleagues [54] reported that after attending a didactic series on the biopsychosocial model and the brain-gut axis, physicians reported increased knowledge and recommended other institutions involve psychologists in physician training. Numerous studies cite psychoeducation about the gut-brain interaction as one of the most crucial aspects the treatment of DGBI [8, 11, 15, 30, 55]. Overall, the existing literature on integration of psychological treatment into GI pediatric medical settings suggests that integration of medical and psychological services can improve patient outcomes and decrease both psychological and GI symptoms. Additionally, integration of services often leads to specific improvements in physician satisfaction by cutting down on the total time required to see GI patients and increasing the opportunities for education about the gut-brain interaction.

Approaches to Integration

Identification of Patients Palsson and Whitehead [56] suggest that psychological treatment should be considered in patients who experience continued moderate or severe symptoms after three to six months of medical management or those who to have stress or emotional symptoms that exacerbate gastrointestinal symptoms, or impairment in coping with their illness. However, it has also been suggested that individuals with significant psychological comorbidity are not the good candidates for BGBT [57, 58]. Specifically, untreated mental health comorbidity that is unrelated to GI diagnosis or severe mental health conditions are considered inappropriate for BGBTs. This includes diagnoses such as major depressive disorder, obsessive compulsive disorder, eating disorders, substance use disorders, psychosis, active posttraumatic-stress disorder [58], or personality disorders [8]. These patients typically do not respond well to therapy focused on GI symptoms and should instead be referred for psychotherapy services focused on mental health concerns [58]. However, once these patients have established psychological treatment for these types of conditions, it is appropriate to refer them for a BGBT consultation [8]. This does not preclude individuals who have mild to moderate mental health diagnoses (generalized anxiety disorder, panic disorder) that are currently in mental health services from also participating in BGBT [58] and many individuals who participate in BGBT are also engaged in long-term therapy for additional concerns [8]. Additional recommendations from Kinsinger include patients who experience symptom-related anxiety or maladaptive coping related to GI conditions, impairment in quality of life related to their GI condition, those who are open to the conceptualization of stress impacting the brain-gut axis, and those who are both willing and motivated to participate in therapy that includes practice outside of visits [58]. Individuals with multiple diagnoses, refractory concerns, significant psychiatric comorbidity, or those requiring tertiary care are likely best cared for by a multidisciplinary team [9].

Tone, Communication, and the Referral Referral for psychological services related to GI conditions can be a sensitive matter for all involved. Stigma of mental health treatment can be particularly difficult for youth with DGBI as a referral to a mental health provider can be interpreted as symptoms not being real, but psychological [59]. It is important for the gastroenterology provider to have tools to effectively communicate a referral for BGBT to help make this a productive discussion. Gastroenterology providers should have patient friendly methods of explaining the gut-brain pathway, how the pathway can become dysregulated, how psychosocial or behavioral factors can maintain or worsen GI symptoms (regardless of etiology), and a clear reasoning for the referral to a mental health provider [57]. Kinsinger [58] recommends four steps to making a successful referral to a GI psychologist: (1) Have the primary rationale for the referral be the role of brain-gut axis; (2) take the time to review scientific support for BGBT; (3) differentiate GI-specific psychological treatment approaches from traditional psychotherapy; and (4) reassure that the gastroenterology provider will stay engaged in the individual's care. Gastroenterologists should be familiar with effective BGBTs and their structure [57] which will be helpful for explaining them to patients. The role of psychological influences and treatment should discussed early in treatment, particularly for those with DBGI. This should help to ensure that a referral for psychological treatment feels like the next step in care, in comparison to being referred following nonresponse to medical intervention which can be perceived as their physician giving up [56] or handing them off to a mental health provider.

Levels of Integration A level of integration framework has been previously proposed by Doherty et al. [60] and has been subsequently updated to include six levels with three main categories [61]. The first level includes the category of coordinated care, which encompasses minimal collaboration (level 1) and basic collaboration at a distance (level 2). This includes behavioral health and medical providers having separate facilities and separate systems with limited communication about patients, typically only focused on gathering information about shared patients [61].

Consistent with this integration category, traditional models of mental health treatment focus on care within a silo. An individual is either referred to mental health services or self-refers, possibly after recommendation from another provider. The provider may facilitate this recommendation by sending a referral or the patient themselves will follow through with finding, contacting, and scheduling an initial appointment. In these circumstances, identification of individuals who would benefit from psychological intervention is placed solely on the gastroenterology provider. However, referring families to find psychological treatment independently is unlikely to be successful as they are likely unfamiliar with types of appropriate therapists and have a limited understanding of what is required [56]. In many areas, the availability of psychologists who specialize in the treatment of DGBI and GI specific health conditions is limited. Gastroenterology providers should have one or more identified suitable mental health providers [56]. Additionally, being able to describe the type of therapy that will be used with an identified mental health provider helps to improve chances of patients following through with the recommendation of mental health services [56].

In the circumstance of locations where specialized psychological providers are not available, there may be benefit to locating the nearest available providers in larger urban centers as patients may be motivated to travel for specialized services [56]. Virtual appointments with an appropriate psychologist may also be a possible option for families. When compared to treatment as usual, children between the ages of eight and 12 years old and diagnosed with a FAPD who were randomly assigned to ten weeks of internet-delivered CBT [62] had significantly larger improvement in symptom severity in addition to improvements in quality of life, avoidance, GI-specific anxiety, and parental responding to symptoms. Gains from CBT persisted through 36 weeks and those in the internet-based CBT group had significantly less health care use than those in the treatment as usual group [62]. Carmody et al. [63] examined a group-based CBT intervention for adolescents with DGBI and reported high retention of participants, improvement on emotional and overall quality of life from pre-intervention to the one month follow-up period. However, no significant differences in somatic symptoms or functional disability were found [63]. Further research into online treatment for children and adolescents with DGBI is needed.

Clinics may also include co-located care, the second integration category with basic collaboration onsite (level 3) and close collaboration with some system integration (level 4) [61]. Basic collaboration onsite includes providers being in the same location, but without sharing a clinic space or having shared systems. Referrals may be more successful due to this shared location and communication may be improved due to provider proximity. However, without clearly defined team roles, providers likely continue to make decisions on patient care on an individual basis. Care that includes close collaboration with some system integration indicates that providers may share the same practice space and some shared systems (scheduling, shared medical record and documentation). Personal communication may occur regarding shared patients and there may be a better understanding of specific roles in patient care [61]. These models may be consistent with larger hospital systems in which mental health providers are collocated at the same location as gastroenterology clinics and they utilize a shared electronic medical record.

The final category of levels of integration includes integrated care (level 5), which includes close collaboration approaching and integrated practice and full collaboration in a transformed/merged practice (level 6). Level 5 is characterized by providers functioning as a team with frequent communication, high levels of collaboration, and understanding of roles on the team. Providers work to alter their practice and care structure with the aim of improving patient care. The highest level of integration occurs at level 6, which includes a single transformed or merged practice where both providers and patients experience a single health system that treats a patient holistically [61]. Eccles et al. [64] included a liaison psychiatrist in their weekly multidisciplinary IBD meeting for adult patients and patient referrals for psychiatric and psychological support were also made by medical staff IBD nurses, pharmacists, and stoma nurses. Participation in psychological intervention services resulted in reduction in IBD symptoms, improvement in depression scores, high satisfaction from both the patient and referrer, and reduction in imaging and outpatient appointments.

Care Team Recommendations for best practice care of management of DBGI patients have been outlined by Burgell and colleagues [9]. Recommended members of an integrated team caring for patients with DBGI should minimally include a medical physician with interest in DBGI, a mental health/behavioral therapist/hypnotherapist, and a dietitian. Additional team members to include or have access to are psychiatrists and pelvic floor physiotherapists. However, all team members working together with an explicit focus on patient-centered care is more important than the specific composition of the team. This care should include an interdisciplinary perspective in which all team members have a solid understanding of the biopsychosocial model. Combined appointments where patients meet with multiple team members or group programs can help to support team collaboration. Burgell and colleagues [9] highlight the importance of communication in interdisciplinary care, either informally or preferably through formal methods such as multidisciplinary meetings, collaborative assessments, or close communication with allied providers following referral.

Conclusion

In this chapter, we have reviewed the role of mental health providers in the care of youth with GI disorders and diagnoses. This has included review of BGBTs and evidence of the impact of psychological care within specific diagnoses. While full integration of psychological services into gastroenterology clinics is still a growing area, there is evidence for a variety of models with differing levels of integration, as reviewed above. As medicine continues to move towards a more holistic model that addresses multiple aspects of functioning with a variety of modalities, there are growing opportunities to help enhance care for children and adolescents with a variety of GI concerns.

References

1. Peery AF, Crockett SD, Murphy CC, Jensen ET, Kim HP, Egberg MD, Lund JL, Moon AM, Pate V, Barnes EL, Schlusser CL, Baron TH, Shaheen NJ, Sandler RS. Burden and cost of gastrointestinal, liver, and pancreatic diseases in the United States: update 2021. Gastroenterol. 2022;F162(2):621–44. https://doi.org/10.1053/j.gastro.2021.10.017.
2. Drossman DA, Hasler WL. Rome IV-functional GI disorders: disorders of gut-brain interaction. Gastroenterol. 2016;150(6):1257–61. https://doi.org/10.1053/j.gastro.2016.03.035.
3. Robin SG, Keller C, Zwiener R, Hyman PE, Nurko S, Saps M, Di Lorenzo C, Shulman RJ, Hyams JS, Palsson O, van Tilburg MAL. Prevalence of pediatric functional gastrointestinal

disorders utilizing the Rome IV criteria. J Pediatr. 2018;195:134–9. https://doi.org/10.1016/j.jpeds.2017.12.012.

4. Rouster AS, Karpinski AC, Silver D, Monagas J, Hyman PE. Functional gastrointestinal disorders dominate pediatric gastroenterology outpatient practice. J Pediatr Gastroenterol Nutr. 2016;62(6):847–51. https://doi.org/10.1097/MPG.0000000000001023.
5. Varni JW, Bendo CB, Nurko S, Shulman RJ, Self MM, Franciosi JP, Saps M, Pohl JF. Pediatric quality of life inventory (PedsQL) gastrointestinal symptoms module testing study consortium. Health-related quality of life in pediatric patients with functional and organic gastrointestinal diseases. J Pediatr. 2015;166(1):85–90. https://doi.org/10.1016/j.jpeds.2014.08.022.
6. Drossman DA. Functional gastrointestinal disorders: history, pathophysiology, clinical features and Rome IV. Gastroenterol. 2016;150(6):1262–1279.e2. https://doi.org/10.1053/j.gastro.2016.02.032.
7. Van Oudenhove L, Crowell MD, Drossman DA, Halpert AD, Keefer L, Lackner JM, Murphy TB, Naliboff BD, Levy RL. Biopsychosocial aspects of functional gastrointestinal disorders. Gastroenterol. 2016;150(6):1355–1367.e2. https://doi.org/10.1053/j.gastro.2016.02.027.
8. Keefer L, Ballou SK, Drossman DA, Ringstrom G, Elsenbruch S, Ljótsson B. A Rome working team report on brain-gut behavior therapies for disorders of gut-brain interaction. Gastroenterol. 2022;162(1):300–15. https://doi.org/10.1053/j.gastro.2021.09.015.
9. Burgell RE, Hoey L, Norton K, Fitzpatrick J. Treating disorders of brain-gut interaction with multidisciplinary integrated care. Moving towards a new standard of care. JGH Open. 2024;8(5):e13072. https://doi.org/10.1002/jgh3.13072.
10. Palsson OS, Ballou S. Hypnosis and cognitive behavioral therapies for the management of gastrointestinal disorders. Curr Gastroenterol Rep. 2020;22(7):1–9. https://doi.org/10.1007/s11894-020-00769-z.
11. Jagielski CH, Riehl ME. Behavioral strategies for irritable bowel syndrome: brain-gut or gut-brain? Gastroenterol Clin N Am. 2021;50(3):581–93. https://doi.org/10.1016/j.gtc.2021.03.006.
12. Lackner JM, Gudleski GD, Radziwon CD, Krasner SS, Firth RS, Naliboff BD, Vargovich AM, Borden AB, Mayer EA. Cognitive flexibility improves in cognitive behavioral therapy for irritable bowel syndrome but not nonspecific education/support. Behav Res Ther. 2022;154:1–14. https://doi.org/10.1016/j.brat.2022.104033.
13. Sugaya N, Shirotsuki K, Nakao M. Cognitive behavioral treatment for irritable bowel syndrome: a recent literature review. Biopsychosoc Med. 2021;15(1):23. https://doi.org/10.1186/s13030-021-00226-x.
14. Chakraborty PS, Daniel R, Navarro FA. Non-pharmacologic approaches to treatment of pediatric functional abdominal pain disorders. Front Pediatr. 2023;11:1–13. https://doi.org/10.3389/fped.2023.1118874.
15. Vasant DH, Whorwell PJ. Gut-focused hypnotherapy for functional gastrointestinal disorders: evidence-base, practical aspects, and the Manchester protocol. Neurogastroenterol Motil. 2019;31(8):1–12. https://doi.org/10.1111/nmo.13573.
16. Noble H, Hasan SS, Simpson V, Whorwell PJ, Vasant DH. Patient satisfaction after remotely delivered gut-directed hypnotherapy for irritable bowel syndrome during the COVID-19 era: implications for future practice. BMJ Open Gastro. 2022;9(1):1–7. https://doi.org/10.1136/bmjgast-2022-001039.
17. Koseki T, Muratsubaki T, Tsushima H, Morinaga Y, Oohashi T, Imafuku M, Suzuki Y, Kanazawa M, Fukudo S. Impact of mindfulness tendency and physical activity on brain-gut interactions. J Gastroenterol. 2023;58(1):158–70. https://doi.org/10.1007/s00535-022-0198-9.
18. Slouha E, Patel B, Mohamed A, Razeq Z, Clunes LA, Kollias TF. Psychotherapy for irritable bowel syndrome: a systematic review. Cureus. 2023;15(12):1–13. https://doi.org/10.7759/cureus.51003.
19. Bishop SR, Lau M, Shapiro S, Carlson L, Anderson ND, Carmody J, Segal ZV, Abbey S, Speca M, Velting D, Devins G. Mindfulness: a proposed operational definition. Clin Psychol Sci Prac. 2004;11(3):230–41. https://doi.org/10.1093/clipsy.bph077.

20. Naliboff BD, Smith SR, Serpa JG, Laird KT, Stains J, Connolly LS, Labus JS, Tillisch K. Mindfulness-based stress reduction improves irritable bowel syndrome (IBS) symptoms via specific aspects of mindfulness. Neurogastroenterol Motil. 2020;32(9):1–10. https://doi.org/10.1111/nmo.13828.
21. Hyams JS, Di Lorenzo C, Saps M, Shulman RJ, Staiano A, van Tilburg M. Functional disorders: children and adolescents. Gastroenterol. 2016;150(6):1456–1468.e2. https://doi.org/10.1053/j.gastro.2016.02.015.
22. Saps M, Velasco-Benitez CA, Langshaw AH, Ramírez-Hernández CR. Prevalence of functional gastrointestinal disorders in children and adolescents: comparison between Rome III and Rome IV criteria. J Pediatr. 2018;199:212–6. https://doi.org/10.1016/j.jpeds.2018.03.037.
23. Youssef NN, Murphy TG, Langseder AL, Rosh JR. Quality of life for children with functional abdominal pain: a comparison study of patients' and parents' perceptions. Pediatrics. 2006;117(1):54–9. https://doi.org/10.1542/peds.2005-0114.
24. Hollier JM, van Tilburg MAL, Liu Y, Czyzewski DI, Self MM, Weidler EM, Heitkemper M, Shulman RJ. Multiple psychological factors predict abdominal pain severity in children with irritable bowel syndrome. Neurogastroenterol Motil. 2019;31(2):e13509. https://doi.org/10.1111/nmo.13509.
25. Hoekman DR, Rutten JM, Vlieger AM, Benninga MA, Dijkgraaf MG. Annual costs of care for pediatric irritable bowel syndrome, functional abdominal pain, and functional abdominal pain syndrome. J Pediatr. 2015;167(5):1103–8.e2. https://doi.org/10.1016/j.jpeds.2015.07.058.
26. Beinvogl B, Palmer N, Kohane I, Nurko S. Healthcare spending and utilization for pediatric irritable bowel syndrome in a commercially insured population. Neurogastroenterol Motil. 2021;33(11):e14147. https://doi.org/10.1111/nmo.14147.
27. Gordon M, Sinopoulou V, Tabbers M, Rexwinkel R, de Bruijn C, Dovey T, Gasparetto M, Vanker H, Benninga M. Psychosocial interventions for the treatment of functional abdominal pain disorders in children: a systematic review and meta-analysis. JAMA Pediatr. 2022;176(6):560–8. https://doi.org/10.1001/jamapediatrics.2022.0313.
28. Chen JY, Chen SN, Lee CH, Huang YJ. A systematic review and meta-analysis of randomized control trials: efficacy of cognitive behavioral therapies for the management of functional and recurrent abdominal pain disorders in children and adolescents. Cogn Behav Ther. 2023;52(5):438–59. https://doi.org/10.1080/16506073.2023.2200562.
29. Ma M, Yang M, Li Y, Hou L, Li M, Wang X, Li Z, Guo K, Liu X, Cheng Y, Niu J, Yang K. Cognitive behavioural therapy for functional abdominal pain disorders in children and adolescents: a systematic review of randomized controlled trials. Behav Res Ther. 2023;169:104397. https://doi.org/10.1016/j.brat.2023.104397.
30. Aliu A, Bosch DHCA, Keszthelyi D, Rezazadeh Ardabili A, Colombel JF, Sawyer R, Törnblom H, Hart A, Jonkers DMAE, Pierik MJ, Mujagic Z. Review article: a practical approach to persistent gastrointestinal symptoms in inflammatory bowel disease in remission. Aliment Pharmacol Ther. 2024;59(12):1470–88. https://doi.org/10.1111/apt.17988.
31. Riggott C, Mikocka-Walus A, Gracie DJ, Ford AC. Efficacy of psychological therapies in people with inflammatory bowel disease: a systematic review and meta-analysis. Lancet Gastroenterol Hepatol. 2023;8(10):919–31. https://doi.org/10.1016/S2468-1253(23)00186-3.
32. Seaton N, Hudson J, Harding S, Norton S, Mondelli V, Jones ASK, Moss-Morris R. Do interventions for mood improve inflammatory biomarkers in inflammatory bowel disease?: a systematic review and meta-analysis. EBioMedicine. 2024;100:1–12. https://doi.org/10.1016/j.ebiom.2023.104910.
33. Vriesman MH, Rajindrajith S, Koppen IJN, van Etten-Jamaludin FS, van Dijk M, Devanarayana NM, Tabbers MM, Benninga MA. Quality of life in children with functional constipation: a systematic review and meta-analysis. J Pediatr. 2019;214:141–50. https://doi.org/10.1016/j.jpeds.2019.06.059.
34. Youssef NN, Langseder AL, Verga BJ, Mones RL, Rosh JR. Chronic childhood constipation is associated with impaired quality of life: a case-controlled study. J Pediatr Gastroenterol Nutr. 2005;41(1):56–60. https://doi.org/10.1097/01.mpg.0000167500.34236.6a.

35. Dos Santos IR, de Abreu GE, Dourado ER, Martinelli Braga AAN, Lobo VA, de Carvalho IWB, Bastos Netto JM, Barroso U Jr. Emotional and behavioural problems in children and adolescents: the role of constipation. J Paediatr Child Health. 2021;57(7):1003–8. https://doi.org/10.1111/jpc.15368.
36. van Dijk M, Benninga MA, Grootenhuis MA, Last BF. Prevalence and associated clinical characteristics of behavior problems in constipated children. Pediatrics. 2010;125(2):e309–17. https://doi.org/10.1542/peds.2008-3055.
37. Joinson C, Grzeda MT, von Gontard A, Heron J. Psychosocial risks for constipation and soiling in primary school children. Eur Child Adolesc Psychiatry. 2019;28(2):203–10. https://doi.org/10.1007/s00787-018-1162-8.
38. Tabbers MM, DiLorenzo C, Berger MY, Faure C, Langendam MW, Nurko S, Staiano A, Vandenplas Y, Benninga MA, European Society for Pediatric Gastroenterology, Hepatology, and Nutrition, North American Society for Pediatric Gastroenterology. Evaluation and treatment of functional constipation in infants and children: evidence-based recommendations from ESPGHAN and NASPGHAN. J Pediatr Gastroenterol Nutr. 2014;58(2):258–74. https://doi.org/10.1097/MPG.0000000000000266.
39. Hankinson JC, Borden L, Allen T, Santo Domingo L, Oliva-Hemker M, Mathews T, Brock K, Perry-Parrish C, Reynolds EK, Specht M, Ostrander R. Outcomes of combined medical and behavioral treatments for constipation within a specialty outpatient clinic. Clin Pract Pediatr Psychol. 2018;6(1):31–41. https://doi.org/10.1037/cpp0000202.
40. Lamparyk K, Mathis M, Piorkowski L, Polasky S, Gross M, Feinberg L. Development and evaluation of an interdisciplinary group intervention for pediatric functional constipation. Clin Pract Pediatr Psychol. 2023;11(1):74–83. https://doi.org/10.1037/cpp0000435.
41. Sartori R, Della Torca A, Bramuzzo M, Barbi E, Tessitore A. Nonpharmacological treatment of rumination syndrome in childhood: a systematic review of the literature. J Pediatr Gastroenterol Nutr. 2024;78(4):763–73. https://doi.org/10.1002/jpn3.12038.
42. Sawada A, Fujiwara Y. Belching disorders and rumination syndrome: a literature review. Digestion. 2024;105(1):18–25. https://doi.org/10.1159/000534092.
43. Kroon Van Diest AM. Intensive outpatient treatment of pediatric rumination syndrome. Clin Pract Pediatr Psychol. 2023;11(4):382–94. https://doi.org/10.1037/cpp0000492.
44. Mayer-Brown S, Downing MA, Webster J, Maxwell EC, Baber KF. Patient education to increase behavioral treatment referrals for rumination syndrome. Clin Pract Pediatr Psychol. 2023;11(4):408–14. https://doi.org/10.1037/cpp0000494.
45. Aziz Q, Fass R, Gyawali CP, Miwa H, Pandolfino JE, Zerbib F. Functional esophageal disorders. Gastroenterol. 2016;150(6):1368–79. https://doi.org/10.1053/j.gastro.2016.02.012.
46. Luo Y, Keefer L. The clinical value of brain-gut behavioral therapies for functional esophageal disorders and symptoms. Neurogastroenterol Motil. 2022;34(6):e14373. https://doi.org/10.1111/nmo.14373.
47. Hurtte E, Rogers BD, Richards C, Gyawali CP. The clinical value of psychogastroenterological interventions for functional esophageal symptoms. Neurogastroenterol Motil. 2022;34(6):e14315. https://doi.org/10.1111/nmo.14315.
48. Bray NA, Koloski NA, Jones MP, Do A, Pang S, Coombes JS, McAllister S, Campos J, Arthur L, Stanley P, DeMaria K, Chao CY, Catague R, Whaley A, Talley NJ, Holtmann GJ. Evaluation of a multidisciplinary integrated treatment approach versus standard model of care for functional gastrointestinal disorders (FGIDS): a matched cohort study. Dig Dis Sci. 2022;67(12):5593–601. https://doi.org/10.1007/s10620-022-07464-1.
49. Basnayake C, Kamm MA, Stanley A, Wilson-O'Brien A, Burrell K, Lees-Trinca I, Khera A, Kantidakis J, Wong O, Fox K, Talley NJ, Liew D, Salzberg MR, Thompson AJ. Long-term outcome of multidisciplinary versus standard gastroenterologist care for functional gastrointestinal disorders: a randomized trial. Clin Gastroenterol Hepatol. 2022;20(9):2102–11.e9. https://doi.org/10.1016/j.cgh.2021.12.005.

50. Schurman JV, Friesen CA. Integrative treatment approaches: family satisfaction with a multidisciplinary paediatric abdominal pain clinic. Int J Integr Care. 2010;10:1–9. https://doi.org/10.5334/ijic.551.
51. Kinsinger SW, Ballou S, Keefer L. Snapshot of an integrated psychosocial gastroenterology service. World J Gastroenterol. 2015;21(6):1893–9. https://doi.org/10.3748/wjg.v21.i6.1893.
52. Winnick JB, Focht DR 3rd, Sukumar K, Kuhn BR, Muldowney R, O'Dell SM. Utilization of pediatric psychology services in outpatient pediatric gastroenterology within a rural health system. J Pediatr Gastroenterol Nutr. 2022;75(1):52–5. https://doi.org/10.1097/MPG.0000000000003468.
53. Chu AS, Torres L, Kao G, Gilbert C, Monico EC, Chumpitazi BP. Multidisciplinary care for refractory pediatric functional abdominal pain decreases emergency and inpatient utilization. J Pediatr Gastroenterol Nutr. 2021;74(2):248–52. https://doi.org/10.1097/MPG.0000000000003305.
54. Turner E, Rodriguez KO, Holbein C, Fussner L, Wilkes C. Enhancing biopsychosocial care for disorders of gut–brain interaction: 10-year growth of an integrated pediatric gastroenterology psychology program. Clin Pract Pediatr Psychol. 2023;11(4):415–22. https://doi.org/10.1037/cpp0000497.
55. Reed-Knight B, Maddux MH, Deacy AD, Lamparyk K, Stone AL. Brain-gut interactions and maintenance factors in pediatric gastroenterological disorders: recommendations for clinical care. Clin Pract Pediatr Psychol. 2017;5(1):93–105. https://doi.org/10.1037/cpp0000166.
56. Palsson OS, Whitehead WE. Psychological treatments in functional gastrointestinal disorders: a primer for the gastroenterologist. Clin Gastroenterol Hepatol. 2013;11(3):208–16. https://doi.org/10.1016/j.cgh.2012.10.031.
57. Keefer L, Palsson OS, Pandolfino JE. Best practice update: incorporating psychogastroenterology into management of digestive disorders. Gastroenterol. 2018;154(5):1249–57. https://doi.org/10.1053/j.gastro.2018.01.045.
58. Kinsinger SW. Practical approaches to working with a gastrointestinal psychologist. Gastroenterol Clin N Am. 2022;51(4):711–21. https://doi.org/10.1016/j.gtc.2022.07.002.
59. Reed B, Buzenski J, van Tilburg MAL. Implementing psychological therapies for gastrointestinal disorders in pediatrics. Expert Rev Gastroenterol Hepatol. 2020;14(11):1061–7. https://doi.org/10.1080/17474124.2020.1806055.
60. Doherty WJ, McDaniel SH, Baird MA. Five levels of primary care/behavioral healthcare collaboration. Behav Healthc Tomorrow. 1996;5(5):25–7.
61. Heath B, Wise Romero P, Reynolds K. A standard framework for levels of integrated healthcare [Internet]. Washington, DC: SAMHSA-HRSA Center for Integrated Health Solutions. 2013. 11/06/2024. https://archive.thepcc.org/resource/standard-framework-levels-integrated-healthcare
62. Lalouni M, Ljótsson B, Bonnert M, Ssegonja R, Benninga M, Bjureberg J, Högström J, Sahlin H, Simrén M, Feldman I, Hedman-Lagerlöf E, Serlachius E, Olén O. Clinical and cost effectiveness of online cognitive behavioral therapy in children with functional abdominal pain disorders. Clin Gastroenterol Hepatol. 2019;17(11):2236–2244.e11. https://doi.org/10.1016/j.cgh.2018.11.043.
63. Carmody JK, Kramer RL, Distel LML, Davidson RD, Snyder JM, Villa M, Nemec GE, Hale AE. Feasibility of a virtual group-based cognitive behavioral therapy intervention for adolescents with disorders of gut–brain interaction. J Pediatr Psychol. 2023;11(4):367–81. https://doi.org/10.1037/cpp0000501.
64. Eccles JA, Ascott A, McGeer R, Hills E, St Clair Jones A, Page LA, Smith MA, Loewenberger A, Gregory J. Inflammatory bowel disease psychological support pilot reduces inflammatory bowel disease symptoms and improves psychological wellbeing. Frontline Gastroenterol. 2020;12(2):154–7. https://doi.org/10.1136/flgastro-2019-101323.

Chapter 13
The Role of Integrated Behavioral Health to Improve Treatment Outcomes of Pediatric Endocrinology Disorders

Megan Moore, Nikoli Nickson, Patricia Vining Maravolo, and Berrin Ergun-Longmire

Introduction

The biopsychosocial model, proposed by psychiatrist George L. Engel, delineates how health and disease are influenced by biological, psychological, and social factors [1]. For example, the progression of a disease impacting physiological function in a patient may be exacerbated by stress or poor mental health. Expanding on this framework, studies of adverse childhood experiences (ACEs) have found that traumatic experiences in childhood increase the risk of developing various physical and mental health conditions [1]. Experiences commonly classified as ACEs include abuse, neglect, exposure to violence, and financial hardships. However, less direct stressors such as severe childhood illness can also be considered as ACEs. These illnesses may cause children to experience a loss of control, leading to adverse health outcomes later in life. Consequently, medical interventions should address not only the biological aspects of disease but also aim to address psychological aspects. The interconnectedness of biological, psychological, and social domains influencing health highlights the importance of interdisciplinary care to address different aspects of disease [1]. A holistic approach facilitated by integrated care models is particularly pertinent to pediatric endocrinology, where the progression of chronic conditions such as diabetes is influenced by both mental health factors.

M. Moore · N. Nickson
Western Michigan University, Homer Stryker M.D. School of Medicine, Kalamazoo, MI, USA

P. V. Maravolo · B. Ergun-Longmire (✉)
Division of Pediatric Endocrinology, Department of Pediatric and Adolescent Medicine, Western Michigan University, Homer Stryker M.D. School of Medicine, Kalamazoo, MI, USA
e-mail: Berrin.Ergun-Longmire@wmed.edu

R. W. Apple et al. (eds.), *Using Integrated Behavioral Health in Pediatric Practice*, https://doi.org/10.1007/978-3-031-85784-3_13

The interplay between medicine and mental health is crucial in managing chronic illnesses like diabetes and obesity [2]. Chronic conditions, as defined by the Centers for Disease Control (CDC), are medical conditions that last for at least one year and impact activities of daily living or require treatment [2]. Chronic conditions are found in 10–30% of youth and often present in childhood or adolescence and are associated with psychological comorbidities such as anxiety, depression, and behavioral disorders, impacting patients throughout their lives. Psychological well-being influences treatment adherence, lifestyle choices, and the ability to cope with the stress of managing a chronic condition [2]. Nonadherence to treatments for chronic conditions results in worse health outcomes [2]. For pediatric endocrinology patients, mental health support is essential to address depression, anxiety, and other conditions that can exacerbate physical symptoms and complicate disease management.

Pediatric endocrinology patients face unique psychological and behavioral challenges related to managing endocrine disorders and coping with chronic diseases. For example, managing diabetes requires consistent blood glucose monitoring, nutrition tracking, insulin administration, and exercise regimen maintenance [3]. These tasks can be particularly difficult for children and adolescents, who may struggle with the daily responsibilities of diabetes management. Social stigma, fear of being different, and the emotional burden of chronic illness can lead to poor treatment adherence, increasing the risk of complications [4]. Adolescents in particular exhibit higher rates of nonadherence and associated psychological issues such as depression and eating disorders, further complicating diabetes management. Diabetes and other chronic endocrine conditions therefore highlight a niche where mental health services are needed.

Soley identifying mental health problems in pediatric endocrinology patients, however, is not enough. Although psychosocial screening tools in pediatric endocrinology clinics can identify psychosocial problems and facilitate referrals to trained mental health providers, barriers persist in the referral process and the actual receipt of mental health services. For instance, a study of pediatric patients at a diabetes clinic found that only 23.7% of patients referred for outpatient mental health care received care [5]. Barriers to care including stigma around mental health, transportation issues, and scheduling difficulties all hinder access to outpatient psychological services [5]. There is therefore both a clear need for mental health services in pediatric patients as well as a gap between the identification of a need for services and the delivery of services.

Further highlighting the importance of addressing the gap in psychological services in pediatric endocrinology is the disproportionate influence of care during childhood and adolescence as compared to adulthood. The importance of providing care during childhood and adolescence is explained by the concept of critical periods (CPs) of development. CPs are particular time periods of elevated brain plasticity when brain development occurs and behavior can be permanently shaped [6]. Childhood and adolescence are critical periods for brain development, during which significant cognitive, emotional, and social changes occur [2]. The developing brain's plasticity during CPs means that experiences can significantly influence behaviors and long-term health outcomes. Children and adolescents are therefore particularly vulnerable to the psychological stressors associated with chronic illness [2].

On top of adolescence being a CP, the nature of adolescence means it is a time of development when health attitudes and behaviors are formed. Adolescence is a period of physical growth and pubertal development, which may be hindered or altered in patients with endocrine disorders. "Off-time" puberty can lead to increased bullying, self-esteem issues, and depression [2]. Adolescence is also a period of psychosocial development where teens seek autonomy, self-identity, and relationships with peers. Teens with chronic health conditions may experience less autonomy due to a reliance on family members for medical treatment and strained relationships with peers due to a feeling of being different [2]. Teens may neglect medical treatment regimens in an effort to fit in with peers, resulting in long-term health consequences. Effective psychological support during this period can promote resilience, improve coping strategies, and enhance overall well-being, which are essential for managing chronic conditions like diabetes [2].

Research has shown the benefit of integrated behavioral health models in treating pediatric endocrinology conditions, with the most extensive data being in the realm of diabetes. Various therapies and counseling provided by mental health professionals including cognitive-behavioral therapy (CBT), family therapy, stress management techniques, and psychoeducation have shown promise in managing endocrine disorders. For type 1 diabetes (T1D), CBT has been proven effective in improving physical and social functioning as well as providing coping skills for youth [2]. CBT helps patients change cognition and behavior in an attempt to reduce negative emotional states that can interfere with disease management [7]. By fostering a more positive outlook and equipping patients with practical coping strategies, CBT can improve both mental health and glycemic control. Motivational interviewing has also shown to be efficacious in treating psychological conditions, which is particularly promising given the minimal cost and time this intervention requires [7]. Motivational interviewing can help adolescents overcome ambivalence about managing their condition through a collaborative relationship between patient and provider that helps evoke a desire for change in patients through a conversation involving open-ended questions, statements of affirmation, and reflective listening. Motivational interviewing for T1D reduces hemoglobin A1c as well as feelings of fear in patients; in the realm of obesity, motivational interviewing is a recommended practice by the American College of Endocrinology [7]. Family therapy is also beneficial, as it addresses the family dynamics that can be strained due to financial challenges, communication problems, and stress associated with managing a chronic condition [7]. Family therapy aims to improve communication, resolve conflicts, and enhance the overall family support system. Integrating these mental health therapies into pediatric endocrinology clinics can provide comprehensive care that addresses both the physical and psychological aspects of diabetes, leading to better health outcomes and quality of life for pediatric patients.

The integration of psychological services into pediatric endocrinology clinics can both address a gap in care for patients with endocrine conditions and overcome barriers to receiving mental health services. Integrated services can improve treatment adherence and ultimately lead to better health outcomes and reduced healthcare costs. Childhood and adolescence represent particularly useful times to implement psychological interventions as they represent critical periods of development when experiences can have permanent impacts on the lives of pediatric patients. By addressing the psychological and behavioral challenges unique to pediatric endocrinology patients, such as treatment adherence and mental health conditions, healthcare providers can improve short- and long-term disease outcomes. This chapter explores the relationship between pediatric endocrinology disorders and mental health conditions, underscoring the importance of psychological services in treating pediatric endocrinology patients. Furthermore, the utilization of integrated behavioral health teams is proposed as a solution to facilitate mental health care for pediatric endocrinology patients. Building from the biopsychosocial model, we advocate for a multidisciplinary approach to pediatric endocrinology care that incorporates psychological services to optimize health outcomes and reduce healthcare costs.

Trends in Psychological Service Usage

Trends in mental health service usage among children and adolescents reveal significant discrepancies between demand for treatment and services received. Approximately half of children with severe mental health conditions receive no treatment, and 63.8% of adolescents with mental health disorders do not receive mental health services [8]. There is also a skew in what conditions tend to be addressed, with pediatric patients being more likely to receive treatment for attention-deficit hyperactivity disorder (ADHD) and less likely to receive treatment for anxiety disorders. Additionally, there is a notable lack of comprehensive national data in the United States regarding the prevalence and treatment of pediatric mental health disorders.

The distribution of entry into mental health services for youth in the United States can be estimated according to the Child and Adolescent Services Assessment (CASA), a survey that assesses the usage of various types of services to treat mental health and behavioral disorders in youth as well as the time point in which the various services are used [9]. These services include services within the sectors of education, specialty medicine, and general medicine. Based on analysis of data from the Child and Adolescent Psychiatric Assessment (CAPA) and the CASA used in the Great Smoky Mountains Study of 1420 children and adolescents, over half of people use some service for mental health treatment in their childhood and adolescent years [9]. The most common entry into mental health care is through services in the education sector. Youth receiving mental health services initially through the education sector tended to have less severe conditions whereas youth initially receiving mental health services in the specialty mental health sector were more likely to have psychiatric diagnoses. Three-quarters of youth received some sort of mental health services in the education sector, indicating the importance of educational services in connecting youth with mental health services, which makes sense as youth have the most access to services in the education sector through attending schools [9]. Interestingly, youth who initially received mental health services through the education sector were less likely to seek mental health treatment from other sectors compared to youth who initially received mental health services outside the education sector, even when controlling for demographic factors and the mental health conditions they received treatment for. This could either positively reflect on the education sector being able to preventatively treat mental health conditions in youth before they progress into more severe problems or highlight issues in the education sector in communicating with services in other sectors to connect youth with more specialized services. Over half of youth were treated by mental health specialists in the mental health sector and a quarter were treated by general medical practitioners in the general medical sector [9].

There has been an increase in mental health care for children and adolescents in pediatric and primary care offices especially. From 1995 to 2010, there was an increase in health care visits for pediatric mental health disorders, particularly in visits outside of the mental health sector with pediatricians not specializing in psychiatry [10]. Mental health disorders encompassed by these visits include behavioral disorders, mood and anxiety disorders, and developmental disorders [10]. This increase in office visits to nonpsychiatrist pediatricians resulted in increased diagnosis and treatment for conditions including ADHD, anxiety and mood disorders, developmental disorders, and psychotic disorders among these physicians. This increase in nonpsychiatrist physicians providing mental health treatment could either be due to a shift in physician roles, a shortage of psychiatrists to refer patients to, or an issue in the referral system for patients whose conditions could benefit from care by mental health specialists [10]. This highlights the importance of connecting pediatricians with mental health professionals to aid in the referral process. In an attempt to remedy barriers in referring pediatric patients to outside mental health services, programs to educate pediatricians or aid in telehealth consultations to nearby mental health centers have been implemented in some states [10].

Traditional methods of psychological service delivery through specialized appointments present challenges for patients related to time constraints and having to juggle attending multiple appointments for different aspects of care. Integrating psychological services into endocrinology appointments presents an attractive alternative with fewer barriers to care. Integrated psychological services allow pediatric endocrinology patients to receive care for both biological and mental health aspects of their conditions. Especially for chronic conditions, where frequent visits to endocrinology clinics are already required, offering integrated services can simplify treatment for patients. Consistent with this, integrated services for diabetes have already proven to be advantageous and cost-effective for pediatric endocrinology clinics [11].

Despite the apparent utility of psychological services to enhance pediatric endocrinology treatments, however, integrated care is still not universally implemented across clinics. One such challenge that must be addressed to allow for more psychological services is the shortage of psychiatrists and pediatric mental health providers. There has been a shortage in child psychiatrists in the USA for decades and despite an approximately 21% increase in the number of child psychiatrists from 2007 to 2016 in the United States, there remains a shortage [12]. Additionally, counties with lower income, lower post-secondary education, and counties outside of metropolitan areas face a disproportionate lack in child psychiatrists [12]. In order to offer psychological services more widely, there must be efforts to increase the number of providers or ability to provide psychological services through other means.

Diabetes

Diabetes is a chronic condition caused by problems in the production or response to the insulin hormone, resulting in hyperglycemia and dysfunction of multiple organ systems [13]. Diabetes can be classified as type 1 diabetes (T1D), an autoimmune condition targeting pancreatic beta cells and preventing insulin production, or type 2 diabetes (T2D), where there is a relative insulin deficiency, or cells become resistant to insulin. T1D is particularly applicable to pediatric endocrinology as it typically presents in childhood and adolescence [13]. In the United States, type 1 diabetes is the second most common chronic illness among pediatric adolescents, accounting for $133.7 billion annually in medical costs [14]. From 2002 to 2018, the incidence of type 1 diabetes in children and adolescents under 20 years old increased, particularly among Non-Hispanic Asian or Pacific Islanders, with the highest incidence observed in Non-Hispanic White children [15].

Hemoglobin A1C (HbA1c) measurements are used to track diabetes management, as they represent blood glucose levels over an 8–12-week period and can better capture glycemic control than acute measurements of blood glucose; regular HbA1c measurements can be used to guide diabetes treatment decisions [3]. The American Diabetes Association (ADA) and the International Society for Pediatric and Adolescent Diabetes (ISPAD) have published guidelines for HbA1c targets that T1D treatments should aim to achieve [16]. The ISPAD target HbA1c is <7.5% for all children and adolescents and the ADA target HbA1c ranges from <8.5% for children 1–6 years old, <8.0% for children 6–13 years old, and <7.5% for children and adolescents 13–20 years old. There are also established treatment guidelines for aiming to have children below the 90th percentile in blood pressure, under the 85th percentile in body mass index (BMI), and fasting LDL <100 mg/dL. Two-thirds of children and adolescents with T1D do not meet these guideline values for HbA1c and around 20–40% of children and adolescents did not meet guideline values for blood pressure, BMI, and other laboratory measurements. This gap in the goal treatment outcomes for children with T1D and the measured values indicates that there is room for improvement in pediatric endocrinology management of T1D in children and adolescents [16].

The goal of diabetes treatment practices is to limit the complications of diabetes as much as possible [3]. This is generally achieved by targeting improved glycemic control, which has been shown by the Diabetes Control and Complications Trial (DCCT) to decrease microvascular complications of diabetes [3]. Specifically, better glycemic control slowed the progression of diabetic retinopathy, nephropathy, and neuropathy [3].

Patients with diabetes have higher rates of various mood and mental health disorders and approximately 32% of youth with T1D have concomitant anxiety [17]. As diabetes is a chronic condition, patients must assume responsibility for managing their diabetes day-to-day and follow complicated treatment regimens including subcutaneous insulin administration, tracking dietary intake, and frequent blood glucose monitoring [3]. Poor adherence to diabetes treatments is a major preventable factor contributing to increased healthcare costs, underscoring the need for enhanced support in managing the disease. The incidence of psychiatric conditions, such as depression and eating disorders, is notably higher in children with T1D, impacting glycemic control and overall health outcomes [17]. Psychological services are therefore important to provide along with the treatment in children with endocrine disorders like diabetes.

Incorporating psychological services in pediatric endocrinology clinics can improve outcomes and reduce healthcare costs for pediatric patients with T1D [11]. Psychological treatments, when integrated with endocrinology services, enhance treatment adherence, leading to better health outcomes and reducing the potential future healthcare costs associated with the long-term effects of poor treatment compliance [11].

Nonadherence to diabetes treatment is particularly high among adolescents when compared to patients in other age groups [4]. Teens with diabetes face a number of barriers to adherence with diabetes treatment regiments. Some teens worry that their friends will respond negatively to their diabetes and social anxiety may cause adolescents to have worse treatment adherence [4]. Teens with T1D are almost twice as likely as teens without diabetes to have depression, which is associated with poor glycemic control and higher HbA1c which are related to less blood glucose monitoring [4].

A cross-sectional case-control study of 356 adolescent girls with T1D and 1098 girls without diabetes found the incidence of eating disorders as high as 10% in adolescent girls with T1D, compared to just 4% in girls without diabetes [18]. Eating disorders also present a significant problem in teens for T1D management, as they are associated with worse glycemic control in adolescents with T1D [19, 20]. Eating disorders are particularly difficult to detect in patients with diabetes as symptoms of eating disorders such as intense monitoring of food intake overlaps with normal diabetes management strategies. Eating disorders can cause teens to exhibit dangerous behaviors such as restricting insulin to lose weight, which increases the risk for diabetes complications as well as mortality [19]. Traditional screening tools for eating disorders are insufficient in detecting eating disorders in adolescents with diabetes as significant focus on food intake is important for diabetes management and traditional tools do not account for insulin restriction as a means of disordered weight management.

In a randomized control trial of adolescents aged 14–17 years in diabetes clinics across South Wales, motivational interviewing techniques were found to significantly lower HbA1c levels in adolescents compared to support visits alone when measured at 12 and 24 months following treatment [21]. Additionally motivational interviewing techniques were associated with higher life satisfaction scores, improved psychosocial functioning, and less anxiety. This shows the potential long-term benefits in glycemic control as well as psychosocial functioning provided by motivational interviewing in teens with T1D and support the adoption of motivational interviewing practices in routine care [21].

Typically, adolescence is a period marked by worse insulin control when compared to childhood and adulthood, which can result in more downstream complications of diabetes. One key factor of this decreased glycemic control is less self-care focus in this age group, leading to less optimal insulin administration practices [3]. Psychological services can help lessen glycemic control challenges and give adolescents tools to improve mental health and, by extension, treatment adherence. Children and adolescents with diabetes have medical appointments almost every three months and frequent clinic visits provide an access point where mental health providers can interact with pediatric patients and provide psychological services [3].

Due to the significant impact of psychosocial factors in influencing glycemic control in children and adolescents, psychological care should be incorporated in the care of children with T1D. The International Society for Pediatric and Adolescent Diabetes (ISPAD) published guidelines for diabetes care and directly recommended that T1D should be managed by an interdisciplinary team including social workers and psychologists in acknowledgement of the major role psychosocial factors have in influencing diabetes management [20].

Motivational interviewing and by extension, other psychosocial interventions may improve outcomes in adolescents with diabetes. Counseling methods such as motivational interviewing have been found to improve glycemic control and quality of life in adolescents with diabetes [21]. Glycemic control is the strongest modifiable factor in the risk of developing diabetes complications in children [22]. Specifically, improved glycemic control decreases the risk and slows the progression of downstream diabetes complications such as microvascular disease [21]. Additionally, better glycemic control is associated with fewer acute complications of T1D in children such as diabetic ketoacidosis and severe hypoglycemia. Motivational interviewing may exert its beneficial psychosocial and physiological effects by helping to shift children from an external locus of control to an internal locus of control where they believe they have the ability to enact changes that will improve their glycemic control [21]. The proposed mechanism behind the efficacy of motivational interviewing in pediatrics with diabetes is that is induces a state of cognitive dissonance in which patients feel a discrepancy between their aspirations and their behaviors that leads to beneficial behavioral changes to help reduce the dissonance [21]. This and other psychological interventions can improve outcomes in pediatric patients with diabetes.

Endocrine Disorders

Congenital Adrenal Hyperplasia

Disorders of sex development (DSDs) are a group of conditions in which external genitalia are discordant with biological gender as a result of genetic mutations, hormone insufficiencies, or hormone excess. Congenital adrenal hyperplasia (CAH) is a collection of genetic disorders affecting the adrenal gland. The adrenal gland produces several types of hormones, mineralocorticoids (aldosterone), glucocorticoids (cortisol), and androgens. The devastating consequences of CAH arise from severe forms of the condition causing inability to produce adequate levels of cortisol and aldosterone and overproduction of androgens leading to ambiguous genitalia and/or virilization.

The survival rate of children born with CAH has increased significantly with the introduction of life-saving hormone replacement in the 1950s and with better newborn screening [23]. However, increases in survival rates have also increased disease burden related to the long-term complications of treatment and disease, affecting growth and development, metabolic and cardiovascular health, and fertility [24]. Furthermore, girls born with virilization of the external genitalia may have additional medical and psychosocial burdens centered on genital restoration surgery or genitoplasty.

Genitoplasty, which includes clitoroplasty and vaginoplasty, optimizes urological function, future sexual function, and establishes congruency of the exterior genitalia with the patient's designated gender. Genitoplasty dates to Classic Roman times (25 BCE-50 CE) when Anulus Cornelius Celsus documented the first congenital vaginal abnormality undergoing surgical treatment for imperforate hymen or transverse vaginal septum [25]. In 1934, Dr. Hugh Hampton Young performed feminizing genitoplasty in a 16-year-old female with CAH [26]. Since Roman times and now in the modern eras, genitoplasty techniques have evolved and continue to be a common approach to alter the appearance of the external genitalia in individuals with DSDs. The current standard of practice for genital reconstruction is to perform these surgeries at an early age rather than delaying until adolescence. The pressures of society centered around body image and gender identity fuel the current practice as a means of surgical and psychosocial treatment for gender rearing [27]. However, the timing of when these surgeries should occur, as well as many other ethical and psychosocial concerns, has been met with much controversy, bias, and lack of consensus adding to the broad challenges and outcomes for patients [27, 28].

Despite the long history of genitoplasty, there are few studies that have examined the long-term outcomes of feminizing procedures, particularly psychosocial outcomes [27]. A review article evaluating feminizing genitoplasty procedures, surgical outcomes, and complications highlights the variability in patient outcomes including patient satisfaction and medical complications that increase risk for continued dysfunction, revision surgeries or procedures, and lower quality of life [26]. Conversely, Gupta et al. analyzed long term outcomes of 163 patients who underwent feminizing genitoplasty and hormone replacement which found the majority of patients evaluated had good outcomes [27]. The authors concluded that the degree of social support, psychosocial adaptation, and coping were important factors that likely contributed to high quality of life despite the impairments associated with CAH [27]. This study, as well as the perceived and anticipated psychosocial barriers for patients born with virilizing conditions, highlights the importance of IBH as a part of routine care in CAH clinics.

Hypopituitarism

The pituitary gland—anatomically split into its anterior and posterior glands—is responsible for the production of numerous hormones, including follicle-stimulating hormone (FSH), luteinizing hormone (LH), adrenocorticotrophic hormone (ACTH), thyroid-stimulating hormone (TSH), growth hormone (GH), prolactin, oxytocin, and antidiuretic hormone. [29] Hypopituitarism is defined as a partial or complete deficiency of the production or release of one, many, or all of these hormones and has numerous etiologies. Hormones released by the pituitary gland are essential for such functions as growth, metabolism, puberty, and stress response. Depending on which hormones are impacted and the extent of pathology, signs of hypopituitarism can vary widely from subtle features to red flag symptoms [30]. Common presenting symptoms are short stature due to GH deficiency; delayed or absent pubertal development with LH and FSH deficiencies; and fatigue, hypotension, or adrenal crisis in patients with ACTH deficiency. Although hypopituitarism can feature more frequently seen sets of symptoms, there is typically no standardized presentation for this pathology.

Patients with hypopituitarism may also have concomitant anxiety and depression [31]. Other neuropsychological features of hypopituitarism can include mood variability and increased perception of pain [32]. Hypopituitarism can also feature disruption of stage II of sleep and therefore negatively impact a patient's sleep efficiency index [33]. Collectively, the neuropsychological stigmata of hypopituitarism can greatly impact a patient's quality of life, even after receiving appropriate treatment. While the treatment for hypopituitarism centers around replacement of relevant hormonal deficiencies, long-standing effects of the pituitary disease process can remain even after hormones are adequately replaced.

One explanation for the neuropsychological features of hypopituitarism is offered from the occurrence of cortisol disruption. Physiologically, cortisol has wide-reaching systemic roles; not only is it an important modulator of sleep-wake cycles, but it is also an important mediator in mood and mental health disorders; abnormalities of the hypothalamic-pituitary-adrenal (HPA) axis—mediated by ACTH released from the anterior pituitary gland—are often associated with neuropsychological abnormalities. Accordingly, one theoretical explanation for the heightened anxiety and increased depression in patients with hypopituitarism is hypercortisolemia resulting from HPA axis dysfunction [33]. While not entirely clear yet, prolonged hypercortisolemia may have an impact on neurogenesis through decreased brain-derived neurotrophic factor (BDNF), a hormone that plays a valuable role in neuronal growth and survival as well as synaptic plasticity [34]. Beyond neurogenesis, decreased function of the pituitary gland in animal models that leads to decreased secretion of hormones negatively impacts critical functions like growth, reproduction, and immunity [34, 35]. More research is required to map these relationships in humans and better understand the role they play in hypopituitarism.

Hypopituitarism featuring anxiety, depression, and other mental health disorders negatively impacts the quality of patients' lives. Even when hormonal axis abnormalities are appropriately corrected, patients with chronic illnesses, such as hypopituitarism, that view their disease process as playing a major role in their life are more likely to experience negative quality of life [32]. Patients with chronic conditions such as hypopituitarism require frequent follow-up with endocrine specialists for the management of long-term hormone replacement therapy; these appointments provide an excellent opportunity for integrated behavioral health where mental health providers can check in with patients and help patients to re-frame their understanding of their chronic illness and the role it plays in their lives, as well as discussing effective strategies for the management of symptoms of anxiety and depression.

Endocrine Cancer

Malignancies involving the endocrine glands, although rare in children and adolescents, can profoundly affect mental health and quality of life. However, the patient's perspective on their cancer diagnosis once in the remission phase, particularly whether they perceive themselves to be a victim or a survivor, greatly impacts their quality of life [36]. It can be difficult to fully understand the role of a cancer diagnosis on a patient's life as each patient's situation is completely different. However, especially in the acute phase following a diagnosis, maladaptive coping, reduced social engagement, and missed educational opportunities may collectively contribute to an increased risk of depression, anxiety, and suicidal ideation [37]. Receiving a cancer diagnosis can often be a tremendous stressor for patients, who require effective stress management to properly regulate their emotions.

Regardless of the patient's outlook on cancer diagnosis, engagement with mental health providers for appropriate treatment is generally supported as an effective intervention for this population [38]. The inclusion of mental health providers in endocrine practices in patients with a current or former cancer diagnosis can provide ample opportunity for ongoing discussion about topics such as stress management. Mental health providers can play an important role in empowering patients with the tools necessary to navigate the complicated feelings surrounding their disease process and prognosis.

Syndromes: Turner, Prader Willi, and Klinefelter

There are numerous chronic endocrine conditions that result from genetic abnormalities, including Turner syndrome, Prader-Willi syndrome, and Klinefelter syndrome. While this is not an extensive list of genetic endocrine conditions featuring concomitant mental health disorders, they are seen in the endocrine practice sufficiently enough to warrant involvement of a mental health provider for integrated behavioral health.

Turner syndrome is the most common sex chromosome abnormality (genotype XO) occurring solely in females, described with an incidence rate of 1/2500 [39]. Common features of Turner syndrome include short stature, primary amenorrhea, cardiovascular malformation, renal abnormalities, and endocrine pathology such as insulin resistance [40]. The neuropsychological stigmata of Turner syndrome can include alterations in visual-spatial, executive, and motor functioning and math skills, among others [41]. Especially in settings such as classrooms, where patients with Turner syndrome would be increasingly assessed by peers, deficits in the aforementioned cognitive functions could negatively impact self-perception and self-esteem, which might offer an explanation for the heightened anxiety and increased depression seen in patients with Turner syndrome. Increased anxiety seen in this condition may also manifest with disruptions of sleep, as insomnia can often serve as an early sign of anxiety [42].

Klinefelter syndrome is a sex chromosome disorder featuring a supernumerary X chromosome paired with a Y chromosome (genotype XXY, XXXY, XXXXY, etc.) Patients with Klinefelter syndrome typically have tall stature, small testes, gynecomastia, broad hips, and hypogonadism [43]. In addition to the aforementioned traditional presentation, Klinefelter syndrome can also feature neuropsychiatric stigmata; patients with Klinefelter syndrome are three times as likely to be hospitalized with a psychiatric disorder [44]. Similar to other chronic endocrine conditions, the most common comorbid mental health conditions associated with Klinefelter syndrome are anxiety and depression [45]. One reason that could help explain this relationship is that patients with Klinefelter syndrome may display low self-esteem, poor social support, and increased psychological stress as a result of their condition. On an anatomical level, patients with Klinefelter syndrome appear to have a decrease in total brain volume (including decreased gray and white matter volume), potentially explaining the mild impairment in neuropsychological function [46–48]. Patients with Klinefelter syndrome also have an increased incidence of conduct disorder and display deficits with attention and impulse control [49]. Although Klinefelter syndrome is typically diagnosed after puberty once endocrine features of the condition become more apparent, there are fewer reported mental health comorbidities when the condition is diagnosed and treated before the age of 10 [50].

Prader-Willi syndrome (PWS) is a genetic condition arising from errors in the imprinting of chromosome 15 typically resulting in maternal disomy. In general, PWS is characterized by infantile hypotonia, hyperphagia with subsequent obesity, short stature, developmental delay, and concomitant behavioral health pathologies

[51]. Commonly featuring neuropsychiatric manifestations such as anxiety, temper outbursts, rigid thinking, and obsessive-compulsive tendencies, PWS can make it difficult to relate to others and present social difficulties, negatively impacting mental health and quality of life [52]. These symptoms may be present early in life, with temper outbursts commonly developing in childhood and anxiety frequently starting around preschool to school age, especially in situations related to routines, food planning, and items of special interest [52, 53]. The impact of these neuropsychiatric features can be tremendous and especially prominent as children reach the young adult stage; the lifetime prevalence of suicidal ideation and suicide attempts is greater in patients with PWS than in the general population [54].

While Turner syndrome, Klinefelter syndrome, and PWS all share varying neuropsychological stigmata that negatively impact patients' mental health and quality of life, these conditions are often diagnosed in childhood or early adolescence and therefore have the potential to be positively impacted by early intervention from a mental health provider. Since the stigmata of these conditions can contribute to difficulties in social situations such as in the classroom or on the playground, impacts on self-esteem and experienced psychological stress can be more effectively managed by the inclusion of mental health providers into regular endocrine specialist visits; these stressors are often dynamic as children progress through various life experiences and multiple integrated behavioral health visits over time will help children and adolescents with these conditions more effectively feel more regulated within their social environments. Integrated behavioral health can also help manage parental expectations, as one study found a discordance between the parent-assessed and child-reported levels of anxiety [55]. While this discordance could be the result of a child's inability to recognize their own anxiety, it may also represent unaddressed parental concerns about their child's day-to-day life. Endocrine practices that are able to incorporate integrated behavioral health can not only help children recognize and manage comorbid mental health conditions like anxiety but can also work with parents on approaches to help their child manage these conditions when present.

Obesity

Obesity is an increasing public health concern among children and adolescents. An estimated one in five children in the Unites States has obesity [56]. Carrying extra weight in childhood is associated with higher rates of anxiety, depression, and adjustment disorders, a trend that is most commonly apparent in adolescents [57]. Mental health comorbidities associated with childhood obesity could be the result of decreased self-esteem and strained relations with peers in the setting of increased weight and stigma [58]. Alternatively, mental health conditions could also precede a child developing an increased BMI and predispose a child to developing obesity through maladaptive coping mechanisms, such as excessive food consumption [59].

Adverse childhood experiences (ACEs), defined as physical, psychological, or sexual abuse; neglect; family members' substance abuse; mental illness; criminal behavior; intimate partner violence; and parental divorce/separation/death, appear to increase the risk of childhood obesity, potentially through their interference with psychosocial and neuroendocrine development [59, 60]. Although it is perhaps intuitive that these experiences early in development can negatively alter a child's life trajectory to some degree, it is difficult to understand the exact role that ACEs play in the development of obesity because ACEs vary widely from person to person, and the impact cannot be assessed as one that is standardized. Despite this interpersonal variation, ACEs offer a connection between childhood obesity and mental health comorbidities, as these negative lived experiences in the formative years can contribute to higher rates of depression in those affected [57].

Focusing on increasing physical activity and limiting screen time are methods for addressing and preventing obesity in childhood, and are also associated with an improvement in mental health [58]. Unfortunately, only a fraction of children meet the recommendations for at least 60 minutes of physical activity a day and limit screen time to less than two hours daily, presenting an opportunity for improvement when it comes to counseling children and adolescents on strategies to prevent obesity. ACEs are widely prevalent and occur in nearly 50% of all children [61, 62]. Approaching childhood obesity from a trauma-informed perspective can help to ensure that patient needs are adequately met to address all appropriate root causes of pathology; in these cases, inclusion of mental health providers in regular endocrine specialist appointments can help center this trauma-informed approach to improve effective management of childhood obesity. Finally, integrated behavioral health creates an opportunity to use up-to-date age-appropriate screening for depression and anxiety, with the necessary follow-up to ensure that children with obesity have comorbid mental health conditions, if present, adequately managed.

Polycystic Ovary Syndrome

Polycystic ovarian syndrome (PCOS) is a relatively common condition that frequently arises during early puberty and is characterized by hyperandrogenism, insulin resistance, and oligomenorrhea [63]. The diagnosis is typically made using the 2003 Rotterdam criteria, which requires two of the following three features to be identified: [1] oligo-ovulation or anovulation, [2] hyperandrogenism, and/or [3] polycystic ovaries [64]. PCOS is estimated to affect 5–20% of women worldwide [65]. Features commonly associated with PCOS, such as acne, hirsutism, and obesity, can play a role in negatively impact mental health and contribute to the development of conditions, such as depression and anxiety [66–68]. While the pathophysiology of PCOS does not necessarily directly cause mental health comorbidities associated with the condition, the increased risk of depression may be associated with obesity and negatively impacted self-perception, often caused by increased weight [69]. While not relevant to the majority of pediatric patients,

patients with PCOS who begin to consider family planning early in the third decade of life may also begin to experience negative impacts on mental health when infertility frequently seen in the condition becomes more relevant to the patient's lived experience [69].

Integrated behavioral health can play an important role in the long-term management of PCOS. Currently, for every three clinical practice guidelines developed for the management of PCOS, only two will recommend inclusion of mental healthcare, despite the frequent occurrence of mental health comorbidities for these patients [70]. This suggests that there is an opportunity to improve the recognition of mental health conditions in patients with PCOS and to work with them to receive the treatment they deserve. Mental health providers included within an integrated behavioral health clinic can frequently discuss with patients with PCOS the importance of finding a strong support network that can help them manage mental health comorbidities [71].

Precocious Puberty

Puberty is a developmental milestone characterized by changes in secondary sexual characteristics that have social and emotional effects on children [72]. As physical appearance changes, children and adolescents must adapt to changing social norms and expectations, which may involve reevaluating their identity [73]. Changes in the timing of pubertal development can increase the risk of emotional and behavioral issues during adolescence [73]. Precocious puberty is a condition that causes earlier pubertal maturation, either due to GnRH acting in the normal hypothalamus-pituitary-gonadal axis (central precocious puberty) or direct overproduction of sex steroids (peripheral precocious puberty) [74]. Precocious puberty results in physical changes including premature hair growth in pubic and axillary areas, rapid growth in height, changes in subcutaneous fat distribution, breast development in females, testicular growth in males, acne, and body odor [74].

Treatment for central precocious puberty generally includes GnRH agonists such as leuprolide acetate every four weeks, which overrides pulsatile GnRH release to suppress the hypothalamic-pituitary-gonadal axis and may cause side effects such as muscle pain and hot flashes [74]. Treatment for peripheral precocious puberty is dependent on the underlying cause and may include surgical resection of a tumor, glucocorticoid medications for Congenital Adrenal Hyperplasia, or aromatase inhibitors like anastrozole for McCune-Albright syndrome. [74]

The onset of menses prior to 11 years of age has been associated with higher rates of conduct disorders, with a higher association with psychosocial causes than genetic causes, according to a cohort study of 708 females [75]. Females who undergo early puberty also tend to drink alcohol and use tobacco more often and earlier than their peers, as well as participate in sexual activities at an earlier age [75].

Explanations for these behavioral differences in females with precocious puberty include that these females do not have adequate coping and social skills to deal with their pubertal changes and thus engage in risky behaviors or that these females tend to associate with older peers and thus are influenced by their peer groups to partake in risky behaviors earlier [75]. Girls with early physical maturation and menses may have difficulty maintaining friendships with their peers to feel emotionally distanced, and older individuals may treat early developing females as more mature, placing girls in situations they may not be emotionally and cognitively prepared for [73].

Early menarche has been linked to symptoms of depression in sixth-grade girls [76]. This was attributed to psychosocial factors rather than menarche itself, as seventh-grade girls undergoing menarche did not experience similarly high rates of depressive symptoms [76]. Females with early menarche are more likely to experience depressive affect, attempt suicide, and have a major depressive disorder [73].

There is a critical need for clinicians to monitor pubertal development in girls, providing an opportunity to address early issues and prevent future psychological problems [77]. Given the increased vulnerability of girls experiencing precocious puberty, psychiatric evaluation and follow-up by mental health professionals are essential [77]. Implementing a multidisciplinary team approach in which pediatric endocrinologists collaborate closely with psychiatrists can significantly improve outcomes. This partnership ensures that girls with early onset puberty receive the most appropriate and effective therapeutic interventions [77].

Hypothyroidism and Hyperthyroidism

Thyroid disorders are conditions characterized by the thyroid gland, either underproducing (hypothyroidism) or overproducing (hyperthyroidism) thyroid hormones [78]. Thyroid hormones influence development of the nervous system including the differentiation patterns, myelination, and connection of neurons. Thyroid hormone production is regulated by the release of thyrotropin-releasing hormone (TRH) in the hypothalamus, which controls the release of thyroid-stimulating hormone (TSH) from the anterior pituitary gland [78]. TSH then stimulates the thyroid to produce thyroid hormones from tyrosine. The main thyroid hormone produced is thyroxine (T4), although triiodothyronine (T3) is also produced or can be formed in peripheral tissue from iodothyronine deiodinase enzymes removing iodine atom from T4. T3 and T4 then travel through the bloodstream mainly bound to serum proteins to reach cells and stimulate cells to increase metabolic rate, and also play a role in a negative feedback loop to inhibit TSH release [78].

Congenital hypothyroidism (CH) historically occurs in 1 in 3–4000 live births, although more recent estimations of CH incidence in the United States approach 1 in 2000, partially due to increased screening rates and, thus, higher detection of disease. CH incidence is particularly high in Asian and Hispanic infants, twins, and preterm births [78]. Congenital hypothyroidism can be caused by defects in thyroid gland development or thyroid hormone production (primary CH), or by defects in pituitary gland function (secondary CH) [79]. Defects in thyroid development are mainly sporadic and permanent [78]. Other etiologies of hypothyroidism may also be reversible, such as maternal autoimmune antibodies or maternal medications, including methimazole or propylthiouracil. Additionally, excess iodine from iodine antiseptics or radiocontrast agents or iodine deficiency can cause hypothyroidism [78]. CH is treated with lifelong synthetic thyroxine [79].

In addition to congenital thyroid disorders, there are acquired thyroid disorders seen in pediatric patients including Hashimoto's thyroiditis causing hypothyroidism [80]. These disorders are caused by the pathological production of anti-thyroid antibodies, which alter the production of thyroid hormones. Autoimmune thyroid disorders tend to occur during puberty and are most commonly observed in females [80].

Hypothyroidism can present with numerous symptoms including slowed growth particularly in limbs, delayed puberty, thin hair, swollen face, goiter, hoarse speech, fatigue, and constipation [79]. Hypothyroidism is also associated with intellectual disabilities, which can increase the risk of mental health disorders in children. This link between intellectual disability and mental health conditions may be explained by the lower cognitive reserve of patients with CH. Cognitive reserve theory postulates that higher educational attainment and cognitively stimulating activities or jobs alter the brain in such a way that it is more resistant to subsequent disease or degeneration, and by extension, would be more resistant to the development of mental disorders [81].

Hyperthyroidism is characterized by high T3 and T4, measured as the concentration of free unbound T3 and T4 in the serum [82]. Graves' disease (GD) is the most common cause of hyperthyroidism in pediatric patients. GD is more common in females and has a prevalence of 1 in 10,000 in the United States, although rare in children. It is caused by the production of antibodies that bind to and stimulate the TSH receptor in thyroid follicular cells [82]. Pediatric GD can be treated with at least three years of antithyroid drugs (carbimazole or methimazole), thyroidectomy, or radioiodine [82].

Hyperthyroidism can present with weight loss and increased appetite, goiter, tachycardia, moodiness, anxiety, exercise intolerance, hyperreflexia, exophthalmos, and tremor [82]. GD is generally more severe in pediatric patients than in adult patients, and is associated with more side effects from antithyroid medications [83]. Patients with GD who receive curative surgery or radioiodine treatment still require long-term levothyroxine administration. In adults, levothyroxine replacement therapy is associated with decreased psychological well-being even when thyroid hormone levels are restored to normal [83].

GD is associated with intellectual disability and low IQ levels. A 2020 survey of young patients aged 8–30 years with GD found that GD is associated with lower psychosocial well-being perceived by GD patients in the school and work context, which may be partially explained by lower academic achievement [83]. Even following definitive surgical treatment for GD, pediatric patients report feeling not recovered from the disease, potentially related to the requirement to regularly still receive medical care for blood monitoring post-surgery [83].

Barriers to Implementing Integrated Services

Although psychological services have been shown to be vital for diabetes management in pediatrics, there are numerous challenges that make it difficult to receive psychological services [11]. One major barrier is the lack of time and logistical issues with attending appointments for specialized psychiatric care. Integrating psychological services into pediatric endocrinology clinics can bridge this gap by streamlining communication between endocrinologists and mental health professionals. This would also lessen the burden faced by pediatric patients and their caregivers in finding care, as wholistic care could be provided in the same office and additional appointments could be cut down on [11].

Benefits of Integrated Behavioral Health

Integrated care is being explored as a promising plan for its benefits in improving patient outcomes, offering one-stop shopping, decreasing stigma, and decreasing overall health care costs. Integrated care is helpful in reducing stigma, because it endorses the message that health is multifaceted and cannot be separated into physical and psychological health conditions. This unified approach to addressing health ensures that importance is placed on all the aspects of health.

The integration of trained mental health professionals into pediatric endocrinology clinics can decrease healthcare costs and improve outcomes in children and adolescents receiving treatment at endocrinology clinics. This can be observed in pediatric patients with a range of endocrinological disorders, including diabetes, obesity, various endocrine syndromes, and thyroid disorders. These endocrine disorders are associated with particular mental health conditions, including anxiety, depression, decreased self-esteem, and behavioral disorders. The treatment of these mental health conditions, whether caused by or only associated with endocrine disorders, can improve treatment outcomes for endocrinology disorders. Therefore, it is important to recognize mental health conditions and provide psychological services to help pediatric endocrinology patients.

There is also a cost-benefit to integrated behavioral health in endocrinology clinics, with reduced medical expenditure associated with children who receive psychological services. Patients who received care at the endocrinology clinic that included a meeting with a psychologist were found to have 0.16% lower HbA1c levels than patients who did not meet with a psychologist [11]. This decrease in HbA1c levels results in fewer complications and, thus, decreases future healthcare costs. Specifically, based on findings from adult patients with diabetes, the savings from improving glycemic control are $1000 per 1% decrease in HbA1c [11]. Weighting the cost of integrating psychological services into endocrinology clinics with the savings from increasing glycemic control in patients who receive psychological services, the cost analysis supports the implementation of integrated endocrinology clinics [11].

Conclusion

Integrated Behavioral Health in Pediatric Endocrinology Clinics

Advancements in diagnosis, management, and treatment of once life-threatening conditions have dramatically increased the number of children now living with a chronic medical condition [84, 85]. According to the Centers for Disease Control and Prevention (CDC), more than 40% of US children and adolescents have at least one chronic medical condition, and this number is expected to increase [86, 87]. The stress of a new diagnosis and the demand for chronic medical care increase the risk of mental and behavioral issues [17, 88]. Youth with chronic endocrine medical conditions are not immune to the risk of developing psychological morbidities such as depression and anxiety. It is widely recognized that mental health issues are an independent predictor of poor health outcomes, increasing poor self-efficacy and self-management, and poor adherence to medical care and treatment. In the past decade and a half, there has been an increased focus on mental health issues owing to their impact on the overall well-being of children and adolescents. The CDC estimates that 13–20% of US children and adolescents aged 18 years or younger have some form of mental health disorder [89]. The rise in mental health concerns has demanded more urgency to address mental health issues [90]. In 2009, and reaffirmed in 2019, the American Academy of Pediatrics, (AAP) published a policy statement that proposed competencies to improve knowledge, skills, and access to mental health care at all levels and across all platforms including advocacy, legislature, and insurance coverage [91, 92]. Similarly, the AACAP initially published a guide for collaborative mental health partnerships in 2010, with an update published in 2023 [93, 94]. More specifically, the International Society for Pediatric and Adolescent Diabetes recommends a multidisciplinary approach to provide preventative and interventional care to improve coping skills and self-management to patients with diabetes [17].

Integrating behavioral health (IBH) services as part of initial and routine follow up visits can provide timely screening and intervention to reduce psychosocial issues that may impact the patient and family's ability to accept a new diagnosis, and to adapt and cope with demands of chronic medical care. Additionally, integrating behavioral health evaluation as part of routine follow-up visits reduces barriers, such as access to care and stigma, normalizing mental and behavioral health screenings, and interventions as part of the patient's chronic care [95]. In an ideal setting, integrated behavioral health providers would be onsite during diabetes and endocrine clinics and fully integrated as part of the multidisciplinary team. The role of mental health professionals in multidisciplinary teams, particularly diabetes clinics, is well established. Their expertise in child development and family dynamics allows for intervention and preventative strategies, thus making them an invaluable part of the multidisciplinary team [87, 96].

Integrating behavioral health within the endocrine clinic requires thoughtful planning and support to ensure that the integration approach meets the needs of the multidisciplinary team and patient population. This begins with a thorough assessment of care providers and team readiness, how the clinic is currently handling the mental health needs of their patients, and its capacity to address mental health needs, including the comfort level of providers to discuss mental health issues with their patients and existing relationships with mental or behavioral health providers. Additionally, addressing changes in policy or protocol, infrastructure, charting, and reimbursement are also important areas to consider [94, 97]. Given the variability of resources available to many clinics and the shortage of mental and behavioral health providers, endocrine clinics may use a combination of approaches to integrate IBH. Integrated approaches include consultation/coordinated care, on-site services, and integrated services.

Consultation or coordinated care has the benefit of utilizing resources that may not be available within the geographic proximity of patients and clinics. Utilizing technology such as telemedicine and "curbside" consultation between IBH and endocrine providers can provide supportive services to meet the immediate and timely psychosocial needs of patients that otherwise may encounter barriers related to access to care [93]. In addition, consultation/coordinated care can also provide benefits for person evaluation. Despite the advantages of this approach, consultation/coordinated care may lead to gaps in care and increase barriers to care owing to technology, travel, work schedules, or insurance coverage [87, 93]. Consultation/coordinated care may also decrease opportunities for timely discussion between the subspecialist and the IBH provider, which may affect the most effective approach to patient care and disease management [93].

Mental and behavioral health services located in the same location, but not within shared space of the endocrine clinic, of the endocrine clinic provided in the same location, provide a proximity of care that is lacking with consultation or coordinated services. This approach may reduce wait times to receive IBH services, reduce access to care barriers, and increase the likelihood that patients and families will follow through with evaluation [93]. Additionally, this approach facilitates more frequent "warm hand offs" between endocrine and IBH providers. Despite the advantages to this approach, limited availability of IBH providers may not reduce wait time or may prevent patients to be seen same day, does not guarantee collaboration, and lack of insurance reimbursement may prohibit patients from receiving timely IBH services [93, 97].

Integrated or collaborative mental and behavioral health services, as part of a multidisciplinary team, is the most comprehensive approach, allowing for a full continuum of IBH services. In this approach, collaborative care allows for formalized and standardized evaluation and assessment, multidisciplinary care conferences, partnering in care management, and care coordination [87, 93, 97]. Additionally, IBH providers can support providers and staff by providing cross-training in mental and behavioral issues in alignment with AAP and AACAP statements to improve mental health care. Similar to the former options, integrated or collaborative care may face challenges related to financial sustainability and reimbursement.

Children and adolescents with chronic medical conditions often experience mental and behavioral challenges, starting with diagnosis and extending well beyond the transition to adulthood. Providing timely mental and behavioral assessments, evaluations, and interventions plays a crucial role in the patient's and family's ability to adapt and cope with the demands of complex, chronic medical care. The AAP and AACP have published position statements recommending and urging the need to improve access to mental health care, training, education, and reimbursement. Integrating behavioral health into subspecialty clinics, particularly endocrine clinics, not only answers this urgency but also ensures that mental and behavioral health concerns are addressed as part of the chronic medical condition, providing a holistic and comprehensive approach to improve patient outcomes.

Key Points

- Integrated behavioral services can be cost effective in pediatric endocrinology clinics.
- Psychological services can help pediatric patients to improve their adherence to treatment regimens for endocrine disorders.
- Psychological services improve outcomes in pediatric patients with endocrine conditions including, but not limited to, diabetes, congenital adrenal hyperplasia, hypopituitarism, cancer, obesity, endocrine syndromes, precocious puberty, and thyroid disorders.

References

1. Førde S, Herner LB, Helland IB, Diseth TH. The biopsychosocial model in paediatric clinical practice – an interdisciplinary approach to somatic symptom disorders. Acta Paediatr. 2022;111(11):2115–24.
2. Russo K. Assessment and treatment of adolescents with chronic medical conditions. J Heal Serv Psychol. 2022;48(2):69–78.
3. Hampson SE, Skinner TC, Hart J, Storey L, Gage H, Foxcroft D, et al. Effects of educational and psychosocial interventions for adolescents with diabetes mellitus: a systematic review. Health Technol Assess. 2001;5(10):1–79.
4. Borus JS, Laffel L. Adherence challenges in the management of type 1 diabetes in adolescents: prevention and intervention. Curr Opin Pediatr. 2010;22(4):405–11.
5. Vassilopoulos A, Valenzuela JM, Tsikis J, Reitblat L, Blanco EJ, Nicholls S, et al. Pediatric diabetes patients infrequently access outpatient psychology services following screening and referral: implications for practice. Child Heal Care. 2020;49(2):202–17.
6. Larsen B, Luna B. Adolescence as a neurobiological critical period for the development of higher-order cognition. Neurosci Biobehav Rev. 2018;94:179–95.
7. Friedberg RD, Paternostro JK, editors. Handbook of cognitive behavioral therapy for pediatric medical conditions. Cham: Springer International Publishing; 2019.

8. Olfson M, Blanco C, Liu S-M, Wang S, Correll CU. National trends in the office-based treatment of children, adolescents, and adults with antipsychotics. Arch Gen Psychiatry. 2012;69(12):1247–56.
9. Farmer EMZ, Burns BJ, Phillips SD, Angold A, Costello EJ. Pathways into and through mental health services for children and adolescents. Psychiatr Serv. 2003;54(1):60–6.
10. Olfson M, Blanco C, Wang S, Laje G, Correll CU. National trends in the mental health care of children, adolescents, and adults by office-based physicians. JAMA Psychiatry. 2014;71(1):81–90.
11. Caccavale LJ, Bernstein R, Yarbro JL, Rushton H, Gelfand KM, Schwimmer BA. Impact and cost-effectiveness of integrated psychology services in a pediatric endocrinology clinic. J Clin Psychol Med Settings. 2020;27(3):615–21.
12. McBain RK, Kofner A, Stein BD, Cantor JH, Vogt WB, Yu H. Growth and distribution of child psychiatrists in the United States: 2007–2016. Pediatrics. 2019;144(6):e20191576.
13. Los E, Wilt AS. Type 1 diabetes in children. In: StatPearls [Internet]. Treasure Island: StatPearls Publishing; 2024.
14. Tao B, Pietropaolo M, Atkinson M, Schatz D, Taylor D. Estimating the cost of type 1 diabetes in the U.S.: a propensity score matching method. PLoS One. 2010;5(7):e11501.
15. Wagenknecht LE, Lawrence JM, Isom S, Jensen ET, Dabelea D, Liese AD, et al. Trends in incidence of youth-onset type 1 and type 2 diabetes in the USA, 2002–18: results from the population-based SEARCH for Diabetes in Youth study. Lancet Diabetes Endocrinol. 2023;11(4):242–50.
16. Wood JR, Miller KM, Maahs DM, Beck RW, DiMeglio LA, Libman IM, et al. Most youth with type 1 diabetes in the T1D Exchange Clinic Registry do not meet American Diabetes Association or International Society for Pediatric and Adolescent Diabetes clinical guidelines. Diabetes Care. 2013;36(7):2035–7.
17. de Wit M, Gajewska KA, Goethals ER, McDarby V, Zhao X, Hapunda G, et al. ISPAD clinical practice consensus guidelines 2022: psychological care of children, adolescents and young adults with diabetes. Pediatr Diabetes. 2022;23(8):1373–89.
18. Jones JM, Lawson ML, Daneman D, Olmsted MP, Rodin G. Eating disorders in adolescent females with and without type 1 diabetes: cross sectional study. BMJ. 2000;320(7249):1563–6.
19. Goebel-Fabbri AE, Fikkan J, Franko DL, Pearson K, Anderson BJ, Weinger K. Insulin restriction and associated morbidity and mortality in women with type 1 diabetes. Diabetes Care. 2008;31(3):415–9.
20. Delamater AM. Psychological care of children and adolescents with diabetes. Pediatr Diabetes. 2009;10(suppl 1):175–84.
21. Channon SJ, Huws-Thomas MV, Rollnick S, Hood K, Cannings-John RL, Rogers C, et al. A multicenter randomized controlled trial of motivational interviewing in teenagers with diabetes. Diabetes Care. 2007;30(6):1390–5.
22. Shibeshi MS, Daba AK, Meiso KM, Tadesse BT. Glycemic control among children and adolescents with diabetes in Southern Ethiopia: a cross-sectional study. BMC Endocr Disord. 2022;22(1):161.
23. Miller WL, White PC. A brief history of congenital adrenal hyperplasia. Horm Res Paediatr. 2022;95(6):529–45.
24. Auer MK, Nordenström A, Lajic S, Reisch N. Congenital adrenal hyperplasia. Lancet (London, England). 2023;401(10372):227–44.
25. Buyukunal C, Zeller KA, Emre S, Nakayama DK. The history of surgery in disorders of sexual development. J Pediatr Surg. 2021;56(2):429–33.
26. Hurwitz RS. Feminizing surgery for disorders of sex development: evolution, complications, and outcomes. Curr Urol Rep. 2011;12(2):166–72.

27. Gupta DK, Shilpa S, Amini AC, Gupta M, Aggarwal G, Deepika G, et al. Congenital adrenal hyperplasia: long-term evaluation of feminizing genitoplasty and psychosocial aspects. Pediatr Surg Int. 2006;22(11):905–9.
28. Kremen J, Harris RM, Aston CE, Perez M, Austin PF, Baskin L, et al. Exploring factors associated with decisions about feminizing genitoplasty in differences of sex development. J Pediatr Adolesc Gynecol. 2022;35(6):638–46.
29. Fleseriu M, Christ-Crain M, Langlois F, Gadelha M, Melmed S. Hypopituitarism. Lancet (London, England). 2024;403(10444):2632–48.
30. Yeliosof O, Gangat M. Diagnosis and management of hypopituitarism. Curr Opin Pediatr. 2019;31(4):531–6.
31. Wei I-H, Huang C-C. Risk of mental illnesses in patients with hypopituitarism: a nationwide population-based cohort study. Psychiatry Investig. 2022;19(6):418–26.
32. Slagboom TNA, Deijen JB, Van Bunderen CC, Knoop HA, Drent ML. Psychological well-being and illness perceptions in patients with hypopituitarism. Pituitary. 2021;24(4):542–54.
33. Künzel H, Kluge M, Zeising M, Schopohl J, Yassouridis A, Stalla G-K, et al. Sleep in pituitary insufficient patients compared to patients with depression and healthy controls at baseline and after challenge with CRH. J Psychiatr Res. 2020;129:124–8.
34. Karachaliou F-H, Karavanaki K, Simatou A, Tsintzou E, Skarakis NS, Kanaka-Gatenbein C. Association of growth hormone deficiency (GHD) with anxiety and depression: experimental data and evidence from GHD children and adolescents. Hormones (Athens). 2021;20(4):679–89.
35. Aberg ND, Brywe KG, Isgaard J. Aspects of growth hormone and insulin-like growth factor-I related to neuroprotection, regeneration, and functional plasticity in the adult brain. ScientificWorldJournal. 2006;6:53–80.
36. Chevalier LL, Zwemer EK, Casey R, Recklitis CJ. The effect of pediatric cancer on identity in young adult survivors: results from Project REACH. J Adolesc Young Adult Oncol. 2022;11(3):297–303.
37. McGrady ME, Willard VW, Williams AM, Brinkman TM. Psychological outcomes in adolescent and young adult cancer survivors. J Clin Oncol. 2024;42(6):707–16.
38. Brinkman TM, Recklitis CJ, Michel G, Grootenhuis MA, Klosky JL. Psychological symptoms, social outcomes, socioeconomic attainment, and health behaviors among survivors of childhood cancer: current state of the literature. J Clin Oncol. 2018;36(21):2190–7.
39. Bondy CA. Care of girls and women with Turner syndrome: a guideline of the Turner Syndrome Study Group. J Clin Endocrinol Metab. 2007;92(1):10–25.
40. Steiner M, Saenger P. Turner syndrome: an update. Adv Pediatr Infect Dis. 2022;69(1):177–202.
41. Hutaff-Lee C, Bennett E, Howell S, Tartaglia N. Clinical developmental, neuropsychological, and social-emotional features of Turner syndrome. Am J Med Genet C Semin Med Genet. 2019;181(1):126–34.
42. Carl A, Good M, Haag E, Hutaff-Lee C, Swain D, Tartaglia N, et al. Anxiety in Turner syndrome: engaging community to address barriers and facilitators to diagnosis and care. Am J Med Genet A. 2024;194(8):e63564.
43. Bonomi M, Rochira V, Pasquali D, Balercia G, Jannini EA, Ferlin A. Klinefelter syndrome (KS): genetics, clinical phenotype and hypogonadism. J Endocrinol Investig. 2017;40(2):123–34.
44. Bojesen A, Juul S, Birkebaek NH, Gravholt CH. Morbidity in Klinefelter syndrome: a Danish register study based on hospital discharge diagnoses. J Clin Endocrinol Metab. 2006;91(4):1254–60.
45. Skakkebæk A, Moore PJ, Pedersen AD, Bojesen A, Kristensen MK, Fedder J, et al. Anxiety and depression in Klinefelter syndrome: the impact of personality and social engagement. PLoS One. 2018;13(11):e0206932.

46. DeLisi LE, Maurizio AM, Svetina C, Ardekani B, Szulc K, Nierenberg J, et al. Klinefelter's syndrome (XXY) as a genetic model for psychotic disorders. Am J Med Genet Part B, Neuropsychiatr Genet Off Publ Int Soc Psychiatr Genet. 2005;135B(1):15–23.
47. Bryant DM, Hoeft F, Lai S, Lackey J, Roeltgen D, Ross J, et al. Neuroanatomical phenotype of Klinefelter syndrome in childhood: a voxel-based morphometry study. J Neurosci. 2011;31(18):6654–60.
48. Skakkebæk A, Gravholt CH, Rasmussen PM, Bojesen A, Jensen JS, Fedder J, et al. Neuroanatomical correlates of Klinefelter syndrome studied in relation to the neuropsychological profile. NeuroImage Clin. 2014;4:1–9.
49. Giagulli VA, Campone B, Castellana M, Salzano C, Fisher AD, de Angelis C, et al. Neuropsychiatric aspects in men with Klinefelter syndrome. Endocr Metab Immune Disord Drug Targets. 2019;19(2):109–15.
50. Samango-Sprouse C, Lasutschinkow P, Powell S, Sadeghin T, Gropman A. The incidence of anxiety symptoms in boys with 47,XXY (Klinefelter syndrome) and the possible impact of timing of diagnosis and hormonal replacement therapy. Am J Med Genet A. 2019;179(3):423–8.
51. Butler MG, Miller JL, Forster JL. Prader-Willi syndrome – clinical genetics, diagnosis and treatment approaches: an update. Curr Pediatr Rev. 2019;15(4):207–44.
52. Schwartz L, Caixàs A, Dimitropoulos A, Dykens E, Duis J, Einfeld S, et al. Behavioral features in Prader-Willi syndrome (PWS): consensus paper from the International PWS Clinical Trial Consortium. J Neurodev Disord. 2021;13(1):25.
53. Shelkowitz E, Gantz MG, Ridenour TA, Scheimann AO, Strong T, Bohonowych J, et al. Neuropsychiatric features of Prader-Willi syndrome. Am J Med Genet A. 2022;188(5):1457–63.
54. Peleggi A, Bohonowych J, Strong TV, Schwartz L, Kim S-J. Suicidality in individuals with Prader-Willi syndrome: a review of registry survey data. BMC Psychiatry. 2021;21(1):438.
55. Alexandrou E, Corathers S, Gutmark-Little I, Casnellie L, Gerstle M, Tatum J, et al. Improving anxiety screening in patients with Turner syndrome. Horm Res Paediatr. 2022;95(1):68–75.
56. Ogden CL, Carroll MD, Fakhouri TH, Hales CM, Fryar CD, Li X, et al. Prevalence of obesity among youths by household income and education level of head of household – United States 2011–2014. MMWR Morb Mortal Wkly Rep. 2018;67(6):186–9.
57. Carroll R, Bice AA, Roberto A, Prentice CR. Examining mental health disorders in overweight and obese pediatric patients. J Pediatr Heal Care. 2022;36(6):507–19.
58. Jerome GJ, Fink T, Brady T, Young DR, Dickerson FB, Goldsholl S, et al. Physical activity levels and screen time among youth with overweight/obesity using mental health services. Int J Environ Res Public Health. 2022;19(4):2261.
59. Schroeder K, Schuler BR, Kobulsky JM, Sarwer DB. The association between adverse childhood experiences and childhood obesity: a systematic review. Obes Rev. 2021;22(7):e13204.
60. Felitti VJ, Anda RF, Nordenberg D, Williamson DF, Spitz AM, Edwards V, et al. Relationship of childhood abuse and household dysfunction to many of the leading causes of death in adults. The Adverse Childhood Experiences (ACE) study. Am J Prev Med. 1998;14(4):245–58.
61. Bellis MA, Hughes K, Leckenby N, Jones L, Baban A, Kachaeva M, et al. Adverse childhood experiences and associations with health-harming behaviours in young adults: surveys in eight eastern European countries. Bull World Health Organ. 2014;92(9):641–55.
62. Soares ALG, Howe LD, Matijasevich A, Wehrmeister FC, Menezes AMB, Gonçalves H. Adverse childhood experiences: prevalence and related factors in adolescents of a Brazilian birth cohort. Child Abuse Negl. 2016;51:21–30.
63. Siddiqui S, Mateen S, Ahmad R, Moin S. A brief insight into the etiology, genetics, and immunology of polycystic ovarian syndrome (PCOS). J Assist Reprod Genet. 2022;39(11):2439–73.
64. The Rotterdam ESHRE/ASRM-Sponsored PCOS Consensus Workshop Group. Revised 2003 consensus on diagnostic criteria and long-term health risks related to polycystic ovary syndrome (PCOS). Hum Reprod. 2004;19(1):41–7.
65. Teede HJ, Misso ML, Costello MF, Dokras A, Laven J, Moran L, et al. Recommendations from the international evidence-based guideline for the assessment and management of polycystic ovary syndrome. Fertil Steril. 2018;110(3):364–79.

66. Jones GL, Hall JM, Balen AH, Ledger WL. Health-related quality of life measurement in women with polycystic ovary syndrome: a systematic review. Hum Reprod Update. 2008;14(1):15–25.
67. Veltman-Verhulst SM, Boivin J, Eijkemans MJC, Fauser BJCM. Emotional distress is a common risk in women with polycystic ovary syndrome: a systematic review and meta-analysis of 28 studies. Hum Reprod Update. 2012;18(6):638–51.
68. Cooney LG, Dokras A. Depression and anxiety in polycystic ovary syndrome: etiology and treatment. Curr Psychiatry Rep. 2017;19(11):83.
69. Karsten MDA, Wekker V, Groen H, Painter RC, Mol BWJ, Laan ETM, et al. The role of PCOS in mental health and sexual function in women with obesity and a history of infertility. Hum Reprod Open. 2021;2021(4):hoab038.
70. Al Wattar BH, Fisher M, Bevington L, Talaulikar V, Davies M, Conway G, et al. Clinical practice guidelines on the diagnosis and management of polycystic ovary syndrome: a systematic review and quality assessment study. J Clin Endocrinol Metab. 2021;106(8):2436–46.
71. Wang G, Liu X, Zhu S, Lei J. Experience of mental health in women with polycystic ovary syndrome: a descriptive phenomenological study. J Psychosom Obstet Gynaecol. 2023;44(1):2218987.
72. Copeland W, Shanahan L, Miller S, Costello EJ, Angold A, Maughan B. Outcomes of early pubertal timing in young women: a prospective population-based study. Am J Psychiatry. 2010;167(10):1218–25.
73. Mendle J, Turkheimer E, Emery RE. Detrimental psychological outcomes associated with early pubertal timing in adolescent girls. Dev Rev. 2007;27(2):151–71.
74. Kota AS, Ejaz S. Precocious puberty. In: StatPearls [Internet]. Treasure Island: StatPearls Publishing; 2024.
75. Burt SA, McGue M, DeMarte JA, Krueger RF, Iacono WG. Timing of menarche and the origins of conduct disorder. Arch Gen Psychiatry. 2006;63(8):890–6.
76. Rierdan J, Koff E. Depressive symptomatology among very early maturing girls. J Youth Adolesc. 1991;20(4):415–25.
77. Temelturk RD, Ilcioglu Ekici G, Beberoglu M, Siklar Z, Kilic BG. Managing precocious puberty: a necessity for psychiatric evaluation. Asian J Psychiatr. 2021;58:102617.
78. Di Cosmo C, Tonacchera M. Congenital hypothyroidism. In: Vitti P, Hegedüs L, editors. Thyroid diseases: pathogenesis, diagnosis, and treatment. Cham: Springer International Publishing; 2018. p. 333–71.
79. Al-Qahtani MH, ElYahia SA, AlQahtani AS, AlQahtani AJ, Alamer AA, AlQahtani SM, et al. Thyroid disorders spectrum in pediatric endocrine clinic; seven-year experience of a teaching hospital in Saudi Arabia. Child (Basel, Switzerland). 2023;10(2):390.
80. Calcaterra V, Nappi RE, Regalbuto C, De Silvestri A, Incardona A, Amariti R, et al. Gender differences at the onset of autoimmune thyroid diseases in children and adolescents. Front Endocrinol (Lausanne). 2020;11:229.
81. Mathiassen B, Brøndbo PH, Waterloo K, Martinussen M, Eriksen M, Hanssen-Bauer K, et al. IQ as a moderator of outcome in severity of children's mental health status after treatment in outpatient clinics. Child Adolesc Psychiatry Ment Health. 2012;6(1):22.
82. Metwalley KA, Farghaly HS. Graves' disease in children: an update. Clin Med Insights Endocrinol Diabetes. 2023;16:11795514221150616.
83. Lane LC, Rankin J, Cheetham T. A survey of the young person's experience of Graves' disease and its management. Clin Endocrinol. 2021;94(2):330–40.
84. Mokkink LB, van der Lee JH, Grootenhuis MA, Offringa M, Heymans HSA. Defining chronic diseases and health conditions in childhood (0–18 years of age): national consensus in The Netherlands. Eur J Pediatr. 2008;167(12):1441–7.
85. van der Lee JH, Mokkink LB, Grootenhuis MA, Heymans HS, Offringa M. Definitions and measurement of chronic health conditions in childhood: a systematic review. JAMA. 2007;297(24):2741–51.

86. Centers for Disease Control and Prevention. Managing chronic health conditions. https://www.cdc.gov/healthyschools/chronicconditions.htm. 2021.
87. Clemente E, Liu G, Cabral MD. Integrated behavioral health in pediatric subspecialty clinics. Pediatr Clin N Am. 2021;68(3):633–49.
88. Compas BE, Jaser SS, Dunn MJ, Rodriguez EM. Coping with chronic illness in childhood and adolescence. Annu Rev Clin Psychol. 2012;8:455–80.
89. Suryavanshi MS, Yang Y. Clinical and economic burden of mental disorders among children with chronic physical conditions, United States, 2008–2013. Prev Chronic Dis. 2016;13:E71.
90. Whitney DG, Peterson MD. US national and state-level prevalence of mental health disorders and disparities of mental health care use in children. JAMA Pediatr. 2019;173(4):389–91.
91. Coleman WL, Dobbins MI, Garner AS, Siegel BS, Wood DL, Earls MF, et al. Policy statement–the future of pediatrics: mental health competencies for pediatric primary care. Pediatrics. 2009;124(1):410–21.
92. Foy JM, Green CM, Earls MF, et al. Mental health competencies for pediatric practice. Pediatrics. 2019;144(5):e20192757.
93. Schlesinger A, Sengupta S, Marx L, Hilt R, Martini DR, DeMaso DR, et al. Clinical update: collaborative mental health care for children and adolescents in pediatric primary care. J Am Acad Child Adolesc Psychiatry. 2023;62(2):91–119.
94. Demaso D, Martini DR, Sulik LR, Hilt R, Marx L, Pierce K, et al. A guide to building collaborative mental health care partnerships in pediatric primary care. Am Acad Child Adolesc Psychiatry. 2010:1–27. Available from: https://www.aacap.org/App_Themes/AACAP/docs/clinical_practice_center/guide_to_building_collaborative_mental_health_care_partnerships.pdf
95. Rybak TM, Herbst RB, Stark LJ, Samaan ZM, Zion C, Bryant A, et al. Provider perspectives on an integrated behavioral health prevention approach in pediatric primary care. J Clin Psychol Med Settings. 2023;30(4):741–52.
96. Lu S, O'Halloran T, Soares N. The many roles of pediatric integrated behavioral health specialists. Pediatr Clin N Am. 2021;68(3):541–9.
97. Ginsburg S, Foster S. Strategies to support the integration of mental health into pediatric primary care National Institute for Health Care Management. 2009:1–40. Available from: https://www.brightfutures.org/wellchildcare/toolkit/nevada/PediatricMH-FINAL.pdf

Chapter 14
Health and Allergic Diseases

Yahia A. Khanfar, Elizabeth G. Wang, and Steven P. Proper

Abbreviations

AIT	Allergy immunotherapy
ARFID	Avoidant/restrictive food intake disorder
CRSwNP	Chronic rhinosinusitis with nasal polyposis
CSU	Chronic spontaneous urticaria
DBPC	Double blind, placebo-controlled
ED	Emergency department
EGPA	Eosinophilic granulomatosis with polyangiitis
EoE	Eosinophilic esophagitis
HES	Hypereosinophilic syndrome
IL	Interleukin
OIT	Oral immunotherapy
OFC	Oral food challenge
q	Every
SCIT	Subcutaneous immunotherapy
SQ	Subcutaneous

Y. A. Khanfar · S. P. Proper (✉)
Homer Stryker MD School of Medicine, Western Michigan University, Kalamazoo, MI, USA

Department of Pediatrics and Adolescent Medicine, Kalamazoo, MI, USA
e-mail: yahia.khanfar@wmed.edu; steven.proper@wmed.edu

E. G. Wang
Homer Stryker MD School of Medicine, Western Michigan University, Kalamazoo, MI, USA
e-mail: elizabeth.wang@wmed.edu

R. W. Apple et al. (eds.), *Using Integrated Behavioral Health in Pediatric Practice*, https://doi.org/10.1007/978-3-031-85784-3_14

Introduction

Some of the most common chronic conditions in the pediatric population are allergic in nature. Asthma is the most common chronic lung disease in children in the United States, affecting 1 in 12, and is the leading cause for Emergency Department (ED) visits in children [1]. Atopic dermatitis is the most common chronic skin condition in children, affecting an estimated 10.7% in the United States [2], with worldwide prevalence as high as 20% [3]. Food allergy affects up to 8% of US children [4]. Allergic rhinitis (environmental allergies) can affect over 10% of US children [5]. With so many allergic diseases affecting children, it is also important to know that incidence of these allergic diseases also is highly dependent on age (Fig. 14.1). Understanding these age relationships provides a framework to manage expectations for patients with allergic conditions (what diseases they may have, and when). Also, allergic conditions, especially when uncontrolled, have long been associated with poorer mental health and quality of life measures, and awareness of these associations is fundamental to both the practice of allergy and behavioral health [6]. In this chapter, we will review the most relevant associations of allergic disease and mental health.

Allergy practice requires the regular use of skin prick testing and needles, and as such, procedural anxiety about these devices is a foremost concern for allergists and an area where we interact most with behavioral health colleagues. For diagnosis of allergic sensitization (identifying one's allergies), skin prick testing is probably the

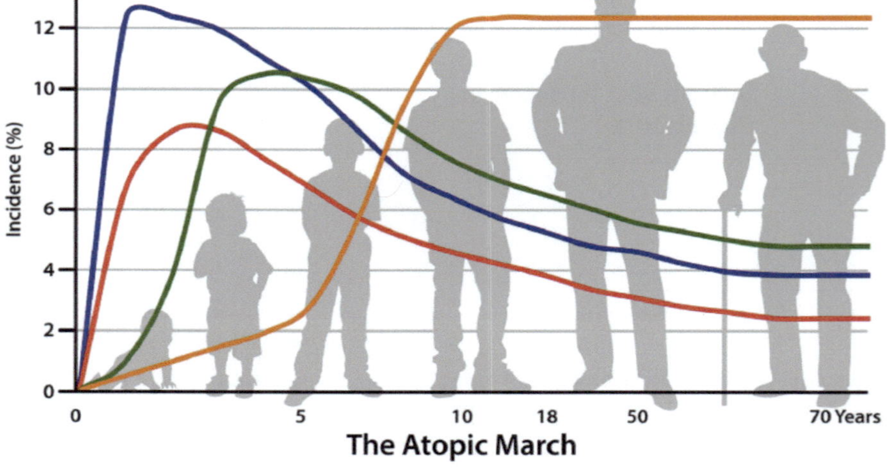

Fig. 14.1 Age-related prevalence of allergic disease: As age increases, allergic diseases become more or less prevalent, with initial spike in eczema, then food allergy, then asthma, followed lastly by allergic rhinitis (Czarnowicki et al. 2017)

most common initial procedure, where a small droplet of allergen extract is applied to the skin while at the same time applying a "prick" or "scratch" with a device, most often made of plastic. In addition to skin prick testing, blood testing is another way to identify allergic sensitizations, which requires the use of needles to obtain the blood sample. Not only are needles used for diagnosis, but also treatment of allergic conditions. Allergy immunotherapy (AIT), where gradually increasing concentrations of allergens are delivered to the patient in an effort to induce tolerance (the ability to be exposed to the allergen without developing symptoms), is the most effective treatment of classic environmental allergies. The delivery of allergens is most often achieved by subcutaneous injections (subcutaneous immunotherapy, or SCIT, also known more commonly as "allergy shots"). Other targeted therapies can include biologics, an ever-expanding category of medications which are antibodies directed against specific inflammatory targets/pathways involved in allergic disease, and require injection either subcutaneously or intravenously. It is not difficult to see that patient acceptance of the required procedures, both to accurately diagnose and treat allergic disease, is critical to successfully managing these conditions and providing good outcomes. As such, treatment of procedural anxiety and needle phobias is of utmost importance and extremely common cause for behavioral health referral in allergy practice.

Another emerging need for behavioral health in allergic practice relates to food ingestion. Children with food allergy require periods of food avoidance, and while this avoidance can be achieved in most instances without behavioral management, this can at times translate into unnecessary avoidance behaviors, anxiety, or present complications when reintroduction to previously avoided foods is required, for example, either with "outgrowing" a food allergy or regular, gradually increasing ingestion of allergenic foods (as is practiced in oral immunotherapy (OIT)). Furthermore, anxiety related to food allergies (whether these allergies are validated by an allergist or not) is often well out of proportion to actual risks food allergies pose. Aside from being a mental health disorder all on its own, the anxiety from food allergies further drives food avoidance behaviors, which can contribute to avoidant/restrictive food intake disorder (ARFID) or related conditions. Awareness of the basics of food allergy management is needed for behavioral health professionals to adequately navigate issues of food avoidance, especially given the increasing prevalence of OIT in the US and elsewhere. We will review some of these treatments for, and issues arising from, food allergy management in this chapter.

Finally, we will discuss the many opportunities and challenges pertaining to behavioral health in allergy practice. One opportunity fundamental to all patients is access to behavioral health. Any methods connecting patients with needed behavioral health resources would contribute to better health equity for pediatric patients with coexisting allergic and behavioral health concerns. Further advancements in allergy treatment may allow less invasive procedures than our current reliance on needles and scratching devices, which will allow for smoother implementation of AIT. While there are many promising therapies on the horizon, regulatory challenges and limited implementation (either from insurance barriers or lack of allergists trained in these newer techniques) remain and should not be underestimated.

Despite the challenges, there are more effective options today for allergy treatments than ever before, and effective collaboration with behavioral health partners will ensure better outcomes for both allergic disease and behavioral comorbidities.

Association of Mental Health and Allergic Disease

Ever since the emergence of allergic disease literature, there have been recognized relationships between allergic disease and neuropsychiatric symptoms. The term "allergy" itself was coined by pediatrician Clemens von Pirquet in 1906 and further elaborated in "Allergie," a book he published in 1910, to describe adverse immunologic reactions, including serum sickness [7]. Shortly after this, one description of the after-effects of an attack of hay fever (allergic rhinitis/conjunctivitis) by W.P. Dunbar in 1913 was described as "… a condition of weakness and enervation which may be so severe that the patient is unable to sit upright in his chair; at the same time the loss of all energy produces a profound mental effect" [8]. These symptoms have also been described as poor memory, slowness of thought, "brain fog," etc., and continue to persist even today in our everyday allergy practice.

Aside from the temporary symptoms surrounding acute episodes of allergic disease, other studies have solidified the relationships between specific allergic diseases and mental health conditions such as psychological stress, depression, or mood disorders [9, 10]. For example, a large cross-sectional study of over 16,000 adults in Korea showed higher odds ratio (OR) for depression compared with non-allergic controls (OR: 2.1 and 1.83, respectively) as well as severe psychological stress (OR: 1.41 and 1.35, respectively) [11]. Another study showed that people with seasonal allergies had significantly higher odds of having a mood disorder (adjusted OR [aOR]: 1.28, $p < 0.01$). The mechanisms of these associations are not yet well understood, but some lines of current research are focused on the possible direct biochemical inflammatory crosstalk between allergy and neuropsychiatric symptoms [12, 13]. This research is still in its early stages, but we are beginning to see that allergic and neuropsychiatric comorbidities vary depending on the particular allergic diseases involved. For example, allergic conditions with a strong itch component (urticaria, atopic dermatitis/eczema) often have significant reduction in quality of life and sleep disturbances [11, 14–16]. It is beyond the scope of this chapter to review all allergic and mental health comorbidities, but we would refer you to the expert review by Conway et al. on this topic [6].

Allergists can play a significant role in screening for these comorbid conditions if their practice allows. This can be informal, through the normal course of eliciting a comprehensive history and physical exam, or more formal screening tools could be implemented. For example, use of the GAD-7 has reasonably good sensitivity and specificity for anxiety disorders (https://www.hiv.uw.edu/page/mental-health-screening/gad-7). Use of these screening tools must also be balanced by the time it takes to administer them. In some cases, shorter screening tools may be appropriate (e.g., using GAD-2, the first 2 questions of the GAD-7, to save time), as excessive use of screening tools may prolong visits considerably. The standard Allergy office visit, which also includes skin prick testing, requires a 15 min waiting period from the time the pricks are placed to the time when they can be interpreted. In our Allergy clinic, we use this time spent waiting for skin testing to work on patient education, for things like inhaler/spacer technique for asthmatics, or try to elicit other parts of the history that may not be as relevant for the testing but are still crucial to comprehensive consultations and evaluations. Doing this also helps to distract the patient from their skin testing, which likely improves their overall procedural anxiety. Most offices include some of these screenings in the standard pre-visit check-in process or other forms of patient communication. It is imperative that allergists and behavioral health practitioners alike be familiar with patients who may be experiencing both kinds of disorders, and strive for a holistic approach to their management, and arrange referrals when needed [17].

Use of Skin Prick Testing and Needles in Allergy Practice

Whether patients develop environmental allergies, food allergies, or both, diagnosis of these conditions is first based on thorough history and physical. Environmental allergies will cause symptoms related in time to allergen exposure that typically involve eyes, nose, throat, and lungs. Allergic triggers often cause rhinitis, conjunctivitis, hives, flares of eczema, as well as exacerbate asthma symptoms. Environmental triggers do not usually cause anaphylaxis. Food allergy will tend to be more likely to cause hives, flushing, swelling (typically lips, face, mouth), upset stomach, and vomiting and is more likely to cause anaphylaxis (involvement of multiple body systems). Regardless of the organ systems involved, if an IgE-mediated allergy is suspected, the first best test to identify allergic triggers is a skin prick test (SPT). In this test, a droplet of allergen extract is placed on the skin and scratched through by a scratch device. Most of these devices are made of plastic and are disposable in the sharps container. They make a very small abrasion in the upper layers of the epidermis, and the practitioner waits for 15 min. Introduction of these allergens to the skin, in sensitized individuals, will make a wheal (raised area that is typically lighter in color than surrounding skin due to the edema, and dependent on histamine), surrounded by a "flare" (area around the wheal that appears red in lighter-skinned individuals, and can be hard to see or sometimes darker purple in color in darker-skinned individuals). Wheals, and not flares, are measured in millimeters of the largest diameter distance to determine the size (see Fig. 14.2). There are many different skin testing devices available, and some comparative studies have been done to determine best practices, though most allergists have preferences that depend on many factors, including training and experience with certain devices, availability and pricing, reliability, and pain or tolerance of devices. Generally skin prick testing is well tolerated and does cause mild sharp pain at the site of the prick temporarily. Our clinic uses UniTest PC® (Lincoln Diagnostics) as this met our needs in the clinic for a single test device and seemed to perform well in published comparisons

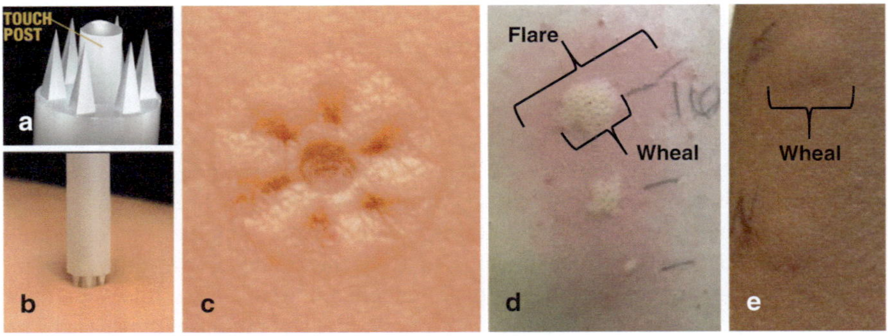

Fig. 14.2 Skin prick testing. (**a**) Shape of UniTestPC tip, with central post which makes initial contact with the skin and brings droplet of extract with it. (**b**) Approximate depth of direct downward application of the UniTest PC. (**c**) Typical indentation (magnified) of the UniTest PC. (**d**) Image of wheal and flare in light-skinned patient. (**e**) Wheals in dark-skinned patient (no clear flare visible), image from Ching et al. (2015). **a–c** images from Lincoln Diagnostics (https://www.lincolndiagnostics.com/products/unitest-pc/) and **d** from our Allergy clinic (with patient consent)

[18]. Anecdotally this device also seemed to be the best tolerated when we tested them in our clinic (unpublished). Typically a 3 mm wheal or larger (above the negative control) is considered positive. This test is preferred because it is a more "real world" introduction of the allergen to the body, whereas blood IgE levels have a much higher rate of false positives, and only tend to tell you whether an allergic reaction is possible, and allergen-specific IgE levels will not usually tell you if you will actually have a clinical reaction to exposure to the allergen [19]. In many instances, for environmental allergies, only a skin prick test positivity is needed. For foods, we will often validate any positive skin prick testing with blood IgE levels specific for the foods of interest. Some allergists also employ intradermal skin testing, and it has shown increased sensitivity, though in our practice the use of needle injections was not preferred for our clinical work flow or patient population (many pediatric patients), so we forego intradermal injection testing.

By far the most impactful intervention in the practice of pediatric allergy is overcoming anxiety related to injection-based therapies and needle phobias [20]. There are many techniques that can be used in the allergy practice setting to help alleviate fears and help mitigate anxiety and fear, many of which are practiced by nurses who perform the majority of the injections in these settings [21]. Implementation of many of these pain-alleviating strategies is crucial in everyday allergy practice, and most children tolerate multiple injections over a long period when adequately delivered [22]. Needle use and exposure is by no means limited to allergic disease, but many treatments for allergic diseases, most notably delivering life-saving doses of epinephrine (intramuscular) for treatment of anaphylaxis, typically require use of needles to deliver allergens or medications. While not all patients with allergic disease require intervention that includes needle injections, the more severe cases often will. The first use of needles in the management of allergic disease was described by Noon and Freeman in 1911 for management of hay fever (allergic rhinoconjunctivitis to pollens) [23]. While it would take another 56 years before the discovery of IgE [24], this practice has continued to be refined by practicing allergists, and subcutaneous immunotherapy continues to be a mainstay of management of environmental allergies [25]. In this practice, increasing doses of allergen are injected subcutaneously, usually weekly (though this can vary) over a period of months, and eventually a maintenance dose is reached, where the patient only receives injections once per month, but this continues often for 3–5 years to achieve maximum benefit and prolong the effect of desensitization to allergens. Figure 14.3 shows our practice's immunotherapy schedule (which is typical). This protocol is not unlike treatment of patients with stinging insect venom allergy. Patients of essentially any age can undergo subcutaneous immunotherapy for allergic rhinitis and asthma safely, though risks, benefits, and practical considerations all must be weighed carefully [26, 27].

There are some protocols which utilize multiple injections in a single day/clinic visit, referred to typically as "cluster" if multiple per day or "rush" protocol if trying to achieve even more rapid control of symptoms (patients planning to be pregnant, or other time constraints). Some studies of these accelerated protocols revealed increased risks of severe reactions including anaphylaxis (reaction rates typically 0.2% for standard protocols but can be as high as 34% in rush protocols) [25,

STANDARD BUILD-UP SCHEDULE				
	GREEN VIAL 1:1,000 v/v	BLUE VIAL 1:100 v/v	YELLOW VIAL 1:10 v/v	RED VIAL 1:1 v/v
Weekly until reaching 0.5 mL of Red Vial (Maintenance)	0.05 mL	0.05 mL	0.05 mL	0.05 mL
	0.1 mL	0.1 mL	0.1 mL	0.1 mL
	0.2 mL	0.2 mL	0.2 mL	0.15 mL
	0.3 mL	0.3 mL	0.3 mL	0.2 mL
	0.4 mL	0.4 mL	0.35 mL	0.25 mL
	0.5 mL	0.5 mL	0.4 mL	0.3 mL
			0.45 mL	0.35 mL
			0.5 mL	0.4 mL
				0.45 mL
				0.5 mL
				0.5 mL (2 wk)
				0.5 mL (3 wk)
				0.5 mL (4 wk)

Fig. 14.3 Standard build-up SCIT protocol, where each volume represents a single visit approximately 1 week apart starting with lowest dose of green vial (most dilute) through highest dose of red vial (most concentrated).

28–31], though these variations are vast, and the overwhelming majority of comparative studies show no difference in severe adverse reaction rates between standard and accelerated protocols, even among pediatric patients [32, 33]. Other ways in which immunotherapy is innovating is in developing allergen extracts that are hyper-concentrated (reducing the volume required for injection), of which one example is acetone-precipitated dog epithelium (often called AP-dog). Many extracts are being developed where the allergen is complexed with aluminum hydroxide (Alum) which allow for slow release of allergen (like a depot)—this reduces the release rate, and thus these extracts are not useful for testing, but only for treatment, requiring less injections overall. Costs and access to these preparations are a factor limiting their widespread use. Many variables still need to be studied, as there are vast differences in extracts used and timing of protocols, but optimization of a faster injection schedule would certainly reduce overall procedural anxiety as well as increase adherence.

The most promising advance in allergy immunotherapy that is needleless is sublingual immunotherapy (SLIT), where extracts are applied orally, under the tongue, for a period of time without swallowing, and patients can apply on their own at home after they undergo instruction and demonstrate tolerance of the dose in the clinic. Three SLIT tablets have FDA approval in the United States: dust mite, ragweed, and grass. The limitations on these methods are that they only apply for single allergens—most patients have several allergens they wish to be desensitized to. Further, Medicare and Medicaid do not typically cover the cost of these tablets, which can be over $150 per month. In Europe, a birch pollen tablet has secure approval through European Marketing Authorization. One method that would address multiple allergens by the sublingual route is use of sublingual drops. In Europe, this practice is widespread, and while they do not have formal approval, their use in Europe is allowed if overseen personally by a physician. The FDA does not currently approve the drops, and the ACAAI and AAAAI Joint Task Force do not recommend their use, which is in contrast with the American Academy of Otolaryngic Allergy which does offer guidance to their members. The studies on SLIT drops are varied, with multiple different extracts and protocols, and studies that would allow convincing evidence leading to FDA approval are lacking [34].

Other uses of needles in allergy (and many other specialties) are a result of using medications which are themselves proteins, which require they be delivered intact into the body (could not be oral). In the case of primary immune deficiency, regular injection of IgG is required to maintain immunity against common pathogens. This is achieved usually through monthly IV infusions (half-life of IgG is approximately 21 days), or subcutaneously approximately weekly (due to limitations on the amount of fluid that can be comfortably injected into the subcutaneous space). Most patients would prefer the subcutaneous infusion route, because over time, repeated IV access can be more difficult, but this also requires more episodes of infusion, which could increase procedural anxiety. Efforts are underway to try to make subcutaneous infusions more tolerable and less invasive, including wearable infusion equipment, which has shown promise [35]. What is most unfortunate about the current state of insurance approvals in the United States is that most patients don't really have a choice about which treatment is covered. Medicaid plans in the state of Michigan essentially require monthly IV infusions at infusion centers for IgG replacement in primary immunodeficiency, even when other preferred options are available. This is similar with patients who have Hereditary Angioedema (HAE), which is most commonly a deficiency in C1-esterase inhibitor (often just called C1-inhibitor), who can have life-threatening episodes of swelling if not regularly receiving medication; essentially, we have the option of subcutaneous treatment, which has shown some evidence of superior reductions in attack rates compared to IV replacement, and is also preferred by patients, but we have difficulty implementing this in our healthcare system due to insurance barriers [36–38].

Other medications common in allergy practice are also antibodies, but rather than replacing a deficient protein, they target specific inflammatory processes to reduce disease activity (referred to as "biologics"). The oldest example of this in allergy practice is omalizumab (Xolair), an IgG1 kappa antibody targeting all human IgE antibodies, which has been FDA approved since 2003 (starting with indication of moderate to severe asthma, but indications have since expanded due to IgE's role in most allergic processes). Biologics in allergy practice now include seven [7] agents as of publication of this chapter (Table 14.1).

It is important to note that intolerance of needles may not be related to a specific diagnosable phobia to needles in all patients, but rather, a broader umbrella of procedural anxiety that is extremely common. Definitions of these fears and phobias have varied over time, and careful understanding of the approach to patients with these fears, especially in pediatrics, is paramount [39]. It is beyond the scope of this chapter to summarize the behavioral interventions for fear of needles, but it typically involves cognitive behavioral therapy and gradual desensitization, reviewed expertly by McMurtry et al. [40]. Efforts aimed at reducing the stress of testing and treatment in Allergy, such as minimizing the requirement of needles, or the frequency of injections, are always ongoing in Allergy research.

Needleless systems are an area of active research and innovation and hold tremendous promise. One type of needleless system, utilizing springs and pressure, can deliver medicine through a fine jet through skin into the subcutaneous space and are referred to more commonly as "jet injectors." A recent study by Traina et al. used a needleless delivery system (Injex 30) for subcutaneous immunotherapy in children, yielding promising results for future advancement in this field, though it needs to be replicated on a larger scale [41]. Literature on these systems in allergy are lacking and should continue to be studied. Another kind of needleless device was approved in August 2024 for epinephrine, which delivers it to the nasal mucosa as a nasal spray (Neffy). This was approved for treatment of anaphylaxis, but only

Table 14.1 Common biologic medications used in allergy practice: a review of currently approved biologic medications for the treatment of allergic disease

Biologic Agent	Target	Indications	Common Dosing
Omalizumab (Xolair)	IgE	6+ yrs for asthma; 12+ yrs for CSU; 18+ yrs for CRSwNP; 1+ yrs for food allergy.	75, 150 or 300 mg SQ q2-4 weeks (varies by disease, age and total IgE level).
Mepolizumab (Nucala)	IL-5	6+ yrs for asthma; 18+ yrs for EGPA and CRSwNP; 12+ yrs for HES.	Asthma: 6-11 yrs: 40 mg SQ q4 weeks. 12 yrs+: 100 mg SQ q4 weeks. CRSwNP: 100 mg SQ q4 weeks. EGPA, HES: 300 mg SQ q 4 weeks.
Benralizumab (Fasenra)	IL-5 receptor	6+ yrs for severe eosinophilic asthma.	12 yrs+: 30 mg SQ q4 weeks x3, then q8 weeks. Patients 6-11 yrs: <35 kg: 10 mg SQ q4 weeks x3, then q8 weeks. 35+ kg: 30 mg SQ q4 weeks x3, then q8 weeks.
Reslizumab (Cinqair)	IL-5	18+ yrs for severe eosinophilic asthma.	18 yrs +: 3 mg/kg IV q4 weeks; infuse over 20-50 minutes.
Dupilumab (Dupixent)	IL-4 receptor alpha (targets both IL-4/IL-13)	6+ mos for atopic dermatitis; 6+ yrs for eosinophilic or OCS-dependent asthma; 18+ yrs for CRSwNP or prurigo nodularis; 1+ yrs for EoE (must be >15kg).	200-300 mg SQ q2-4 weeks
Tezepelumab (Tezspire)	TSLP	12+ yrs for severe asthma.	210 mg SQ q4 weeks
Tralokinumab-ldrm (Adbry)	IL-13	12+ yrs for moderate-to-severe atopic dermatitis	18+ yrs: 300mg q2 weeks. 12-17 yrs: 150mg q2 weeks.

for patients who weigh >30 kg (66 pounds). While we anxiously await the approval for patients <25 kg, we also must contend with implementation hurdles for these new needleless systems. When trying to switch our Allergy patients from standard epinephrine needle autoinjectors to Neffy, most insurances denied Neffy, stating that our patients had to "demonstrate failure with standard injectable epinephrine" before these would be approved. In the 4 months since its approval, I have yet to successfully have the needle-less option covered by a single patient. Obstacles put into place by insurance companies (requiring prior authorizations and high rates of denials of coverage) are an ongoing barrier for patients experiencing procedural anxiety, and often put significant delays on widespread use of these medications by patients. Given that the most common cause of death from food allergy reactions was delayed epinephrine use [42], and even when properly coached, there is tremendous hesitancy among parents to actually use the epinephrine autoinjector [43], significant challenges remain. Incentive structures should more specifically reward pharmaceutical companies not just for developing less invasive and less painful delivery systems but also facilitating their rapid distribution.

Behavioral Impact of Food Allergy

Food allergy refers to several types of immune-mediated reactions to foods, but most commonly is meant to refer to an IgE-mediated process leading to mast cell release of histamine and other mediators that drive food allergy reactions. Other food allergies that are not IgE-mediated are things such as Food-Protein-Induced Enterocolitis Syndrome (FPIES), which still require avoidance of trigger foods, but their treatment does not require epinephrine. For the remainder of this chapter, we will refer to food allergy as the IgE-mediated form. In the United States, food allergy affects approximately 4% of people, but prevalence varies dramatically with age, and our best estimates are that approximately 8% of children have food allergy, though approximately 11% of parents report a food allergy [4, 44].

The most common nine foods (which are required by law in the United States to be labeled accordingly) that people are allergic to are cow's milk, hen's egg, wheat, soy, peanuts, tree nuts, fish, crustacean shellfish, and sesame. While history, skin prick testing, and food-specific IgE levels from the blood are usually sufficient to make the diagnosis of food allergy, the gold standard test is an oral food challenge (OFC) [45]. In an ideal situation, and what is practiced in all clinical trials of food allergy interventions, these are also double-blind placebo controlled (DBPC), such that the patients as well as physicians and nurses administering the food challenge do not know whether the samples are placebo or not (other team members prepare the doses and they are brought to the patient's room). This level of blinding is not typical in the standard allergy practice, however, and they are performed "open." This does introduce a significant amount of bias in terms of patients understanding the doses they are receiving; however, most of the endpoints of an oral food challenge are not just subjective, and I am typically stopping the oral food challenge only when objective findings are made (rash, vomiting, respiratory or blood pressure changes that are observable/measurable). While it is not required to perform oral food challenges to make the diagnosis of food allergy, they are essentially required to rule them out if there is history or testing suggestive of food allergy, and I highly recommend that my patients undergo these when wishing to confirm an allergy has been outgrown or when testing is equivocal or contradictory. They have tremendous value not just diagnostically but also in helping families deal with anxiety associated with allergenic food exposure [46]. We perform OFC in children as young as 8 months, though this is not a typical age to perform one, and there are special considerations to employ when performing OFCs in different populations, as doses change with age, and there are many alterations that an allergist can make to this approach [47].

Once food allergies are diagnosed, we typically monitor food-specific IgE levels over time, such that it is not unreasonable to expect that a child with food allergy will need yearly or every other year blood draws for this purpose. Office visits for new food allergy diagnosis require a significant amount of patient and family education, not just for food avoidance and reading food labels, but also how to recognize and treat food allergy with medications such as diphenhydramine (Benadryl) for mild reactions to epinephrine for severe reactions, and review a Food Allergy Action Plan. The Food Allergy Research and Education patient advocacy organization for food allergy (FARE, at http://www.foodallergy.org) is a great resource for patients, families, and allergists. IgE-mediated food allergy reactions can vary from mild, which typically only involve the skin (hives, swelling, flushing), or involve other body systems to be more systemic (angioedema, nausea, vomiting, diarrhea, coughing, wheezing, shortness of breath, or hypotension and syncope), and to qualify as anaphylaxis must typically involve two or more body systems [48]. Approximately 50% of children with milk or egg allergy will no longer be allergic by age 5, and we commonly tell parents that their children are likely to "outgrow" these particular food allergies, but this is not always the case with other foods such as peanut, tree nut, shellfish, and others [45]. Another factor that separates milk and egg allergy from other foods is that some patients can tolerate a baked product (cake or muffin) due to the baking breaking down some of the allergenic proteins. This is not possible with other foods, however, and baking/cooking may make some foods more allergenic. When children appear like they might tolerate a baked product, we can do an oral baked milk or baked egg challenge, which usually encourages eventual tolerance.

Due to the possibility of severe reactions to foods, having a food allergy diagnosis and the accompanying requirement of food avoidance causes significant levels of anxiety for both the patients and their families [49–58]. In a global survey study of adults with food allergy or parents of children with food allergy, 67.3% and 77.2%, respectively, reported food-allergy related psychological distress [59]. This anxiety as it pertains to fear of fatal food anaphylaxis is somewhat out of proportion to its actual risk, which is thankfully low, and best estimates have it somewhere near death from lightning strike, though data are sparse (Fig. 14.4) [60]. It is not

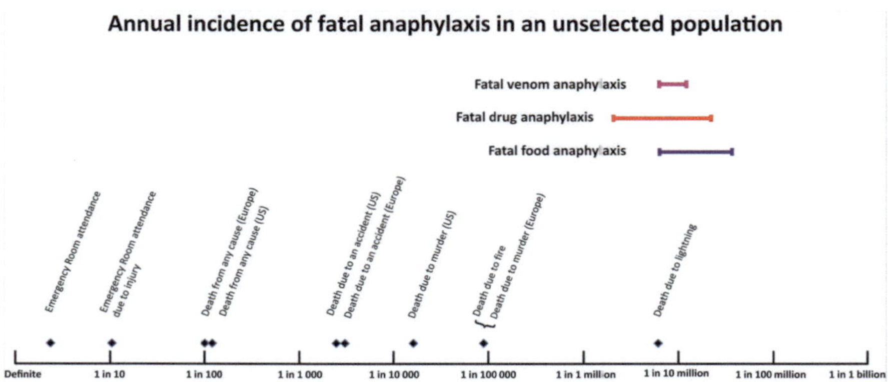

Fig. 14.4 Annual incidence of fatal anaphylaxis. Best estimates have fatal food anaphylaxis, fatal drug anaphylaxis, and fatal venom anaphylaxis approximately at rates of fatal lightning strike. (From Ref. [60])

surprising that anxiety has increased, though many factors may account for this. Ongoing reinforcement from schools and public venues about the potential for severe food allergy reactions is a double-edged sword, as awareness is crucial in identification and prevention (good), but may serve to ramp up anxiety (bad). These messages of possible fatal reaction are not tempered by the data, nor direct experience that families have with these reactions. For this reason, I typically want to perform oral food challenges if there is any diagnostic uncertainty, or we witnessed a gradual decrease of IgE to very low/undetectable levels over time and want to know if the reaction still occurs. One clinical example that we witness frequently is over-testing for food allergies by methods such as IgE levels, prior to introduction of these allergenic foods, often in the context of patients with eczema. The nature of eczema is such that many IgE levels will be positive without necessarily any clinical reactions to ingestion of these IgE-positive foods. It is for this reason (and results of the LEAP trial) that we encourage introduction of allergenic foods before pre-emptively testing for food allergies [61]. The LEAP trial indicated that 70–80% of food allergy (at least to peanut, but presumably all foods) could be prevented by early and frequent introduction of allergenic foods from age 8 months through 5 years. The amount of disease burden, costs, anxiety, and suffering that could be alleviated from this kind of prevention cannot be forgotten. Adopting approaches of frequent and regular exposure of children to allergenic foods is far more likely to improve the behavioral health issues related to food allergy more than other efforts, so we must always encourage appropriate food introduction practices.

More recently it has been posited that conditions requiring strict dietary adherence may be associated with eating disorders [62–66]. In the first systematic review of the association of eating disorders and food allergy, the rates of Avoidant/Restrictive Food Intake Disorder (ARFID) or anorexia nervosa/bulimia nervosa had some alarmingly high rates in the range of 0.8% to 62.9% [67]. While limited by small sample sizes, these associations require further study. While it may seem very logical that dietary restrictions or GI disease would put someone at higher risk for eating disorders, a recent cross-sectional analysis of 289 adults with achalasia, celiac disease, eosinophilic esophagitis, and inflammatory bowel disease by Fink and colleagues revealed that the Nine Item ARFID Screen may overestimate ARFID rates in these patients with these GI disorders [68]. This may be due to broad sample pool from which they were obtaining data, but more targeted study on food allergy, EoE, or FPIES would be helpful.

Oral Immunotherapy

One of the most impactful interventions for food allergy in recent years has been the expansion of oral immunotherapy (OIT) for food allergy. In essence, patients with food allergies begin to ingest once daily doses of their allergenic foods (avoiding all other instances of ingesting these foods other than for their OIT dose for the day), and over time, increase this daily dose until they reach a "maintenance dose." The initial doses are referred to as the "escalation" phase, and typically use only very tiny amounts of food allergen protein, to catch patients with very low thresholds for clinical food allergy reactions. The next phase is the "Build up" phase, and much like with other forms of allergy immunotherapy this is a gradual process. Most patients on OIT protocols increase their doses every 1–2 weeks until reaching the "maintenance" phase. After some time on maintenance dose, some forms of oral challenges are often delivered to assess for clinical reactions. This process is summarized in Fig. 14.5 [69].

In most cases, the patients are required to continue their once daily maintenance doses indefinitely, or risk decreasing their tolerance back to previous lower levels. The ultimate goal of all treatments for food allergy is to achieve is what's referred to as "sustained unresponsiveness," meaning patients will be able to eat the target food after long periods of avoiding it (not taking regular daily doses). There has not been widespread agreement on how long "sustained" really should be, given that the natural state of food tolerance is indefinite, though most studies use intervals of several weeks to months. This nebulous definition of sustained unresponsiveness will continue to confound this topic until such a time as large groups of patients can complete different lengths of maintenance phase followed by oral food challenges over the course of many years of avoidance. Preliminary data suggests that most patients will revert relatively quickly to baseline sensitivity to foods after discontinuing maintenance doses [70]. Thus, while the ultimate cure for food allergy of indefinite sustained unresponsiveness seems out of reach, a growing body of literature shows evidence that some semblance of sustained unresponsiveness is achievable [71].

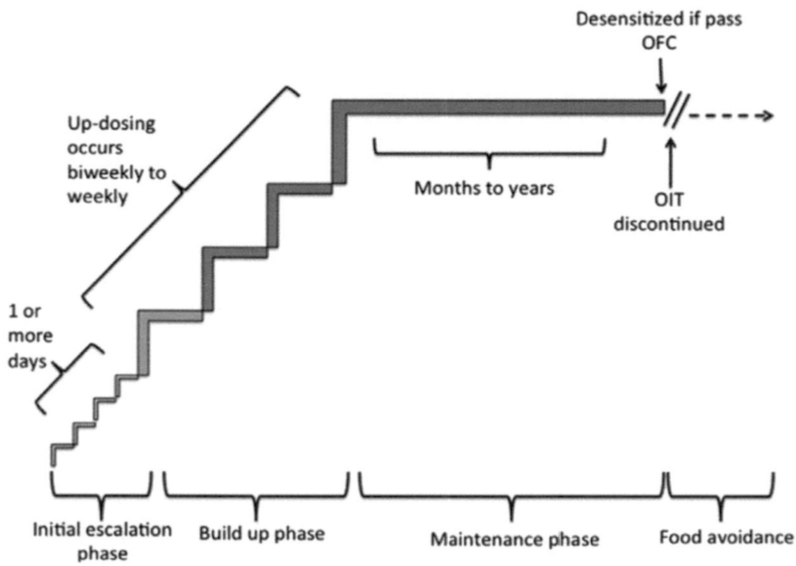

Fig. 14.5 Standard OIT protocol, where food-allergic patients are started from avoidance on the far left through initial escalation, build-up and then maintenance [69]

Risks of OIT include increased rates of anaphylaxis and epinephrine use, in addition to development of eosinophilic esophagitis [70, 72, 73]. It is important to remember that analyses of OIT compare multiple different protocols, and there may be significant variations in rates of adverse reactions during OIT. Despite these risks, many patients on OIT experience significant benefits, including the ability to tolerate accidental exposures and oral food challenges after some periods of maintenance dosing, accompanied by significant reduction in anxiety related to accidental food exposures and increased quality of life [70, 71]. Other methods of immunotherapy for food allergy exist, though OIT appears to be the most effective at present [74]. Due to the nature of OIT being a newer procedure and one that not all allergists were trained how to do, FDA approval for peanut OIT was achieved by Palforzia in 2020, and this has increased the amount of exposure that peanut OIT has achieved in the United States [75]. More recent adjuncts to treatment of food allergy include use of biologics, and omalizumab was the first biologic to achieve FDA approval for treatment of food allergy. While ongoing research is needed to define and compare optimal protocols, it appears that several options for treatment of food allergy are possible [76].

In our clinical experience with peanut OIT using PB2 powder (available at most grocery stores), the most common symptoms in build-up are not anaphylaxis or epinephrine use, but mild abdominal pain. Once on maintenance dose, the most difficult problem was patient adherence, either due to aversion to the daily doses (due to significant oral aversion and hating the taste) or desire to stop taking doses. We tended to see that older teenage patients, perhaps 15–18 years old, when pursuing OIT, had very good outcomes and adherence. We assume that part of this is due to them having more of a personal stake in reducing their own risks of food allergy reactions and anxiety. With younger patients driven largely by parental decisions, the outcomes could be varied. What is interesting about OIT is that it takes messaging about food avoidance that most patients have heard their whole life (which can be summarized by "avoid this or you could die") and instantly changes it—that now we must take a daily dose. Even with the most careful education, this contrast can be jarring for patients, and we certainly run the risk of developing some complex relationships with allergenic foods. Implementation of these OIT protocols should not be taken lightly, and patient/family selection must be careful. If proper precautions are taken, we have found peanut (and mixed tree nut) OIT to be a very rewarding process both for our patients and their families. Further research should aim to optimize the preferred OIT protocols to maximize success and minimize risk and cost.

Opportunities and Future Challenges

In the realm of behavioral health and allergy practice, the largest opportunities arise in minimizing and mitigating procedural anxiety and developing treatments and devices that allow optimal treatment of disease that are as painless as possible.

Further, developing more comprehensive, free preparation materials for patients and families about allergy procedures will also go a long way to make the experience more predictable [77]. Allergy practices must strive to implement the latest and most successful methods if they are to improve outcomes for children with allergic disease. Given the comorbidity of mental health and allergic disease, allergy practices must also have ways of screening and identifying patients that may need more evaluation and treatment for these conditions, whether for procedural anxiety, needle phobias, or other mood disorders. This does not always have to involve additional screening tools, though many are available and useful for this purpose.

The next most important area for opportunity is improving access to behavioral health generally. In-person behavioral health can be difficult for many communities. When adding the extra layer of complexity that Telehealth or other similar technologies require to reach more rural and under-resourced communities, health systems must continue to support and develop the infrastructure and reimbursement schemes needed to make these viable. Despite our best efforts, access via Telehealth has fragmented somewhat in the wake of COVID becoming more endemic (post-lockdowns), and we must continue to encourage creative solutions to connect behavioral health professionals to all specialty practices when needed. When both allergy practices and their behavioral health colleagues work together to minimize procedural anxiety and identify any comorbid conditions, outcomes for children will improve dramatically.

References

1. Zahran HS, Bailey CM, Damon SA, Garbe PL, Breysse PN. Vital signs: asthma in children – United States, 2001–2016. MMWR Morb Mortal Wkly Rep. 2018;67(5):149–55.
2. Shaw TE, Currie GP, Koudelka CW, Simpson EL. Eczema prevalence in the United States: data from the 2003 National Survey of Children's Health. J Invest Dermatol. 2011;131(1):67–73.
3. Odhiambo JA, Williams HC, Clayton TO, Robertson CF, Asher MI, Group IPTS. Global variations in prevalence of eczema symptoms in children from ISAAC phase three. J Allergy Clin Immunol. 2009;124(6):1251–8 e23.
4. Gupta RS, Springston EE, Warrier MR, Smith B, Kumar R, Pongracic J, et al. The prevalence, severity, and distribution of childhood food allergy in the United States. Pediatrics. 2011;128(1):e9–17.
5. Licari A, Magri P, De Silvestri A, Giannetti A, Indolfi C, Mori F, et al. Epidemiology of allergic rhinitis in children: a systematic review and meta-analysis. J Allergy Clin Immunol Pract. 2023;11(8):2547–56.
6. Conway AE, Verdi M, Kartha N, Maddukuri C, Anagnostou A, Abrams EM, et al. Allergic Diseases and Mental Health. J Allergy Clin Immunol Pract. 2024;12:2298.
7. Shulman ST. Clemens von Pirquet: a remarkable life and career. J Pediatric Infect Dis Soc. 2017;6(4):376–9.
8. Dunbar WP. The present state of our knowledge of hay-fever: being a paper presented at the berlin congress of the Royal Institute of Public Health. J Hyg (Lond). 1913;13(2):105–48.
9. Xu X, Li S, Chen Y, Deng X, Li J, Xiong D, et al. Association between allergic diseases and mental health conditions: an umbrella review. J Allergy Clin Immunol. 2024.

10. Oh H, Koyanagi A, DeVylder JE, Stickley A. Seasonal allergies and psychiatric disorders in the United States. Int J Environ Res Public Health. 2018;15(9):1965.
11. Lee GN, Koo HYR, Han K, Lee YB. Analysis of quality of life and mental health in patients with atopic dermatitis, asthma and allergic rhinitis using a nation-wide database, KNHANES VII. Allergy Asthma Immunol Res. 2022;14(2):273–83.
12. Hoggard M, Nocera A, Biswas K, Taylor MW, Douglas RG, Bleier BS. The sinonasal microbiota, neural signaling, and depression in chronic rhinosinusitis. Int Forum Allergy Rhinol. 2018;8(3):394–405.
13. Houghton V, Eiwegger T, Florsheim EB, Knibb RC, Thuret S, Santos AF. From bite to brain: Neuro-immune interactions in food allergy. Allergy. 2024;79:3326.
14. O'Donnell BF, Lawlor F, Simpson J, Morgan M, Greaves MW. The impact of chronic urticaria on the quality of life. Br J Dermatol. 1997;136(2):197–201.
15. Staubach P, Dechene M, Metz M, Magerl M, Siebenhaar F, Weller K, et al. High prevalence of mental disorders and emotional distress in patients with chronic spontaneous urticaria. Acta Derm Venereol. 2011;91(5):557–61.
16. Klinnert MD, Booster G, Copeland M, Darr JM, Meltzer LJ, Miller M, et al. Role of behavioral health in management of pediatric atopic dermatitis. Ann Allergy Asthma Immunol. 2018;120(1):42–8 e8.
17. Oland AA, Booster GD, Bender BG. Integrated behavioral health care for management of stress in allergic diseases. Ann Allergy Asthma Immunol. 2018;121(1):31–6.
18. Tversky JR, Chelladurai Y, McGready J, Hamilton RG. Performance and pain tolerability of current diagnostic allergy skin prick test devices. J Allergy Clin Immunol Pract. 2015;3(6):888–93.
19. Bernstein IL, Li JT, Bernstein DI, Hamilton R, Spector SL, Tan R, et al. Allergy diagnostic testing: an updated practice parameter. Ann Allergy Asthma Immunol. 2008;100(3 Suppl 3):S1–148.
20. McLenon J, Rogers MAM. The fear of needles: a systematic review and meta-analysis. J Adv Nurs. 2019;75(1):30–42.
21. Pfieffer J, Wehmeier K, Gee K, DeSanto T, Yousef E. Evaluation of pain-alleviating strategies during allergy shots (subcutaneous immunotherapy): a randomized controlled pilot study. Eur Ann Allergy Clin Immunol. 2024;56(3):128–36.
22. de Vos G, Shankar V, Nazari R, Kooragayalu S, Smith M, Wiznia A, et al. Fear of repeated injections in children younger than 4 years receiving subcutaneous allergy immunotherapy. Ann Allergy Asthma Immunol. 2012;109(6):465–9.
23. Noon L. Prophylactic inoculation against hay fever (historical document). Ann Allergy. 1955;13(6):713–6. passim
24. Johansson SGO. The discovery of IgE. J Allergy Clin Immunol. 2016;137(6):1671–3.
25. Cox L, Nelson H, Lockey R, Calabria C, Chacko T, Finegold I, et al. Allergen immunotherapy: a practice parameter third update. J Allergy Clin Immunol. 2011;127(1 Suppl):S1–55.
26. Parashar S, Pandya A, Portnoy JM. Pediatric subcutaneous allergen immunotherapy. Allergy Asthma Proc. 2022;43(4):286–91.
27. Schmidlin KA, Bernstein DI. Safety of allergen immunotherapy in children. Curr Opin Allergy Clin Immunol. 2023;23(6):514–9.
28. Cardona R, Lopez E, Beltran J, Sanchez J. Safety of immunotherapy in patients with rhinitis, asthma or atopic dermatitis using an ultra-rush buildup. A retrospective study. Allergol Immunopathol (Madr). 2014;42(2):90–5.
29. Temino VM, Wu P, Konig J, Fahrenholz JM. Safety of multiple aeroallergen rush immunotherapy using a modified schedule. Allergy Asthma Proc. 2013;34(3):255–60.
30. Epstein TG, Liss GM, Murphy-Berendts K, Bernstein DI. AAAAI and ACAAI surveillance study of subcutaneous immunotherapy, Year 3: what practices modify the risk of systemic reactions? Ann Allergy Asthma Immunol. 2013;110(4):274–8. 8 e1
31. Cox L. Accelerated immunotherapy schedules: review of efficacy and safety. Ann Allergy Asthma Immunol. 2006;97(2):126–37. quiz 37–40, 202

32. Traina G, Martelli A, Barberi S, Licari A, Marseglia GL, Tosca MA, et al. Evaluation of safety and tolerability of a rush up-dosing allergen-specific immunotherapy with grass pollen, birch, hazel, and alder allergoid in children with allergic rhinoconjunctivitis, with or without asthma. Acta Biomed. 2021;92(1):e2021037.
33. Pimentel RAGDR, Oliveira G, Ferreira Chaves Loureiro ELCS. Accelerated subcutaneous immunotherapy in pediatric population – systematic review. Pulmonology. 2018;24(3):182–93.
34. Creticos PS, Gunaydin FE, Nolte H, Damask C, Durham SR. Allergen immunotherapy: the evidence supporting the efficacy and safety of subcutaneous immunotherapy and sublingual forms of immunotherapy for allergic rhinitis/conjunctivitis and asthma. J Allergy Clin Immunol Pract. 2024;12(6):1415–27.
35. Wasserman RL, Cunningham-Rundles C, Anderson J, Lugar P, Palumbo M, Patel NC, et al. Systemic IgG exposure and safety in patients with primary immunodeficiency: a randomized crossover study comparing a novel investigational wearable infusor versus the Crono pump. Immunotherapy. 2022;14(16):1315–28.
36. Lumry W, Craig T, Anderson J, Riedl M, Li H, Tachdjian R, et al. Patient outcomes associated with subcutaneous C1INH prophylaxis for hereditary angioedema: a retrospective analysis. Allergy Asthma Clin Immunol. 2023;19(1):105.
37. Bernstein JA, Li HH, Craig TJ, Manning ME, Lawo JP, Machnig T, et al. Indirect comparison of intravenous vs. subcutaneous C1-inhibitor placebo-controlled trials for routine prevention of hereditary angioedema attacks. Allergy Asthma Clin Immunol. 2019;15:13.
38. Lumry WR, Craig T, Zuraw B, Longhurst H, Baker J, Li HH, et al. Health-related quality of life with subcutaneous C1-inhibitor for prevention of attacks of hereditary angioedema. J Allergy Clin Immunol Pract. 2018;6(5):1733–41 e3.
39. Orenius T, LicPsych SH, Mikola K, Ristolainen L. Fear of injections and needle phobia among children and adolescents: an overview of psychological, behavioral, and contextual factors. SAGE Open Nurs. 2018;4:2377960818759442.
40. McMurtry CM, Taddio A, Noel M, Antony MM, Chambers CT, Asmundson GJ, et al. Exposure-based Interventions for the management of individuals with high levels of needle fear across the lifespan: a clinical practice guideline and call for further research. Cogn Behav Ther. 2016;45(3):217–35.
41. Traina G, De Vuono A, Valluzzi R, Fierro V, Dahdah L, Artesani MC, et al. Tolerance of needle-less subcutaneous immunotherapy in children. Pediatr Allergy Immunol. 2020;31(5):582–5.
42. Lieberman P. Biphasic anaphylactic reactions. Ann Allergy Asthma Immunol. 2005;95(3):217–26. quiz 26, 58
43. Narchi H, Elghoudi A, Al Dhaheri K. Barriers and challenges affecting parents' use of adrenaline auto-injector in children with anaphylaxis. World J Clin Pediatr. 2022;11(2):151–9.
44. Gupta RS, Warren CM, Smith BM, Blumenstock JA, Jiang J, Davis MM, et al. The public health impact of parent-reported childhood food allergies in the United States. Pediatrics 2018;142(6).
45. Sampson HA, Aceves S, Bock SA, James J, Jones S, Lang D, et al. Food allergy: a practice parameter update-2014. J Allergy Clin Immunol. 2014;134(5):1016–25 e43.
46. Bird JA, Leonard S, Groetch M, Assa'ad A, Cianferoni A, Clark A, et al. Conducting an oral food challenge: an update to the 2009 adverse reactions to Foods Committee Work Group Report. J Allergy Clin Immunol Pract. 2020;8(1):75–90 e17.
47. Upton JEM, Bird JA. Oral food challenges: special considerations. Ann Allergy Asthma Immunol. 2020;124(5):451–8.
48. Golden DBK, Wang J, Waserman S, Akin C, Campbell RL, Ellis AK, et al. Anaphylaxis: a 2023 practice parameter update. Ann Allergy Asthma Immunol. 2024;132(2):124–76.
49. Greiwe J. Quality of life and psychological issues associated with food allergy. J Food Allergy. 2023;5(2):43–8.
50. Casale TB, Warren C, Gupta S, Schuldt R, Wang R, Iqbal A, et al. The mental health burden of food allergies: insights from patients and their caregivers from the Food Allergy Research & Education (FARE) Patient Registry. World Allergy Organ J. 2024;17(4):100891.

51. Drakouli AE, Kontele I, Poulimeneas D, Saripanagiotou S, Grammatikopoulou MG, Sergentanis TN, et al. Food allergies and quality of life among school-aged children and adolescents: a systematic review. Children (Basel). 2023;10(3).
52. Feng C, Kim JH. Beyond avoidance: the psychosocial impact of food allergies. Clin Rev Allergy Immunol. 2019;57(1):74–82.
53. Ferro MA, Van Lieshout RJ, Ohayon J, Scott JG. Emotional and behavioral problems in adolescents and young adults with food allergy. Allergy. 2016;71(4):532–40.
54. Herbert L, Shemesh E, Bender B. Clinical management of psychosocial concerns related to food allergy. J Allergy Clin Immunol Pract. 2016;4(2):205–13. quiz 14
55. Maciag MC, Herbert LJ, Sicherer SH, Young MC, Schultz F, Westcott-Chavez AA, et al. The psychosocial impact of food protein-induced enterocolitis syndrome. J Allergy Clin Immunol Pract. 2020;8(10):3508–14 e5.
56. Quigley J, Sanders GM. Food allergy in patients seeking mental health care: what the practicing psychiatrist should know. Curr Psychiatry Rep. 2017;19(12):99.
57. Ravid NL, Annunziato RA, Ambrose MA, Chuang K, Mullarkey C, Sicherer SH, et al. Mental health and quality-of-life concerns related to the burden of food allergy. Psychiatr Clin North Am. 2015;38(1):77–89.
58. Rubeiz CJ, Ernst MM. Psychosocial aspects of food allergy: resiliency, challenges and opportunities. Immunol Allergy Clin N Am. 2021;41(2):177–88.
59. Knibb RC, Herbert LJ, Jones CJ, Protudjer JLP, Screti C, Roleston C, et al. Global availability and uptake of psychological services for adults, caregivers and children with food allergy. Allergy. 2024;79(10):2787–97.
60. Turner PJ, Jerschow E, Umasunthar T, Lin R, Campbell DE, Boyle RJ. Fatal anaphylaxis: mortality rate and risk factors. J Allergy Clin Immunol Pract. 2017;5(5):1169–78.
61. Du Toit G, Roberts G, Sayre PH, Bahnson HT, Radulovic S, Santos AF, et al. Randomized trial of peanut consumption in infants at risk for peanut allergy. N Engl J Med. 2015;372(9):803–13.
62. Jafri S, Frykas TL, Bingemann T, Phipatanakul W, Bartnikas LM, Protudjer JLP. Food allergy, eating disorders and body image. J Affect Disord Rep. 2021:6.
63. Patrawala MM, Vickery BP, Proctor KB, Scahill L, Stubbs KH, Sharp WG. Avoidant-restrictive food intake disorder (ARFID): a treatable complication of food allergy. J Allergy Clin Immunol Pract. 2022;10(1):326–8 e2.
64. Proctor KB, Volkert VM, Klin A, Vickery BP, Sharp WG. The intersection of autism spectrum disorder, food allergy, and avoidant/restrictive food intake disorder: a clinical case study. J Pediatr. 2024;269:113965.
65. Su KW, Patil SU, Stockbridge JL, Martin VM, Virkud YV, Huang JL, et al. Food aversion and poor weight gain in food protein-induced enterocolitis syndrome: a retrospective study. J Allergy Clin Immunol. 2020;145(5):1430–7 e11.
66. Wroblewska B, Szyc AM, Markiewicz LH, Zakrzewska M, Romaszko E. Increased prevalence of eating disorders as a biopsychosocial implication of food allergy. PLoS One. 2018;13(6):e0198607.
67. Ciciulla D, Soriano VX, McWilliam V, Koplin JJ, Peters RL. Systematic review of the incidence and/or prevalence of eating disorders in individuals with food allergies. J Allergy Clin Immunol Pract. 2023;11(7):2196–207 e13.
68. Fink M, Simons M, Tomasino K, Pandit A, Taft T. When is patient behavior indicative of avoidant restrictive food intake disorder (ARFID) vs reasonable response to digestive disease? Clin Gastroenterol Hepatol. 2022;20(6):1241–50.
69. Burbank AJ, Sood P, Vickery BP, Wood RA. Oral immunotherapy for food allergy. Immunol Allergy Clin N Am. 2016;36(1):55–69.
70. Chu DK, Wood RA, French S, Fiocchi A, Jordana M, Waserman S, et al. Oral immunotherapy for peanut allergy (PACE): a systematic review and meta-analysis of efficacy and safety. Lancet. 2019;393(10187):2222–32.
71. Lodge CJ, Waidyatillake N, Peters RL, Netting M, Dai X, Burgess J, et al. Efficacy and safety of oral immunotherapy for peanut, cow's milk, and hen's egg allergy: a systematic review of randomized controlled trials. Clin Transl Allergy. 2023;13(7):e12268.

72. Lucendo AJ, Arias A, Tenias JM. Relation between eosinophilic esophagitis and oral immunotherapy for food allergy: a systematic review with meta-analysis. Ann Allergy Asthma Immunol. 2014;113(6):624–9.
73. Wilson BE, Sacta MA, Wright BL, Spergel J, Wolfset N. The relationship between eosinophilic esophagitis and immunotherapy. Immunol Allergy Clin N Am. 2024;44(2):281–91.
74. Alghamdi R, Alshaier R, Alotaibi A, Almutairi A, Alotaibi G, Faqeeh A, et al. Immunotherapy effectiveness in treating peanut hypersensitivity: a systemic review. Cureus. 2022;14(2):e21832.
75. Borne GE, Daniel CP, Wagner MJ, Plaisance CJ, Nolen A, Kelkar RA, et al. Palforzia for peanut allergy: a narrative review and update on a novel immunotherapy. Cureus. 2023;15(12):e50485.
76. Riggioni C, Oton T, Carmona L, Du Toit G, Skypala I, Santos AF. Immunotherapy and biologics in the management of IgE-mediated food allergy: systematic review and meta-analyses of efficacy and safety. Allergy. 2024;79(8):2097–127.
77. Farkas C, Solodiuk L, Taddio A, Franck L, Berberich FR, LoChiatto J, et al. Publicly available online educational videos regarding pediatric needle pain: a scoping review. Clin J Pain. 2015;31(6):591–8.

Chapter 15
Integrated Behavior Therapy in the Management of Childhood Obesity

Mahesh Shrestha, Maria Asif, and Conrad Czejdo

Obesity in Children and Its Contributors to Development

The incidence of childhood obesity has been increasing worldwide. The 2017–2018 National Health and Nutrition Examination Survey (NHANES) data showed that an estimated 19.3% of US children and adolescents aged 2–19 years have obesity [1]. Obesity among children and adolescents has increased significantly over the past few decades [2].

The causes are multifaceted and include a combination of genetic, environmental, and social factors. Key genes associated with increased obesity risk, including FTO (fat mass and obesity-associated), MC4R (melanocortin 4 receptor), and LEP (leptin). These genes have been linked to the regulation of satiety and the body energy balance [3–5]. Estimates of the heritability of obesity are as high as 70%, with a higher genetic influence during childhood [6, 7]. However, the rapid increase in recent years underscores how an "obesogenic" environment, characterized by excessive caloric intake and reduced physical activity, amplifies the genetic predisposition to obesity, creating a synergistic effect that drives the escalating rates of childhood obesity.

Socioeconomic factors also play a role in childhood obesity, with lower family income restricting access to healthy foods and safe places to be physically active [8]. Sleep pattern disparities among those with lower socioeconomic status (SES) are an additional risk factor for obesity development [9]. Exposure to pollution can also play a role, with the presence of endocrine-disrupting chemicals (e.g., phthalates) linked to metabolic disturbances, such as increased fat storage [10].

M. Shrestha (✉) · M. Asif · C. Czejdo
Department of Pediatrics and Adolescent Medicine, Western Michigan University School of Medicine, Kalamazoo, MI, USA
e-mail: Mahesh.shrestha@wmed.edu

R. W. Apple et al. (eds.), *Using Integrated Behavioral Health in Pediatric Practice*, https://doi.org/10.1007/978-3-031-85784-3_15

The impacts of childhood and adolescent obesity are profound, affecting not only physical health, but also psychological and social well-being. Among the many medical conditions associated with childhood obesity are type 2 diabetes, hypertension, sleep apnea, and non-alcoholic fatty liver disease [11]. Childhood obesity is also a risk factor for mental health issues including anxiety and depression [12]. Furthermore, obesity can affect a growing child's ability to interact with their peers and is associated with higher rates of being bullied and loneliness [13]. Distress from social exclusion can drive children towards unhealthy eating behaviors and continued weight gain.

An effective approach to childhood and adolescent obesity requires a comprehensive understanding of its many contributors as well as its wide-ranging impacts. An important component of strategies to reduce childhood obesity is collaboration among healthcare providers, policymakers, families, and schools. Such a multifaceted approach is necessary to prevent and treat childhood obesity comprehensively.

Obesity and Mental Health Disorders

Obesity is closely associated with mental health. Children and adolescents with obesity are significantly more likely to experience anxiety and depression [14–16]. Depression can lead to physical inactivity and disordered eating habits, resulting in an increase in body weight and mass. There is also a possibility that people don't feel like eating with a low mood and can sometimes lose weight. This is also seen with anxiety and panic attacks. Food intake is inherently associated with mood. Changes in mood especially depression and severe anxiety can really affect food intake. It is very important to address changes in mood when managing obesity. This is especially important when you are planning to start anti-obesity drugs. Targeting just rapid weight loss through use of anti-obesity medications without addressing the issues of severe anxiety and/or depression can lead to disordered eating habits and in future could lead to eating disorders.

There is a close association between increased incidence of ADHD in people with obesity and disordered eating [17]. Children with ADHD may not eat regular meals, especially skipping breakfast especially adolescents. Their hyperactivity and inattention coupled with impulsivity may act as a roadblock for ensuring proper time given to eating balanced food. Children especially adolescents tend to snack a lot limiting nutritious food intake and eating more junk foods leading to weight gain and obesity. Stimulants, which are the first-line medications for ADHD, also cause decreased appetite. Poor appetite due to suppressive nature of stimulants to decrease hunger is one of the main side effects of simulants. Appetite suppression is the most severe when the effect of medication is at its peak which usually happens during lunch. One of the advice physicians gives to their patients who use stimulants for ADHD knowing that it will suppress lunch at a good dose that they should be eating heavy breakfast and dinner with high calorie foods and the morning medication should always be taken after breakfast. Weight loss with stimulant use is expected, so some physicians use stimulants off-label for weight reduction in obese patients Esp Vyvanse (Lis-dexamphetamine) due to its approval for binge-eating disorder. Emotional eating, which refers to eating due to increased stress or emotions, also increases in people with significant obesity. This is very common in females, but it can happen to both sexes. People with emotional eating are not aware what they are eating, and it usually leads to eating high calorie foods leading to obesity.

A longitudinal relationship exists between eating disorders and mental health. Binge eating, which involves eating rapidly until feeling too full or sick, is prevalent in at least 30% of obese patients [18–19]. In contrast, bulimia nervosa, which is characterized by body shape distortion, weight, and self-induced vomiting, has a high incidence in the adolescent population [20]. Anorexia nervosa is another eating disorders where the patients do not eat food due to fear of being overweight. Anorexia nervosa can be so severe that it can lead to emaciation and rarely could lead to death due to starvation. Night eating syndrome and sleep-related eating disorders are other eating disorders are closely associated with mental health and obesity. Both binge eating and bulimia are both common in adolescents. Adolescence is a special phase of life and growth where they are very conscious of self-image and peer pressure. The desire to be slim and fit is very common at this age especially among female adolescents leading to eating too full or do self-induced vomiting or use laxatives to lose weight. There is a great role of behavioral therapy in treating eating disorders, as it is the only way to change disordered concepts of body shape and weight.

A child or an adolescent living with obesity can have different psychosocial consequences in the form of adverse childhood experiences and an increased level of stress. There is an increased incidence of bullying at school among obese patients. Weight-associated bullying is the most common form of bullying at school and can lead to negative emotional consequences, academic failure, and peer rejection. The overall quality of life is poor in patients with obesity.

Though not mental health related, obesity is now established to be causing more than 100 diseases. Common among them are due to endocrine changes called adiposopathy and due to physical response to increased weight called fat mass disease. The diseases that occur due to endocrine changes due to obesity are impaired fasting glucose, metabolic syndrome, hypertension, type 2 diabetes, non-alcoholic fatty liver disease (NAFLD), dyslipidemia, and gynecomastia. The diseases that are due to physical forces due to increased fat mass are asthma, sleep apnea, GERD, stress in weight bearing joints, slipped capital femoral epiphysis (SCFE), Blount's disease, osteoarthritis, and scoliosis. There are also psychological changes due to obesity besides the above-mentioned causes like eating disorders and anxiety/depression are isolation from peers, decreased ability to participate in normal childhood activities, and lack of social relationships.

Position Statements on Obesity from the American Academy of Pediatrics (AAP) and American Psychology Association (APA)

The guidance developmental panel after American Psychological Association in 2020 recommended that any patient from ages 2 to 20 years obesity or overweight, there were strong recommendation for provision of family-based multi component behavioral interventions with a minimum of 26 contact hours initiated at the earliest age possible [21]. Same views for echoed by the American Academy of Pediatrics in 2023 for having 26 contact hours which was shown in several different research to be effective for effective weight loss [22]. The AAP Also gave guidelines about creating intensive health behavior and lifestyle treatment centers named IHBLT centers which provided treatment programs that provided engaging, group-based physical activity, and nutritional programs. These programs are delivered either through academic medical centers or hospitals primary care offices or through local community partners like YMCA or parks. AAP also suggested that these programs should be face to face, multimodal, family based to be effective.

AAP and FDA have highlighted several lifestyle programs that could be helpful in reduction of weight. Some of the programs are Healthy weight clinic, Fit together, MEND (Mind, Exercise, Nutrition…Do It!) Program, Building Healthy Families, Family-based behavioral Treatment, Smart Moves for Kids/Bright Bodies, healthy weight and your child [23].

MEND Program is for families with children aged 2–13 years with 60–120-min sessions for ages 6–13 years and 90-min session for ages 2–5 years for 10 weeks where there is physical activity, healthy eating, and behavioral change sessions. Healthy Weight and your Child program is adapted from MEND, and it is given usually in YMCA locations as 25 2-h session spread over 4 months. Healthy Weight Clinic program covers more age ranges from 2 year still 18 years and have combination of individual visits, group sessions, and telephone check in for a year. Smart Moves for Kids includes age range 7–18 years, 2 45-min exercise sessions, and 1 40-min nutrition or behavior session in 12-week program. FBT is described above with 26 contact hours with psychologist virtually in-person visits or family visits. Building healthy Families is tailored for children aged 6–12 years with smaller communities and has 2 hourly weekly session for total 12 times over 3 months but can have refresher sessions up to a year. These programs are researched to be used in communities and have shown reasonable weight loss from different studies [22, 23].

Use of Complementary and Alternative Methods Associated with Mental Health in Managing Obesity

There are different complementary and alternative (CAM) methods tried in managing obesity. We will only discuss CAM methods that have associations with mental health. We will talk about few mind body interventions which were done through self-hypnosis, slow deep breathing, emotional freedom techniques (EFTs), and stress management techniques. Self-hypnosis also called relaxation mental imagery was studied by Cohen et al. [24] in 505 children and adolescents aged 3–20 years for behavioral encounters which ranged from obesity to bed-wetting and found it helps in resolving 51% of their problems and 32% shows a great improvement in their symptoms. Emotional freedom techniques (EFTs) are techniques that stimulate acupressure points by pressuring, tapping, or rubbing while focusing on situations that represent personal fear or trauma [25]. Stapleton et al. [26] compared 44 students (aged 12–18 years) with emotional freedom techniques versus controls for 6 weeks and found it improved eating habits and self-esteem which may ultimately help in weight-associated psychopathology. Another new mind-body intervention model is the Mandolean method whose principle is based on how people eat rather than how much by focusing on slow eating and small portion sizes. Hinton et al. [27] randomized 24 obese (BMI > 95 percentile) adolescents (aged 11–18 years) into standard care for 6 months in an obesity clinic versus standard care with short-term Mandolean training. Functional MRI data showed that the Mandolean training group had less activation of brain regions associated with food cue reactivity after a glucose meal and 22% less portion size, with no change in food satiety. Mindfulness and stress management have emerged as important ways to maintain healthy life with people with stressors and it also has shown promise with someone with chronic conditions like obesity. Paltoglou et al. [28] studied six Randomized Control Trials (RCTs) on mindfulness and stress management in children and adolescents with obesity. There were 112 subjects in the intervention group and 137 subjects in the control group aged 8–17.9 years and interventions for mindfulness-based stress reduction therapy for 8 weeks (3 studies), mindfulness-based group program for adolescents (1 study), and mindful eating program for 6 and 10 weeks (1 study each). They found reduced adiposity markers such as BMI and waist-to-hip ratio in four out of six studies and supported that mindfulness-based interventions can play a role in decreasing BMI. The Samueli Institute coined the term *Optimal Healing Environment* (OHE) in 2004 to describe a healthcare system designed to stimulate and support the inherent healing capacity of patients, families, and their care providers [29]. Freedman et al. [30] focused on the role and components of OHE that help in managing pediatric obesity: healing intention, healing relationships, health promotion and disease prevention, and healing spaces. Exergaming has been advocated by AAP as one of the strategies to do more activities in obese children. Exergaming, which is exercise while doing gaming, can be video game based, dance based, or other methods. Wagoner et al. [31] performed an RCT on group dance-based exergaming for 10 weeks on 40 obese adolescents aged 12 to 18 years and showed a significant increase in self-reported competence to exercise regularly and significant improvement in relations with parents. The National Center of Complementary and Integrative Health defines acupuncture as a technique in which practitioners insert fine needles into the skin to treat health problems. The needles used may be manipulated manually or stimulated with small electrical currents (electroacupuncture) [32]. Quan et al. [33] examined 1288 overweight/obese children and teenagers between 7 and 16 years using a RCT in China and Korea and found improved metabolic indicators with the use of acupuncture in BMI, body weight, and serum leptin. Hong Zhang et al. [34] evaluated acupuncture therapy in 10 healthy obese children and adolescents between ages 10 and 13 years daily for a month and observed statistically significant improvements in Body Mass Index (BMI) and abdominal visceral abdominal tissue using magnetic resonance imaging (MRI) scans. Yoga is an ancient Indian science that emphasizes the attainment of complete health and well-being through various physical postures (*asanas*), breathing techniques (*pranayama*), and meditation [35]. Jain et al. [36] conducted an RCT in 165 obese children (aged 8–15 years) and concluded that yoga with dietary modification was effective in reducing BMI and systolic blood pressure (BP) compared to the control group and was as effective as standard weight management for BMI reduction. Forseth et al. [37] conducted a pilot study with 30 adolescents aged 8–18 years with obesity and incorporated PHIT (promoting health in teens) yoga into a 12-week pediatric weight management intervention. Fifty-four percent of the children in the PHIT yoga cohort and 65% of the children in the PHIT Kids cohort attended 75% or more of the intervention sessions. The survey results support the view that PHIT yoga is acceptable to both caregivers and children. Improvements in BMI were observed in 50% of the children in each cohort, and five of the seven health habits improved in both groups.

Role of Integrated Behavioral Health in Obesity

Obesity is caused by multiple factors, including genetic disposition, lifestyle preferences, chronic diseases, and socioeconomic and environmental factors. Owing to its multifactorial nature, treatment requires an integrated approach that includes different modalities. The management of obesity involves preventive, diagnostic, and therapeutic strategies. According to the recent AAP guidelines, integrated behavioral therapy remains the mainstay of obesity management [22].

According to the Lexicon for Behavioral Health and Primary care integration, Integrated Behavioral health (IBH) is defined as "a practice team of primary care and behavioral health clinicians working together with patients and families, using a systematic and cost-effective approach to provide patient-centered care for a defined population" [38]. This approach is utilized to address multiple health issues, including health behaviors. Integrated behavioral therapy has shown successful results in managing childhood obesity, with the success rate of these therapies largely dependent on the number of hours spent per week. Most psychological treatments focus on the combination of three components: dietary modifications, increasing physical activity, decreasing sedentary lifestyle, and using behavioral strategies to expedite these changes.

Behavioral interventions include self-monitoring, goal setting, problem-solving, reinforcement of goal achievement, stimulus control, social support, and motivational techniques [39].

Integrated behavioral therapies are conducted in special clinics but studies have shown better outcome when performed in the primary care clinic [40]. Childhood obesity is an endemic health condition and integrated therapies have shown promising results in its management, specifically if it involves the patient, family, and siblings.

Different psychological approaches using IBH that can be used in management of obesity include motivational interviewing (MI), family-based behavioral treatment (FBT), cognitive behavior therapy (CBT), acceptance and commitment therapy (ACT), and dialectal behavior therapy (DBT).

Motivational Interviewing (MI)

Motivational interviewing is a method of counseling in which we identify the patient's motivation to change and work toward making that behavior change. Traditionally, it is the counselor or caregiver who illustrates the reason to change and how the change helps the patient, but in MI, we ask the patient why change is necessary, how motivated he is to make the change, and what are the things the patient himself can do to make the change. In pediatric obesity, MI has emerged as a good way for caregiver to start "change talk" and motivate patient to change key behaviors like decreasing sugary beverages, increasing physical activity, and targeting adequate sleep [41].

One of the important recommendations of the AAP obesity position statement in 2023 was to have 26 contact hours with more patients and caregivers for implementing a healthy lifestyle, which has been shown to be very effective in losing weight. MI could be a useful tool for caregivers to motivate them to follow up regularly [22].

Various techniques are used in motivational interviewing, most of which are based on resolving ambivalence. Some techniques used include asking open-ended questions, reflective listening, affirming, summarizing, and exploring discrepancies. It is a powerful tool when used properly and can cause significant behavioral changes in adolescents.

There are many ways for a physician to start the change talk for children and adolescents, and we are ready to start losing weight. One of the strategies used is to start engaging by getting to know the patient and understanding his issues and establishing a doctor-patient relationship using open-ended questions and not judgmental affirmations. The next step would be to focus on where there is a desire to change and the readiness of the adolescent. The process after focusing would be evoking when a behavior change is warranted where there is a lot of motivation provided. Finally, the last process would be planning where both the doctor and the patient have an effective plan formulated, ensuring that the patient understands the plan using a teach-back method and forms a smart goal, which means the goal should be specific, measurable, achievable, realistic, and timely [42].

Family-Based Behavioral Treatment (FBT)

Family-based behavioral treatment has emerged as an efficient method for providing weight-reducing interventions through counseling and education of patients and their caregivers. The counselor or coach teaches healthy eating habits and lifestyle changes through a series of visits with patients and their caregivers. It is recognized as one of the Intensive Health Behavioral Lifestyle treatments (IHBLT) programs approved by CDC and AAP to lose weight by encouraging 26 or more contact hours with providers face to face or virtually to teach and practice new behaviors in variety of setting to sustain healthy changes and lose weight [23]. Since most medical care occurs in primary care, it is important that these family-based behavioral treatments, which mostly occur in specialty clinics and psychologist offices, be integrated into primary care offices.

Several studies have been conducted to demonstrate its effectiveness. Epstein et al. studied 452 child-parent dyads in RCT trails over 24 months and found a statistically significant reduction of over 6% BMI reduction [40]. Staiano et al. studied barriers to programs like FBT with caretakers who listed lack of time, frustration with previous weight-loss unsuccessful attempts, and cost of healthy foods as barriers [43].

Cognitive Behavioral Therapy (CBT)

CBT works with the concept of making one aware of their own inaccurate distortions in thought processes and helps them cope and manage problems more effectively. Obesity is sometimes a result of disorganized food habits caused by poor perception of food and calories; therefore, CBT may be helpful. Obesity is associated with many other mental issues, such as anxiety, depression, and eating disorders, for which CBT has proven to be very effective.

Ricardo Dallo Grave et al. in 2020 discussed a RCT of 77 patients who used personalized CBT in obesity (CBT-OB) in real-world setting achieved 9.9% weight loss in 18 months [44]. Katja Kurnik Mesaric et al. did a meta-analysis of CBT for lifestyle changes in patients with obesity and type 2 diabetes and found a medium, significant effect of CBT interventions for weight loss and weight maintenance [45].

Acceptance and Commitment Therapy (ACT)

ACT works by accepting stressors as it is and learning to embrace them; however, it is unpleasant through mindfulness and commitment [46]. It is helpful in situations such as workplace stress, anxiety, and depression, which can be associated with obesity [47]. ACT could be beneficial in obesity management by helping a person gain acceptance of being obese rather than being anxious about it and then working towards reducing weight slowly.

Evan M Forman et al. studied 190 participants with overweight and obesity and randomized them to 25 sessions of ACT versus standard behavioral treatment (SBT) for a year and found greater 12-month weight loss versus SBT(13.3% vs. 9.8%) and more likely to maintain weight loss at 12 months (64% vs. 48.9%, $p = 0.04$) [48].

Dialectical Behavioral Therapy (DBT)

DBT combines aspects of CBT and ACT and is an evidence-based talk therapy that helps people cope with extreme scenarios, such as self-injurious behavior, by helping strategies and building new skills they feel are worth living. The four skills used in DBT were mindfulness, interpersonal effectiveness, emotion regulation, and distress tolerance. It is effective in conditions such as anxiety, borderline personality disorder, and depression, which may be associated with obesity.

DBT has been intensively studied for the treatment of eating disorders. Emily N Vogel et al. did a systematic review of CBT and DBT in adolescent eating disorders and found both studies ($n = 50$) were reasonably feasible, acceptable, and effective [49].

Models of Delivery of Integrated Behavioral Health (IBH)

IBH is the mode of providing behavioral therapy through clinical collaboration between physicians and mental health providers in an outpatient primary care setting. There are various ways to provide integrated behavioral health as described by Sullivan et al. [50].

IBH is usually provided either by having an independent or separate office location or by having the same office location, also called the collocation model.

The most common model currently in use is the separate office location with independent functions. In this model, the physician makes a referral, and the psychologist accepts the referral and provides consultation and management of the patient at a separate office location. The patient goes back to the original primary care provider once management is incomplete on the form of communication between the caregivers, usually in the form of written medical notes. Although it is easy to operate this model of care for IBH, it has the least integration among caregivers.

Another model of care where the office locations are separate but there is more integration in the care is the indirect consultation model. In this model, the psychologist provides advice and guidance to the physician about how to take care of the patient, along with the resources needed. Physicians are responsible for patient care and management. Communication between the psychologist and physician can occur in the form of telephone calls and collaborative venues. Christopherson et al. have discussed different ways physicians can use this indirect consultation model for issues such as sleep, eating, toileting, and other behavioral compliance issues [51, 52].

Collocation models can be performed in many ways, where the physician and psychologists are working in the same office space.

One is a specialty collocation model, similar to the separate office model described above; both physicians and psychologists see the patient at different times. There could be room for faster referral in the same office space, but there is little collaboration between the two. This model could also work for many conditions, such as substance abuse, but it could also be used for conditions such as pediatric obesity.

Another could be a chronic disease program that involves the management of chronic conditions such as diabetes or obesity. There could be more integration where the physician helps with the management of the disease, and the psychologist helps with education and motivation.

The third could be a collaborative team model with a high level of integration between psychologists and physicians by sharing responsibilities and making joint decisions. Commonly used in oncology programs, there could be a role in the integration of other conditions such as ADHD and obesity. This model champions the ideology of integrated behavioral health, which could be helpful for the effective management of complex conditions.

There could be a reverse collocation model in which the physician could be present in a mental health office with many psychologists [50].

Our pediatric academic center has a lot of experience in using integrated behavioral health in a specialty colocation model, where the physician makes a referral to the psychologist and sees the patient in the same office at different times. However, the most important model that we have used and had a good success is the chronic disease program model, where the patient is seen right after the physician visit to discuss any mental issues encountered during well child visits, such as obesity, chronic diseases like diabetes, and cystic fibrosis.

Conclusion

The incidence of obesity has been increasing worldwide. Obesity can cause many mental, physical, and social issues and contribute to mental health disorders such as anxiety, depression, and eating disorders. Integrated behavioral health, which combines primary care physicians and behavioral therapists, can be helpful in the management of obesity. Both AAP and APA endorse lifestyle behavioral programs with 26 contact hours with providers be mainstay of obesity management. Various CAM methods associated with mental health have been studied in managing obesity in children. IBH in the form of motivational interviewing, family-based behavioral therapy, CBT, ACT, and DBT could be implemented for obesity management. IBH can be provided via different delivery models using separate office locations or in the same collocation model. Working in the same collocation office with a collaborative team, where the primary care physician first sees the patient with obesity, followed by family-based behavioral therapy with a therapist, seems to be the ideal model for IBH care in obesity.

Acknowledgments We thank psychologists Dr. Katherine Beenen and Dr. Rebecca Rausch for their help in providing some resources for this chapter.

References

1. Fryar CD, Carroll MD, Afful J. Prevalence of overweight, obesity, and severe obesity among children and adolescents aged 2–19 years: United States, 1963–1965 through 2017–2018. NCHS Health E-Stats. p. 2020.
2. Abarca-Gómez L, Sein AA, Savva S, et al. Worldwide trends in body-mass index, underweight, overweight, and obesity from 1975 to 2016: a pooled analysis of 2416 population-based measurement studies in 128·9 million children, adolescents, and adults. Lancet. 2017;390:2627–42.
3. Farooqi IS, Langmack G, Prentice AM, Lawrence E, O'Rahilly S, Jebb SA, et al. Effects of recombinant leptin therapy in a child with congenital leptin deficiency. N Engl J Med. 1999;341:879–84.
4. Frayling TM, Groves CJ, Melzer D, et al. A common variant in the FTO gene is associated with body mass index and predisposes to childhood and adult obesity. Science. 2007;316:889–94.
5. Montague CT, Barnett AH, Soos MA, et al. Congenital leptin deficiency is associated with severe early-onset obesity in humans. Nature. 1997;387:903–8.
6. Herrera BM, Keildson S, Lindgren CM. Genetics and epigenetics of obesity. Maturitas. 2011;69:41–9.
7. Elks CE, Ong KK, Loos RJF, et al. Variability in the heritability of body mass index: a systematic review and meta-regression. Front Endocrinol. 2012;3:29. https://doi.org/10.3389/fendo.2012.00029.
8. Singh GK, Siahpush M, Kogan MD. Rising social inequalities in US childhood obesity, 2003–2007. Ann Epidemiol. 2009;20:40–52.
9. Jehan S, Myers AK, Zizi F, et al. Sleep health disparity: the putative role of race, ethnicity and socioeconomic status. Sleep Med Disord. 2018;2(5):127–33. https://doi.org/10.1016/j.sleep.2018.03.002.

10. Janesick A, Blumberg B. Endocrine disrupting chemicals and the developmental programming of adipogenesis and obesity. Birth Defects Res C. 2011;93:34–50.
11. Balasundaram P, Krishna S. Obesity effects on child health. StatPearls [Internet]. 2023; Available from: https://www.ncbi.nlm.nih.gov/books/NBK570613/
12. Kokka I, Bacopoulou F, Mourikis I. Psychiatric disorders and obesity in childhood and adolescence – a systematic review of cross-sectional studies. Children. 2023;10:285.
13. Harrist AW, Shriver LH, Swindle TM, et al. The social and emotional lives of overweight, obese, and severely obese children. Child Dev. 2016;87:1564–80.
14. Quek YH, Tam WWS, Zhang MWB, Ho RCM. Exploring the association between childhood and adolescent obesity and depression: a meta-analysis. Obes Rev. 2017;18:742–54.
15. Sanders RH, Han A, Baker JS, et al. Childhood obesity and its physical and psychological co-morbidities: a systematic review of Australian children and adolescents. Eur J Pediatr. 2015;174:715–46.
16. Schwartz BS, Glass TA, Pollak J, et al. Depression, its co-morbidities and treatment, and childhood body mass index trajectories. Obesity. 2016;24:2585–92.
17. Cortese S, Moreira-Maia CR, St. Fleur D, et al. Association between ADHD and obesity: a systematic review and meta-analysis. Am J Psychiatry. 2016;173:34–43.
18. Burrows T, et al. Food addiction, binge eating disorder, and obesity: is there a relationship? Behav Sci. 2017;7(3):40.
19. De Giuseppe R, et al. Pediatric obesity and eating disorders symptoms: the role of the multidisciplinary treatment. A systematic review. Front Pediatr. 2019;7:123.
20. Hail L, Le Grange D. Bulimia nervosa in adolescents: prevalence and treatment challenges. Adolesc Health Med Ther. 2018;9:11–6.
21. Guideline Development Panel for Treatment of Obesity, American Psychological Association. Summary of the clinical practice guideline for multicomponent behavioral treatment of obesity and overweight in children and adolescents. Am Psychol. 2020;75(2):178–88. https://doi.org/10.1037/amp0000530.
22. Hampl S, Sharifi M, Eneli I, et al. Clinical practice guideline for the evaluation and treatment of children and adolescents with obesity. Pediatrics. 2023;151 https://doi.org/10.1542/peds.2022-060640.
23. Centers for Disease Control and Prevention. CDC-recognized family healthy weight programs. Available from: https://www.cdc.gov/family-healthy-weight/php/recognized-programs/index.html
24. Kohen DP, Olness KN, Colwell SO, Heimel A. The use of relaxation-mental imagery (self-hypnosis) in the management of pediatric behavioral encounters. J Dev Behav Pediatr. 1984;5:21–5.
25. Wikipedia Contributors. Emotional freedom techniques. Wikipedia. The Free Encyclopedia. Available from: https://en.wikipedia.org/w/index.php?title=Emotional_Freedom_Techniques&oldid=1244239671. Accessed 6 Sept 2024.
26. Stapleton P, Chatwin H, William M, et al. Emotional freedom techniques in the treatment of unhealthy eating behaviors and related psychological constructs in adolescents: a randomized controlled pilot trial. Explore (NY). 2016;12:113–22. https://doi.org/10.1016/j.explore.2015.12.001.
27. Hinton EC, Birch LA, Barton JM, et al. Using neuroimaging to investigate the impact of Mandolean® training in young people with obesity: a pilot randomized controlled trial. BMC Pediatr. 2018;18:366. https://doi.org/10.1186/s12887-018-1342-1.
28. Paltoglou G, Chrousos GP, Bacopoulou F. Stress management as an effective complementary therapeutic strategy for weight loss in children and adolescents with obesity: a systematic review of randomized controlled trials. Children (Basel). 2021;8:670. https://doi.org/10.3390/children8080670.
29. Sakallaris BR, MacAllister L, Voss M, et al. Optimal healing environments. Glob Adv Health Med. 2015;4:40–5. https://doi.org/10.7453/gahmj.2015.043.

30. Freedman MR, Stern JS. The role of optimal healing environments in the management of childhood obesity. J Altern Complement Med. 2004;10(Suppl 1):S231–44.
31. Wagener TL, Fedele DA, Mignogna MR, et al. Psychological effects of dance-based group exergaming in obese adolescents. Pediatr Obes. 2012;7:e68–74. https://doi.org/10.1111/j.2047-6310.2012.00065.x.
32. National Center for Complementary and Integrative Health. Acupuncture: What You Need to Know. Available from: https://www.nccih.nih.gov/health/acupuncture-effectiveness-and-safety#:~:text=Acupuncture%20is%20a%20technique%20in,for%20at%20least%202%2C500%20years. Accessed 4 Aug 2024.
33. Quan T, Su Q, Luo Y, et al. Does acupuncture improve the metabolic outcomes of obese/overweight children and adolescents? A systematic review and meta-analysis. Medicine (Baltimore). 2023;102:e34943. https://doi.org/10.1097/MD.0000000000034943.
34. Zhang H, Peng Y, Liu Z, et al. Effects of acupuncture therapy on abdominal fat and hepatic fat content in obese children: a magnetic resonance imaging and proton magnetic resonance spectroscopy study. J Altern Complement Med. 2011;17:413–20. https://doi.org/10.1089/acm.2010.0322.
35. Nayak NN, Shankar K. Yoga: a therapeutic approach. Phys Med Rehabil Clin North Am. 2004;15:783–vi. https://doi.org/10.1016/j.pmr.2004.04.004.
36. Jain V, Kumar B, Sharma A, et al. A comprehensive yoga programme for weight reduction in children & adolescents with obesity: a randomized controlled trial. Indian J Med Res. 2022;155(3&4):387–96. https://doi.org/10.4103/ijmr.IJMR_525_20.
37. Forseth B, Hampl S, Dreyer Gillette M, et al. Incorporating yoga into a pediatric weight management program: a pilot study. Child Obes. 2022;18(1):67–71. https://doi.org/10.1089/chi.2021.0114.
38. Peek CJ. National Integration Academy Council. Lexicon for behavioral health and primary care integration: concepts and definitions developed by expert consensus. AHRQ Publication No. 13-IP001-EF. Rockville: Agency for Healthcare Research and Quality; 2013.
39. Altman M, Wilfley DE. Evidence update on the treatment of overweight and obesity in children and adolescents. J Clin Child Adolesc Psychol. 2015;44(4):521–37. https://doi.org/10.1080/15374416.2014.963854.
40. Epstein LH, Wilfley DE, Kilanowski C, et al. Family-based behavioral treatment for childhood obesity implemented in pediatric primary care: a randomized clinical trial. JAMA. 2023;329(22):1947–56. https://doi.org/10.1001/jama.2023.8061.
41. Resnicow K, Davis R, Rollnick S. Motivational interviewing for pediatric obesity: conceptual issues and evidence review. J Am Diet Assoc. 2006;106(12):2024–33.
42. Miller WR, Rollnick S. Motivational interviewing: helping people change. 3rd ed. New York: Guilford Press; 2013.
43. Staiano AE, Marker AM, Comeaux J, et al. Family-based behavioral treatment for childhood obesity: caretaker-reported barriers and facilitators. Ochsner J. 2017;17(1):83–92.
44. Dalle Grave R, Calugi S, Sartirana M. Personalized cognitive-behavioural therapy for obesity (CBT-OB): theory, strategies and procedures. BioPsychoSocial Med. 2020;14:5. https://doi.org/10.1186/s13030-020-00177-9.
45. Mesarič KK, Pajek J, Zakrajšek BL, et al. Cognitive behavioral therapy for lifestyle changes in patients with obesity and type 2 diabetes: a systematic review and meta-analysis. Sci Rep. 2023;13:2987. https://doi.org/10.1038/s41598-023-49838-z.
46. Plumb JC, Stewart I, Dahl J, et al. In search of meaning: values in modern clinical behavior analysis. Behav Anal. 2009;32(1):85–103. https://doi.org/10.1007/BF03392177.
47. White K, Stetson L, Hussain K. Integrated behavioral health role in helping pediatricians find long-term mental health interventions with the use of assessments. Pediatr Clin N Am. 2021;68(3):685–705. https://doi.org/10.1016/j.pcl.2021.02.006.
48. Forman EM, Wyckoff EP, Thomas JG, et al. Acceptance-based versus standard behavioral treatment for obesity: results from the mind your health randomized controlled trial. Obesity. 2016;24:2050–6.

49. Vogel EN, Singh S, Accurso EC. A systematic review of cognitive behavior therapy and dialectical behavior therapy for adolescent eating disorders. J Eat Disord. 2021;9:131. https://doi.org/10.1186/s40337-021-00461-1.
50. Sullivan AW, Lozowski-Sullivan S. The continuum of intervention models in integrated behavioral health. Pediatr Clin N Am. 2021;68:551–61.
51. Christophersen E, Mortweet SL. Treatments that work with children: empirically supported strategies for managing childhood problems. Washington, DC: American Psychological Association; 2001.
52. Christophersen E. Pediatric compliance: a guide for the primary care physician. New York: Plenum; 1994.

Chapter 16
Integrated Behavioral Health in a Sleep Subspecialty Clinic

Katie White, Caroline Miller, and Carlynn Gasser

Introduction

It is widely known, across medical and mental health disciplines, and it is the position of the American Academy of Sleep Medicine "that sleep is essential to health" and the lack thereof can negatively affect an individual's daily life [1–3]. Poor sleep can impact cognitive functioning, behavior, mood, and mental health and can lead to a higher risk of being involved in accidents [1, 3]. Sleep problems are further complicated when they occur in the pediatric population, as these symptoms can be caused or influenced by a number of factors from a child's microsystem, mesosystem, and macrosystem [4]. This illustrates why assessing sleep health and providing appropriate sleep interventions are vital for the well-being of all [1]. These concerns will likely be encountered first by a patient's primary care physician (PCP), with pediatric patients' symptoms usually being reported by parents. However, PCP's often do not feel comfortable discussing, treating, and managing sleep related disorders due to a lack of sleep-related medical training, complicated by a difficulty with prioritizing information gathered during appointments [3, 5]. When a PCP does not feel these symptoms can be resolved within a general pediatric office, or

K. White (✉)
Division of Pediatric Psychology, Western Michigan Homer Stryker M.D. School of Medicine, Kalamazoo, MI, USA
e-mail: Kathryn.white@wmed.edu

C. Miller
Fielding Graduate University, Santa Barbra, CA, USA
e-mail: carolinemiller@fielding.edu

C. Gasser
Western Michigan Homer Stryker M.D. School of Medicine, Kalamazoo, MI, USA
e-mail: carlynn.gasser@wmed.edu

R. W. Apple et al. (eds.), *Using Integrated Behavioral Health in Pediatric Practice*, https://doi.org/10.1007/978-3-031-85784-3_16

feel more specialized assessment is needed, a referral to a sleep specialty clinic is warranted.

The existence of sleep specialty clinics began around the 1970s and is now a core component of almost all major US medical centers [6]. Treatment of sleep disorders is best coordinated through an interdisciplinary approach, wherein physicians diagnose the observed medical disorder and psychologists evaluate and provide treatment for the sleep concerns [7]. Because sleep disturbances co-occur with other mental health disorders and are often maintained by behavioral elements in young children, behavioral and cognitive interventions are first line approaches to addressing these symptoms [3]. An Integrated Behavioral Health (IBH) specialist can be integrated into any subspecialty clinic. Because many of the interventions used for sleep-related concerns are behavior and/or psychology based, we suggest these therapeutic interventions are best provided by psychologists. Research suggests that having a multidisciplinary approach within a sleep specialty setting provides the most well rounded care to patients and their families, though not all centers utilize this method [6, 7]. Including psychologists into the medical setting can help bridge the gap between what physicians are lacking in the identification, prevention, and treatment of sleep disorders [5]. This chapter will provide information on the role of integrated behavioral health in a sleep subspecialty clinic, an overview of pediatric sleep, a few common pediatric sleep disorders, and associated interventions/therapies among children and adolescents.

Overview of Pediatric Sleep

Children spend nearly 40% of their day asleep, and an estimated 25–40% of the pediatric population experience some type of sleep difficulty [2]. However, research has determined that sleep disorders diagnosed in a primary care setting are lower than prevalence rates would suggest [5]. Sleep patterns change rapidly from infancy, through adolescence, and into adulthood; as such, sleep in a pediatric population conceptually differs from adult sleep [4]. Further, this population typically has varying levels of control over their sleep hygiene, with less control occurring early in life [4]. The American Academy of Pediatrics endorsed the following recommendations from the American Academy of Sleep Medicine regarding pediatric sleep: within a 24 h period, infants ages 4–12 months need 12–16 h of sleep (including naps); toddlers ages 1–2 years need 11–14 hours (including naps); toddlers ages 3–5 years need 10–13 h (including naps); children ages 6–12 years need 9–12 h; and teenagers ages 13–18 years need 8–10 h of sleep [8]. Specifically with the pediatric population, deficits in sleep can result in problems with attention, behavioral issues, and learning problems, and can increase the risk of injuries, accidents, depression, obesity, and diabetes [5, 8].

Beginning at infancy, sleep is one of the most robust contributors of health and development. Newborn infants sleep around 12 hours per day, with those born premature sleeping even more. Newborns do not have an established sleep pattern and will therefore wake and sleep many times throughout the day and night [9]. Sleep is especially important during the first 2 years of life, with a robust body of research demonstrating that sleep contributes significantly to cognitive development, particularly in the areas of memory, language, and executive functioning, as well as physical growth [9]. By the time the child enters school, they should no longer require a daytime nap but do still need approximately 10 h of sleep per night for adequate functioning and health. In this population, there are many barriers to adequate sleep. Environmental factors, like noise and light pollution, parental factors, like work schedules and bedtime interactions, and individual factors, like temperature and sense of safety, can all contribute to disturbances in sleep [10]. For this age group, parents are heavily involved in all aspects of their child's sleep routine, from setting the bedtime, ensuring appropriate hygiene, observing sleep onset, and participating in sleep disruptions and awakenings [4]. Therefore, parental involvement in ensuring quality sleep is paramount.

As a child approaches adolescence, a strive for autonomy becomes greater and social, cognitive, behavioral, and academic demands increase, which directly impacts their sleep [11, 12]. Between middle and high school, an adolescent will lose around 90 min of sleep each year [12]. The CDC reports on average, $\frac{2}{3}$ of 9–12th graders get around 7 h of sleep a night [12]. Emerging research has also suggested that sleep is likely important for an adolescents brain development [12]. Specifically for adolescents, insufficient sleep is associated with poor emotional functioning, an increase in depressive symptoms including feelings of hopelessness, an increase in anxiety, and an increase in risk taking behavior to include substance use (e.g., nicotine and alcohol) and behaviors that could impact driving (e.g., texting) [12]. A meta-analysis found that good sleep hygiene results in shortened sleep latency, earlier bedtimes when combined with physical activity, and longer sleep length when combined with parental set bedtimes [13]. The same research found a myriad of factors that contribute to poor sleep hygiene, to include internet use, video gaming, and computer/phone usage, with negative home environments and evening light serving as general sleep hygiene risk factors [13]. Together, these factors threaten the quality and duration of sleep. Negative factors of sleep can begin as insufficient sleep and without intervention, it is possible that these disturbances may become a sleep-related disorder causing long-term impacts on functioning into adulthood.

Role of an Integrated Behavioral Health Specialist in Sleep Subspecialty Clinic

Sleep disorders are common in childhood and adolescence, and behavioral interventions should be a core component of any treatment plan targeting sleep disturbances. Many behavioral interventions can and should be delivered by the patient's primary care or sleep medicine physician, but may also be delivered by nurses, occupational therapists, and other trained staff [1, 11]. Behavioral interventions can also be delivered in a variety of modes, including printed material, video meetings, phone calls, and group classes [11]. At their most basic, strategies for improving sleep should provide education about the importance of sleep on the child's health and instructions for implementing behavioral interventions [11]. These features are well within the scope of a sleep medicine physician to deliver. However, mental and behavioral health considerations should also be a key element of all sleep-related disturbances given the significant overlap between sleep and mood, functioning, neurodevelopment, and cognitive and behavioral problems [1]. As such, sleep medicine physicians should recognize when a patient requires a higher level of psychological care and make the appropriate referral. Most pediatric sleep disturbances are resolved in a relatively short time period, with significant improvement observed in six meetings or less [11]. Because of this, the integration of behavioral health specialists (i.e., psychologists) into this setting is suggested. Integrated Behavioral Health (IBH) is achieved in 0–6 sessions with solution-focused interventions designed to help improve presenting concerns. IBH can be an integral part of a multidisciplinary team approach in developing appropriate interventions for patients as they provide input in other factors that may influence sleep problems. They can also give and interpret psychological assessments to determine an appropriate diagnosis, assess for any comorbid factors and/or diagnoses, and provide follow-up data to determine intervention efficacy.

Because there are numerous factors that impact sleep across a child's lifespan, with psychological and behavioral factors being highly comorbid, sleep disturbances are best treated using an interdisciplinary approach. Addressing sleep concerns from both a medical and behavioral health perspective can be accomplished when psychology services are readily available in the sleep subspecialty clinic. Referrals to outpatient psychological services may be an option, but this can result in lengthy wait lists or barriers to finding providers that are within the family's insurance network. If these services are available through co-located consultation or fully integrated care, parents and families will receive same-day assistance and be provided with tangible interventions that they can implement that very night. Although a full review of the literature examining efficacy of IBH in sleep subspecialty clinics is outside the scope of this review, a meta-analysis of 16 studies representing 2133 participants (ages 1–17.9) evaluated behavioral interventions for pediatric insomnia and found robust statistical evidence for the efficacy of these interventions for improving sleep-onset latency, diminishing night time wakening, and reducing night time wakening duration, for very young children (ages 0–5 years) [14]. This meta-analysis also found that behavioral intervention diminished night time wakening duration and improved sleep efficiency for children and adolescents (ages 6–17.9 years), though the quality of studies is low for older children and adolescents. Further, a 2015 meta-analysis found that integrating behavioral health services into primary care led to an improvement in overall behavioral health outcomes for youth [15]. This evidence indicates that behavioral interventions for children with sleep disorders, receiving subspecialty care, would result in improved sleep quality and quantity. This illustrates the importance of psychology within a sleep subspecialty clinic. The remainder of this chapter will discuss common sleep disorders, syndromes and disturbances from infants to early childhood and into adolescence, and evidenced-based psychological interventions.

Infant and Early Childhood

Sleep Disorders and Disturbances

Many of the most common sleep disturbances experienced by children do not have a corresponding diagnosis in the DSM-V-TR, but are nonetheless significantly impactful to child development. Furthermore, disturbances in sleep can be extremely disruptive to the entire family and impact parent and sibling emotional and functional wellbeing. As such, sleep disturbances are clinically evaluated on the basis of age, development, severity, frequency, and degree of functional impairment to both the child and the family unit [14]. Because many sleep disturbances and disorders may have an underlying medical pathology, considerations for physical health must be examined when first evaluating changes or challenges in sleep behavior. In the absence of a medical cause, sleep disturbances and disorders are best conceptualized as behavioral concerns.

Understanding the nature of sleep disturbances and disorders first requires the clinician to evaluate where in the sleep cycle the disturbance occurs. To this end, there are two main categories of sleep disturbances: dyssomnia, which includes difficulties with initiating sleep, maintaining sleep, or excessive sleepiness; and parasomnia, which are disturbances that occur predominantly while the child is sleeping but can also occur during the transition between sleep and wake and include physical behaviors or phenomena like sleepwalking and night terrors [16]. Determining where in the sleep cycle the disturbance occurs is necessary for the proper conceptualization of the nature of the sleep concern and will guide intervention strategies. A central challenge to recognizing and correctly identifying sleep disturbances for infants and young children is their diminished ability to accurately self-report their sleep experiences [4]. Therefore, evaluations of adequate and appropriate sleep for this population are almost entirely observations made by parents and other adults.

Frequent Awakening with Excessive Crying (Infants)

Sleep patterns established during infancy can predict and influence sleep behavior throughout early childhood, so addressing sleep disturbances during infancy is important for preventing longer term sleep problems. For infants, frequent nighttime awakening, which is often accompanied by excessive crying, is a common issue experienced by up to 30% of infants [17, 18]. After 6 months of age, frequent awakening with excessive crying is associated with significant impairment in infant and family functioning [18]. Because frequent awakening requires parental intervention, like rocking or holding the infant, this disturbance is conceptualized as a disorder of sleep-onset [19]. For the purposes of this review, this disturbance is characterized by an absence of an obvious need (e.g., food, diaper change) and a rule out of a medical pathology (e.g., acid reflux). Furthermore, the frequency of typical nighttime awakening varies based on the age of the infant, such that the majority of infants aged 6 months wake more than once per night, but by 18 months the majority of infants experience no nocturnal wakening [20]. Therefore, there is no numerical threshold of nighttime awakening which constitutes describing this phenomenon as a disorder; rather, evaluation of this disturbance includes not just how frequently the infant awakens, but the intensity of their distress, the time duration until sleep is again obtained, and the functional impairment of the family.

Bedtime Resistance

Bedtime resistance, sometimes referred to as bedtime stalling or bedtime refusal, is understood to be maintained by inadequate limit-setting by the parent or caregiver [19]. Beginning at around 2 years of age, this disturbance is characterized by a broad range of behavior exhibited by children, from verbal protests to tantrum-throwing [19]. Bedtime resistance includes delay tactics, like requesting another bedtime story or prolonging the bedtime routine, and removal tactics after lights out, like getting out of bed to request water [19]. Bedtime resistance typically occurs when parents maintain poor or inconsistent expectations for bedtime [19]. For example, parents that allow their children to engage in a preferred activity (e.g., watching television) until bedtime, or allow children to stay up later on weekends, risk establishing poor boundaries for bedtime, which children find difficult to follow and even confusing to understand. While not all children in these environments develop bedtime resistance, understanding the bedtime expectations in the home which maintain resistance for children with this disturbance is key to appropriately conceptualizing this pathology.

Nightmares, Night Terrors, and Bedtime Fears

Nightmares are disorders of partial arousal and occur during REM sleep. Repeated and frequent nightmares that are severe enough to cause sleep disturbances affect up to 15% of children, with as many as 85% of children ages 7–9 endorse experiencing occasional nightmares [16, 21]. Nightmares are different from night terrors because they are accompanied by less panic, the child is more easily awakened, the child is more likely to be able to recall the subject/nature of the dream, and are typically observed during the last third of the sleep cycle [16]. Nightmares are disruptive to sleep because they cause significant emotional distress that can preclude the resumption of sleep, and fear of experiencing nightmares can delay sleep onset.

Night terrors are disorders of arousal and are typically experienced as intense and dramatic displays of panic, screaming or crying, extreme agitation, and autonomic responses, typically lasting 3–5 min [16]. As many as nearly 40% of children ages 2.5–6 years old experience night terrors [16]. These disturbances typically occur within the first third period of the sleep cycle during slow-wave sleep and are characterized by a lack of alertness, responsiveness, and memory of the event [16, 21]. The frequency of night terrors tends to decrease with age, with approximately 0.6% of children experiencing night terrors past the age of 11 [16].

While bedtime fears are exceedingly common, with as many as approximately 85% of children ages 7–9 experiencing at least mild bedtime fears, for about 20% of children, bedtime fears are severe enough to cause sleep disturbances [22]. Bedtime fears include a variety of worries that children experience prior to falling asleep. These worries include fear of the dark, fear of "monsters," fear of nightmares, and anxiety about being separated from parents. Bedtime fears are associated with diminished sleep quality, more frequent nocturnal awakening, and decreased overall sleep time [22]. Furthermore, bedtime fears are distressing to the child, who may experience significant anticipatory anxiety in the hours prior to bedtime and elevated anxiety throughout the night, and can also be disruptive to the family [22]. Conceptualization of this disturbance should include consideration for the subjective level of distress reported by the child and parent, degree of functional impairment, and impact on sleep quality and quantity.

Nocturnal Enuresis (Bedwetting)

Nighttime bedwetting, or nocturnal enuresis, occurs when a child repeatedly voids their bladder into their bed or clothes during sleep [23]. Importantly, a child must be at least 5 years of age to diagnose nocturnal enuresis, as intermittent involuntary nighttime elimination is developmentally typical prior to age five [23]. Bedwetting typically occurs during the first one-third period of sleep, during slow-wave sleep. To be formally diagnosed with nocturnal enuresis, a child must have at least two instances of bedwetting per week for at least three consecutive months [23]. If a child does not meet this frequency criteria, a diagnosis may still be warranted if significant impairment in an important area of functioning, like social or academic performance, is reported. This sleep disorder is common, with 5%–10% of 7 year old children experiencing regular bedwetting [24]. As with other sleep disturbances, nighttime bedwetting may be caused by an underlying medical disorder like diabetes or a seizure disorder, so nocturnal enuresis can only be diagnosed after a potential medical cause has been ruled out.

Interventions

Because parents are heavily involved in all areas of their child's sleep routine, it follows that behavioral interventions for sleep disturbances are carried out by the parents. As such, clinicians must provide adequate education to the parents to ensure their ability to implement interventions in the home. This may include providing rationale for behavior interventions, emphasizing the importance of consistency and follow through, providing detailed instructions for integrating interventions into the established routine, providing suggestions for modifying interventions to suit parents' unique needs or circumstances, and allowing the parent to ask clarifying questions.

Extinction

Extinction emphasizes reducing inadvertent parental reinforcement of problematic child sleep behavior by targeting the behaviors that are maintained through positive or negative parental attention. To be clear, this intervention requires the parent to change their own behavior. For example, infant and child bedtime resistance in the form of excessive crying or screaming is reinforced by the parent entering the child's room and talking to or soothing the child. The extinction process therefore requires the parent to put the child to bed and ignore the child's cries or screams unless the parent determines that attention is absolutely necessary [17]. This process is sometimes referred to as "planned ignoring." By not responding to the child's inappropriate bids for attention, the parent stops reinforcing poor behavior. A significant drawback to this intervention is that this method can be distressing to both children and parents. Unless the parent can withstand the increasingly intense attempts by the child to receive attention, there is a risk that the parent will reinforce more intense behavior. In addition, post-extinction response bursts are common, and some literature suggests that planned ignoring can be harmful and therefore it is unethical [21]. To this end, a practitioner can integrate several modifications into the extinction process to mitigate risk for harm. These strategies include minimal checking, where a parent will check on their child at regular intervals (5–20 min apart) for brief moments to ensure the child's safety and to ease parental anxiety; parental presence, where a parent physically sleeps in the child's room but in a separate bed for the first week of extinction but refrains from interacting with the child at all, even if the child awakens at night; and graduated extinction with fading, where a parent either systematically increases their response latency to infant and child crying (5 min intervals recommended) or they systematically decrease the time they spend with the child after responding and decreasing the reward value for behavior [17]. These modifications improve intervention efficacy and reduce harm.

Scheduled Awakening

Another intervention strategy is scheduled awakening. This intervention can be used in treatment of a broad range of sleep disturbances, to include night terrors, bedwetting, and frequent nighttime arousal. For infants and children who frequently wake through the night, this strategy can help reduce the frequency and duration of child awakening. The parent must first have an understanding of when their child typically awakens or when their sleep disturbance (e.g., night terrors, bedwetting) occurs, so the clinician should instruct the parent to observe and document the times that their child awakens through the night [16]. After this data is known, the parent is then instructed to awaken their child 15–30 min before the child usually awakens themselves [16]. This involves rousing the child to the point of full consciousness, followed by allowing the child to return to sleep. For bedwetting, the parent directs the child to eliminate in the bathroom before returning to sleep. For night terrors, which can be precipitated by overtiredness, there is a risk that scheduled awakening can actually worsen night terrors, though in most cases improvement is achieved in 4–8 weeks [16, 21]. With time, the frequency of scheduled awakening is gradually decreased to zero, whereupon the child is sleeping regularly through the night.

Stimulus Control

Stimulus control is used to address bedtime resistance, bedtime fears, delays in sleep onset, and excessive daytime sleepiness due to poor sleep quality. This strategy involves evaluating the physical environment and bedtime routine, and modifying both to prompt sleep onset in a more predictable and regular pattern [11]. There are several different methods of integrating stimulus control. For infants and toddlers with excessive delays in sleep onset, parents are suggested to observe the child and document the average sleep onset time. Once this data is known, parents are then instructed to begin their sleep routine 15–30 min prior to regular sleep time until the existing bedtime is regularly achieved [11]. Parents are then instructed to progressively begin the bedtime routine earlier, in 30 min increments, until the desired bedtime is reliably achieved. This practice is sometimes referred to as "faded bedtime" [11]. For parents of older children, stimulus control strategies include disallowing the child to lay or be in their bed for activities other than sleep, engaging in only calming activities in the hour before sleep, and removing the child from the bed to engage in a calming activity if sleep onset isn't achieved within 20 min, returning to bed only after the child indicates tiredness [11]. Stimulus control may also be used for children who endorse experiencing bedtime fears. Reducing the salience of nighttime crutches (e.g., dimming nightlights, reducing parental time spent in the room), teaching relaxation techniques, and reducing or removing specific anxiety-inducing objects may all reduce bedtime fears and prompt appropriate sleep onset [11, 25].

Self-Control Strategies and Systematic Desensitization

For parents who have children with excessive bedtime fears, self-control strategies and systematic desensitization help reduce night time anxiety. Self-control strategies refer to a collection of strategies aimed at increasing the child's self-esteem and self-efficacy. This includes things like teaching relaxation techniques (e.g., age-appropriate instruction in diaphragmatic breathing, like "big belly breathing"), guided imagery through storybook characters (e.g., stories of characters facing their fears, etc.), and other pleasant imagery, and positive self-talk (e.g., "I am brave") [16, 21]. These interventions should be accompanied by positive reinforcement, which can be in the form of praise, tokens, stickers, etc. Self-control strategies like guided imagery and relaxation are also recommended for treatment for children who experience nightmares to help prompt a return to sleep [16].

Bedwetting Alarms

There are many behavioral interventions that help reduce the frequency of nighttime bedwetting. Monitoring and restricting a child's fluid intake prior to bedtime, ensuring proper elimination as part of a bedtime routine, and waking the child prior to their typical elimination time and directing bathroom usage are all effective strategies to mitigate the occurrence of bedwetting. Another effective strategy is the use of enuresis alarms. Bedwetting alarms are available in a variety of forms, like mattress pads and specialized underwear [24]. These alarms become activated when urine makes contact with a detector, at which point a strong, typically acoustic, stimulus is activated [24]. The child awakens with the stimulus and becomes aware of their voiding behavior. With time, the child associates the urge to eliminate with sleep arousal, thus diminishing the frequency of nocturnal bedwetting. The efficacy of bedwetting alarms is robustly empirically supported, with some research demonstrating as many as 80% of children overcoming their nighttime enuresis [24, 26]. For best results, parents should be advised to integrate behavioral strategies with bedwetting alarms [26].

Adolescence

Sleep Disturbances and Disorders

Adolescence is characterized by a developmental period where the brain undergoes substantial changes to support cognition, learning, and emotion [27]. These changes aid the transformation to a more mature brain state through strengthening of connections amongst various brain regions [27]. To the detriment of the developing brain, these changes are paralleled by increases in sleep deprivation. Impacts of sleep deprivation include diminished cognition, memory, and academic performance, as well as increased risk-taking behaviors, self-harm, depressed mood, and suicidal ideation [27, 28]. Recent studies suggest that sleeping less than 8 h a night may be associated with an almost threefold increase in suicide attempts, and more significant sleep deficits (less than 4 h a night) are associated with severe forms of suicidality where an adolescent would require treatment following an attempt [28]. Given the alarming nature of these statistics, understanding the factors that contribute to sleep deprivation in adolescents becomes of vital importance.

As previously mentioned, as a child enters adolescence their sleep requirements range from 8 to 10 h per night [8]. Despite an evolving understanding of the vital role that sleep plays in adolescent development, 62–72% of students report an average of less than 8 h of sleep on school nights [29]. Many factors contribute to sleep deprivation in this age group, particularly sleep disorders which frequently emerge during adolescence. The most common sleep disorders experienced by adolescents are delayed sleep-phase disorder (DSPD), insomnia disorder, obstructive sleep-disordered breathing such as obstructive sleep apnea and snoring, and restless leg syndrome [30]. These disorders are outlined in the DSM-V-TR.

It is important to mention the relationship between psychiatric disorders and sleep disturbances. Many psychiatric disorders such as attention-deficit/hyperactivity disorder (ADHD), mood and anxiety disorders, and obsessive-compulsive disorder are comorbid with sleep disorders. Just as patients with psychiatric disorders are predisposed to sleep disturbances, patients with sleep disorders are predisposed to psychiatric disturbances. A study by Ivanenko et al. investigated the relationship of sleep complaints and psychiatric symptoms in 174 children and adolescents. In children with psychiatric disorders, they had a significantly higher frequency of sleep problems compared to non-psychiatric controls, with 61.5% experiencing delayed sleep onset, 66.7% experiencing daytime sleepiness, and 67.8% experiencing restless sleep, among other symptoms. Additionally, they found that complaints of sleep duration and sleep latency were strongly correlated with psychiatric symptoms such as aggression, hyperactivity, and depression, and snoring and witnessed apneas were significantly correlated with aggression, atypicality, hyperactivity, depression, and somatization. What this study conveys is the significant overlap of sleep complaints with psychiatric disorders and it is important to keep this in mind when addressing sleep disorders in children and adolescents [31].

Circadian Rhythm Sleep-Wake Disorders; Delayed Sleep-Phase Type (DSPD)

Adolescents have a natural biological shift towards a schedule that coincides with pubertal development, influenced by both a slower homeostatic drive to sleep and a delay in melatonin secretion [29]. This results in later sleep onset times that then correspond to later sleep offset times, i.e., going to bed later and waking up later. Most adolescents are able to adapt to sleep and wake times outside of their preferred schedules, but individuals with DSPD struggle to adapt [32]. DSPD is the most common circadian rhythm disorder with some sources citing a prevalence as high as 16% amongst adolescents with females impacted greater than males [30, 33]. The International Classification of Sleep Disorders (ICSD) third edition defines DSPD as a "significant delay in the phase of a major sleep episode (as evidenced by inability to fall asleep and difficulty awakening at a desired or required clock time)" that is present for at least 3 months, is not better explained by another disorder, and causes a functional impairment [29, 33]. An important external contributor to DSPD is school start times. Approximately 43% of public high schools in the United States have school start times before 8:00 am, much earlier than the preferred wake time of adolescents [34]. As such, early school start times contribute to chronic sleep loss and its consequences. A 2015 systematic review examined the effects of delaying school start times in adolescent sleep, health, and academic performance. Delays in school start time ranged from 25 to 60 min with a corresponding increase in their total sleep time from 25 to 77 min [35]. Additionally, this review also found that delays in school start times were associated with improved self-reported daytime sleepiness, and significant declines in student tardiness and presenteeism (struggling to stay awake in class) [35]. This review supports the AAP guideline that middle and high schools should delay start times to 8:30 am or later [34].

The use of electronic devices and caffeine intake work similarly in delaying sleep times in adolescents in that they are both stimulating. Electronic devices such as tablets, phones, computers, TVs, and video games are commonly used in bedrooms, but their association with sleep time can negatively affect an adolescent's ability to fall asleep at an appropriate time. A population study with approximately 10,000 adolescents (mean age 17 years old) found that almost all reported using at least one electronic device in the last hour before bedtime [36]. There was a positive association between electronic device usage and increased sleep-onset latency and sleep deficiency, and an inverse dose-response relationship between sleep duration and media use [36], highlighting the detrimental effects that electronic devices have on adolescent sleep. Furthermore, several characteristics of electronic media use facilitate interruptions in sleep patterns via stimulation from incoming messages and calls, melatonin suppression from the bright screen light, and increases in psychophysiological arousal [37]. Similarly, late afternoon or evening consumption of caffeinated beverages contributes to delays in sleep onset, decreases in sleep duration, and increased morning sleepiness [37].

Insomnia Disorder

Insomnia is the most common sleep disorder in childhood with a prevalence of 20–30% [38]. It is defined as "a repeated difficulty with sleep initiation, duration, consolidation, or quality that occurs despite age-appropriate time and opportunity for sleep and results in daytime functional impairment for the child and/or family" [30]. The disturbance has to be present at least three times per week and for at least 3 months [23]. There are two types of insomnia most commonly experienced by children: behavioral and psychophysiologic insomnia, with the latter being more prevalent with adolescents [30]. This type is typically multifactorial and influenced by genetics, psychiatric comorbidities, stress, poor sleep hygiene, caffeine, and more [38]. It is characterized by an exaggerated preoccupation with sleep, including falling asleep and the consequences of not sleeping enough [38]. The development of insomnia involves the complex interplay between genetics, biology, environment, and social pressures [37]. Risk factors for developing insomnia include female sex and puberty, school stress, use of electronic devices, and high caffeine intake [37].

Puberty likely affects the development of insomnia in the same way that it affects other human conditions–via hormones. The exact role that hormonal changes play in the development of insomnia has not yet been fully elucidated; however recent studies have shown that self-reports of insomnia symptoms in adolescents increases significantly as they go through the stages of puberty with females being affected to a higher degree than males [37]. The higher prevalence of insomnia in females could be related to the higher prevalence of depression in females, higher stress levels, and greater stress reactivity [37].

Adolescents endure enormous pressure from the academic sphere. They have to balance academic performance, extracurricular activities, college applications, social groups, and work while trying to satisfy expectations from their parents, teachers, and peers. The weight of these expectations leads to significant stress levels. In a 2014 survey from the American Psychological Association, 27% of teens reported experiencing high levels of stress with school being the most common source of insomnia [37]. A 12-month prospective study examined chronic insomnia and associated factors and found that school related stress in 11–17 year old's was a significant independent predictor of insomnia [37, 39].

Obstructive Sleep-Disordered Breathing: Snoring and Obstructive Sleep Apnea

Primary snoring and obstructive sleep apnea syndrome (OSAS) are part of a larger spectrum of obstructive sleep-disordered breathing disorders. Other diseases on this spectrum include upper airway resistance syndrome and obesity hypoventilation syndrome [30]. Primary snoring, also known as habitual snoring, has a reported prevalence of 10–15% with some studies citing a prevalence as high as 35% and is defined as snoring more than 3 times per week and is not associated with pauses in breathing (apneic episodes) [30]. While primary snoring has previously been considered a benign condition, growing evidence suggests that primary snoring may be associated with increased risk of developing neurocognitive and behavioral problems similar to those experienced by children with OSAS.

The prevalence of OSAS is estimated to be 2–3.5% of children and affects children in a biphasic pattern with the first peak occurring from 2 to 8 years of age [30]. This first peak is associated with enlarged adenoids and/or tonsils [40]. The second peak occurs during adolescence as a result of maturation of an adult body habitus and craniofacial structure, and the growing prevalence of adolescent obesity [40]. Snoring is the most common symptom reported with OSAS with other symptoms such as apneic episodes, gasping, snorting, restless sleep, frequent awakenings, sleeping with the neck hyperextended, and daytime behavioral difficulties [40]. The gold standard for diagnosing OSAS is overnight polysomnography (PSG) [41] as it is able to characterize disease severity and establishes a baseline for postoperative comparison for children who undergo adenotonsillectomy [40]. Identifying this disorder in adolescents is important due to its significant consequences.

A population-based study in Denmark evaluated the long-term health and socioeconomic outcome of sleep apnea in children and adolescents. They found that patients with OSA had a higher mortality rate, lower educational level, lower income, and high healthcare costs compared to controls [42]. A separate study conducting a 20-year follow-up of children with OSAS found that patients with severe OSAS had significantly higher adulthood BMI and cardiovascular complications [43]. Childhood OSAS is also a strong risk factor for neurobehavioral problems such as impaired attention, hyperactivity, learning disorders, and depression, which may correlate to the lower educational level and lower income in this population. These complications and more highlight the importance of prompt diagnosis of OSAS in childhood [43].

Restless Leg Syndrome

Restless leg syndrome (RLS) is a common neurological disorder experienced by children and adolescents. It has an estimated prevalence of 2–4% [44]. Family history is an important influencer of RLS, and approximately 40–92% of children with RLS have a family member who is affected, so care should be taken when gathering patient histories [44]. The diagnostic criteria of RLS are [1] the urge to move the legs, usually accompanied or caused by uncomfortable and unpleasant sensations in the legs, [2] that begins during periods of rest or inactivity, [3] that are worse in the evening compared to the day or occur exclusively at night, and [4] that improves with movement (walking, stretching) [45]. However mild the disorder may seem, though, the impact it has on adolescent sleep can be significant. In a study examining RLS and quality of life in adolescents, they reported that 67% of participants had trouble falling asleep, and that participants with RLS symptoms were more likely to have excessive daytime sleepiness [46]. Furthermore, the study found that adolescents had a lower health-related quality of life [46], highlighting the fact that sleep plays a vital role in individual wellbeing.

Interventions for Adolescents with Sleep Disorders

As adolescents become more independent, so does their involvement in the success of interventions for sleep disturbances/disorders, often needing the teenager to be motivated to make changes [32]. However, as with infants and children, parents continue to be influential in an adolescents environment and are therefore important in the treatment of these disorders [47]. As referenced above, there are many negative immediate and future consequences that are a result of poor sleep, especially among the adolescent population, suggesting that providing intervention as early as possible is a public health priority [47, 48]. Many of the sleep issues described above require several levels of intervention including taking medication, using medical devices, and psychological therapies. For the purposes of this chapter, we will discuss a few common psychological interventions that studies have determined are successful in treating these concerns.

Sleep Hygiene

Poor sleep hygiene is often the cause of poor sleep [47]. This level of intervention requires both behavioral and environmental change to occur [32, 33]. Improving sleep hygiene can be one level of intervention to help with DSPD, restless leg syndrome, and insomnia [32, 33, 38]. There are a number of models, programs, and interventions that have been developed to address sleep hygiene. One tool developed that resulted in improvements in sleep is the Sleep Smart Program [49]. There is evidence that three factors can be targeted in order to improve sleep: avoid going to bed hungry or thirsty; avoid activities that increase anxiety and stress; and make the environment restful [47, 50]. The Sleep Smart Program begins by helping an adolescent identify and articulate what sleep is and why it is important [49]. Next, it educates the adolescent about what healthy sleep habits are. This leads to the adolescent creating their own sleep hygiene schedule [49]. Some examples included in a schedule are establishing a specific bedtime and wake time, creating a bedtime routine, creating a comfortable/restful environment, ensuring that the use of technology is limited prior to bedtime, being cognizant to avoid caffeine and high intense physical activity, and avoiding exposure to things that could be emotionally upsetting [49]. It is important to implement a method for reflection once a schedule has been established so that the adolescent may track their improvements and identify areas for growth. Examples of reflection tools include journals, graph systems, or another type of documenting system, and should be agreed upon by both the provider and the adolescent. Additionally, including parents in the creation of this intervention is important for its success as they may help with motivating and encouraging their child.

Cognitive Behavioral Therapy-Insomnia (CBT-I)

Studies have indicated that Cognitive Behavior Therapy for Insomnia (CBT-I) is an effective intervention for the treatment of insomnia and obstructive sleep apnea in adolescents [51–55]. CBT-I is the first line of treatment for insomnia as it has better long-term effects and less adverse reactions then sleep medication [56]. Additionally, it can help improve other comorbid psychological factors that may co-occur with sleep related issues while increasing one's quality of life [56]. It is notable to consider that when this form of treatment is provided, that the intervention caters to the adolescent as their needs will likely differ from adults [54].

CBT-I encompasses psychoeducation/sleep hygiene, relaxation training, stimulus control therapy, sleep restriction, and cognitive therapy [53]. Psychoeducation focuses on ways to improve sleep hygiene, similar to what is discussed in the above section designated to sleep hygiene. Relaxation training teaches the patient methods of decreasing intrusive thoughts and promoting relaxation of the body (e.g., progressive muscle relaxation techniques) [53]. Sleep restriction therapy first helps to train the patient to stay in bed only when they are asleep. Then, the sleep schedule is adjusted each week by either increasing or decreasing total time in bed in 15–30 min intervals until the desired time is reached [53]. Stimulus control therapy is used to help the patient identify that the bed/bedroom is only for sleep, while also creating a sleep-wake schedule [53]. Cognitive therapy teaches the patient ways to identify, challenge and change misconceptions surrounding sleep [53].

Fitting into the concept of IBH, there is evidence from several studies that brief or other forms of CBT-I are also effective [53]. CBT-I is typically completed within 4–8 sessions and can be delivered through a combination of face to face and phone and/or telehealth platforms [53]. Further, utilizing internet-based programs and group therapy are also effective ways to utilize CBT-I [53]. IBH can provide follow-up and tracking data that can drive changes to the intervention plan that may be necessary, all while keeping the physician informed of any challenges and successes that the patient may experience.

Motivational Interviewing

As reported earlier, adolescence is a time for gaining autonomy. Although an important transition, it can also lead to difficulties in their buy-in to change. Oftentimes adolescents will perceive well-intentioned psychoeducation as being lectured to, resulting in an increase in therapeutic resistance [57]. A way to help promote change is by using motivational interviewing (MI). The purpose of this technique is to help the teen become motivated to change by helping them become less ambivalent about the issue while simultaneously taking into account their goals, values and beliefs [57].

There are three main components of MI: collaboration, evocation, and autonomy [57]. Collaboration emphasizes mutual trust and teamwork between the patient and the clinician, such that the clinician understands that the patient is the expert in their lived experiences while the patient understands that the clinician is the expert in behavior [57]. Evocation is a technique where the clinician uses open ended questions to help the adolescent challenge any ambivalence they may feel about changing and helps them resolve any conflicts they may have surrounding their values, goals, beliefs, and behaviors that may prevent them from making a change [57]. Lastly, the clinician helps the adolescent use their autonomy to decide whether they will or will not make any changes to improve sleep [57].

There are four principles that a clinician must have and do in order for MI to be successful. First, they must express empathy by reflecting the adolescents perspective and refraining from giving advice [57]. Second, the clinician helps identify discrepancies between an adolescents current behavior and their expressed goals. Third, the clinician must be non-confrontational in the face of any resistance that the adolescent may display [57]. Lastly, the clinician must support the client's developing self-efficacy, which occurs when the adolescent realizes there is a problem, by being optimistic and helping them formulate several ways to achieve their goal [57].

MI is a treatment that is effective for helping adolescents transition into a state of change. It is an intervention that can easily be facilitated by IBH and fits into the realm of brief, solution focused interventions. This intervention can be used not only to elicit change from adolescents, but decrease any resistance that may occur in treatment of infants/pre and school aged children, that require the caregiver to implement.

Conclusion

In reviewing this chapter, it was noted that there is little information on exactly how to integrate behavioral health specialists into a sleep subspecialty environment; however, there is literature on how this role has been implemented into a primary care setting. IBH is done in 0–6 sessions with solution focused interventions to help improve the presented concerns. Many of the above mentioned interventions can easily be implemented through this timeline.

Sleep concerns that persist beyond this time frame may require a referral to a psychologist for longer term interventions. Furthermore, when sleep disturbances are especially severe, patients will likely require more structured and clinical interventions than are typically provided by a medical practitioner [11]. Children and adolescents with comorbid psychological concerns, like anxiety or depression, may also benefit from a referral to a psychologist [11]. Finally, the medical practitioner should consider the intensity of the underlying psychological factors when evaluating the patient's sleep disturbance; if the underlying pathology is deemed atypical (e.g., a child's bedtime fear is actually a phobia), a referral to a psychologist should be made [22].

It is also important to consider with any intervention that there may be additional factors that influence implementation. For example, patients that have a co-occurring diagnosis of a developmental disorder (i.e., autism or intellectual disability disorder) may need these interventions tailored to account for how these diagnoses may impact functioning. In addition, more research is needed to examine the efficacy of behavioral interventions for adolescents, children with neurodevelopmental disorders, children with mood disorders, and children with comorbid and chronic illness [14].

References

1. Goetting MG. Role of psychologists in pediatric sleep medicine. Pediatr Clin North Am. W.B. Saunders. 2022;69:989–1002.
2. Meltzer LJP, Mindell JAP. Behavioral sleep disorders in children and adolescents. Sleep Med Clin. 2008;3:269.
3. Ramar K, Malhotra RK, Carden KA, Martin JL, Abbasi-Feinberg F, Aurora RN, et al. Sleep is essential to health: an American Academy of Sleep Medicine position statement. J Clin Sleep Med. 2021;17(10):2115–9.
4. Meltzer LJ, Williamson AA, Mindell JA. Pediatric sleep health: it matters, and so does how we define it. Sleep Med Rev. W.B. Saunders Ltd. 2021;57:101425.
5. Honaker SM, Saunders T. The sleep checkup: sleep screening, guidance, and management in pediatric primary care. Clin Pract Pediatr Psychol [Internet]. 2018;6(3):201–10. https://doi.org/10.1037/cpp0000227.
6. Stepanski EJ, Perlis ML. Behavioral sleep medicine. An emerging subspecialty in health psychology and sleep medicine. J Psychosom Res. 2000;49:343–7.
7. Alessandra G, Vincenza C, Alessandro C. Psychological interventions in behavioral sleep medicine: an overview for clinicians and psychologists. Ann Psychiatry Treat. 2022;6(1):033–48.
8. Jenco M. AAP endorses new recommendations on sleep times. 2016.
9. Tham EKH, Schneider N, Broekman BFP. Infant sleep and its relation with cognition and growth: a narrative review. Nat Sci Sleep. Dove Medical Press Ltd. 2017;9:135–49.
10. Ordway MR, Logan S, Sutton EH. Sleep deficiency in young children. Clin Chest Med. W.B. Saunders. 2022;43:229–37.
11. Lunsford-Avery JR, Bidopia T, Jackson L, Sloan JS. Behavioral treatment of insomnia and sleep disturbances in school-aged children and adolescents. Child Adolesc Psychiatric Clin North Am. W.B. Saunders. 2021;30:101–16.
12. Tarokh L, Saletin JM, Carskadon MA. Sleep in adolescence: physiology, cognition and mental health. Neurosci Biobehav Rev. Elsevier Ltd. 2016;70:182–8.
13. Bartel KA, Gradisar M, Williamson P. Protective and risk factors for adolescent sleep: a meta-analytic review. Sleep Med Rev. W.B. Saunders Ltd. 2015;21:72–85.
14. Meltzer LJ, Mindell JA. Systematic review and meta-analysis of behavioral interventions for pediatric insomnia. J Pediatr Psychol. Oxford University Press. 2014;39:932–48.
15. Asarnow JR, Rozenman M, Wiblin J, Zeltzer L. Integrated medical-behavioral care compared with usual primary care for child and adolescent behavioral health: a metaanalysis. JAMA Pediatr. 2015;169(10):929–37.
16. Owens J, Mohan M. Behavioral interventions for parasomnias. Curr Sleep Med Rep. Springer. 2016;2:81–6.
17. France KG, Blampied NM, Henderson JMT. Infant sleep disturbance. Curr Paediatr [Internet]. 2003;13(3):241–6. https://doi.org/10.1016/S0957-5839(03)00004-6.

18. Singh BSK, Danckaerts M, Van den Bergh BRH. Helping families of infants with persistent crying and sleep problems in a day-clinic. Front Psychiatry. 2021;12:12.
19. Kang EK, Kim SS. Behavioral insomnia in infants and young children. Clin Exp Pediatr. Korean Pediatric Society. 2021;64:111–6.
20. Hysing M, Harvey AG, Torgersen L, Ystrom E, Reichborn-Kjennerud T, Sivertsen B. Trajectories and predictors of nocturnal awakenings and sleep duration in infants. J Dev Behav Pediatr [Internet]. 2014;35:309–16. Available from: www.jdbp.org
21. Owens JL, France KG, Wiggs L. SLEEP MEDICINE reviews behavioural and cognitive-behavioural interventions for sleep disorders in infants and children: a review. Sleep Med Rev. 1999;3:281.
22. Lewis KM, Amatya K, Coffman MF, Ollendick TH. Treating nighttime fears in young children with bibliotherapy: evaluating anxiety symptoms and monitoring behavior change. J Anxiety Disord. 2015;30:103–12.
23. American Psychiatric Association. Diagnostic and statistical manual of mental disorders. American Psychiatric Association Publishing; 2022.
24. Nevéus T. Nocturnal enuresis-theoretic background and practical guidelines. Pediatr Nephrol. 2011;26:1207–14.
25. Abrams Z. Helping children get a good night's sleep. Monit Psychol. 2020;51(5):36.
26. Glazener CM, Evans JH, Peto RE. Alarm interventions for nocturnal enuresis in children. Cochrane Database Syst Rev. 2005.
27. Galván A. The need for sleep in the adolescent brain. Trend Cognit Sci. Elsevier Ltd. 2020;24:79–89.
28. Owens J, Au R, Carskadon M, Millman R, Wolfson A, Braverman PK, et al. Insufficient sleep in adolescents and young adults: an update on causes and consequences. Pediatrics. 2014;134(3):e921–32.
29. Kansagra S. Sleep disorders in adolescents. Pediatrics. 2020;145:2.
30. Trosman I, Ivanenko A. Classification and epidemiology of sleep disorders in children and adolescents. Child Adolesc Psychiatric Clin North Am. W.B. Saunders. 2021;30:47–64.
31. Ivanenko A, McLaughlin Crabtree V, O'Brien, Louise, Gozal D. Sleep complaints and psychiatric symptoms in children evaluated at a pediatric mental health clinic. J Clin Sleep Med [Internet]. 2006;2:42. https://doi.org/10.5664/jcsm.26434.
32. Feder MA, Baroni A. Just let me sleep in: identifying and treating delayed sleep phase disorder in adolescents. Psychiatric Clin North Am. W.B. Saunders. 2024;47:163–78.
33. Narala B, Ahsan M, Ednick M, Kier C. Delayed sleep wake phase disorder in adolescents: an updated review. Curr Opin Pediatr. Lippincott Williams and Wilkins. 2024;36:124–32.
34. Au R, Carskadon M, Millman R, Wolfson A, Braverman PK, Adelman WP, et al. School start times for adolescents. Pediatrics. 2014;134(3):642–9.
35. Minges KE, Redeker NS. Delayed school start times and adolescent sleep: a systematic review of the experimental evidence. Sleep Med Rev. W.B. Saunders Ltd. 2016;28:86–95.
36. Hysing M, Pallesen S, Stormark KM, Jakobsen R, Lundervold AJ, Sivertsen B. Sleep and use of electronic devices in adolescence: results from a large population-based study. BMJ Open. 2015;5(1):e006748.
37. de Zambotti M, Goldstone A, Colrain IM, Baker FC. Insomnia disorder in adolescence: diagnosis, impact, and treatment. Sleep Med Rev. W.B. Saunders Ltd. 2018;39:12–24.
38. Nunes ML, Bruni O. Insomnia in childhood and adolescence: clinical aspects, diagnosis, and therapeutic approach. Jornal de Pediatria. Elsevier Editora Ltda. 2015;91:S26–35.
39. Roberts RE, Roberts CR, Duong HT. Chronic insomnia and its negative consequences for health and functioning of adolescents: a 12-month prospective study. J Adolesc Health. 2008;42(3):294–302.
40. Gileles-Hillel A, Bhattacharjee R, Gorelik M, Narang I. Advances in sleep-disordered breathing in children. Clin Chest Med. W.B. Saunders. 2024;45:651–62.
41. Choi JH, Lee B, Lee JY, Kim HJ. Validating the Watch-PAT for diagnosing obstructive sleep apnea in adolescents. J Clin Sleep Med. 2018;14(10):1741–7.

42. Jennum P, Rejkjær-Knudsen M, Ibsen R, Kiær EK, von Buchwald C, Kjellberg J. Long-term health and socioeconomic outcome of obstructive sleep apnea in children and adolescents. Sleep Med. 2020;75:441–7.
43. Nosetti L, Zaffanello M, Katz ES, Vitali M, Agosti M, Ferrante G, et al. Twenty-year follow-up of children with obstructive sleep apnea. J Clin Sleep Med. 2022;18(6):1573–81.
44. DelRosso LM, Mogavero MP, Baroni A, Bruni O, Ferri R. Restless legs syndrome in children and adolescents. Child Adolesc Psychiatr Clin North Am. W.B. Saunders. 2021;30:143–57.
45. Trenkwalder C, Paulus W. Restless legs syndrome: pathophysiology, clinical presentation and management. Nat Rev Neurol. 2010;6:337–46.
46. Silva GE, Goodwin JL, Vana KD, Vasquez MM, Wilcox PG, Quan SF. Restless legs syndrome, sleep, and quality of life among adolescents and young adults. J Clin Sleep Med. 2014;10(7):779–86.
47. Lin CY, Strong C, Scott AJ, Broström A, Pakpour AH, Webb TL. A cluster randomized controlled trial of a theory-based sleep hygiene intervention for adolescents. Sleep. 2018;41(11):1.
48. Garbers S, Ancheta AJ, Gold MA, Maier M, Bruzzese JM. Sleeping healthy, living healthy: using iterative, participatory processes to develop and adapt an integrated sleep hygiene/mind-body integrative health intervention for urban adolescents. Health Promot Pract. 2023;25:865.
49. Wolfson AR, Harkins E, Johnson M, Marco C. Effects of the Young Adolescent Sleep Smart Program on sleep hygiene practices, sleep health efficacy, and behavioral well-being. Sleep Health. 2015;1(3):197–204.
50. Kor K, Mullan BA. Sleep hygiene behaviours: an application of the theory of planned behaviour and the investigation of perceived autonomy support, past behaviour and response inhibition. Psychol Health. 2011;26(9):1208–24.
51. Dewald-Kaufmann J, de Bruin E, Michael G. Cognitive Behavioral Therapy for Insomnia (CBT-i) in school-aged children and adolescents. Sleep Med Clin. W.B. Saunders. 2019;14:155–65.
52. Koontz KL, Slifer KJ, Cataldo MD, Marcus CL, Koontz K, Health HB. Introduction Obstructive Sleep Apnea (OSA) is a significant cause of morbidity in children with complications, including failure to thrive, developmental delay, and Cor Pulmonale. 1 Improving Pediatric Compliance with Positive Airway Pressure Therapy: the Impact of Behavioral Intervention [Internet]. Vol. 26, Improving Pediatric Compliance with PAP-Koontz et al SLEEP. 2003. Available from: https://academic.oup.com/sleep/article/26/8/1010/2707895
53. Riemann D, Baglioni C, Bassetti C, Bjorvatn B, Dolenc Groselj L, Ellis JG, et al. European guideline for the diagnosis and treatment of insomnia. J Sleep Res. 2017;26(6):675–700.
54. de Bruin EJ, Bögels SM, Oort FJ, Meijer AM. Efficacy of cognitive behavioral therapy for insomnia in adolescents: a randomized controlled trial with internet therapy, group therapy and a waiting list condition. Sleep. 2015;38(12):1913–26.
55. Ma ZR, Shi LJ, Deng MH. Efficacy of cognitive behavioral therapy in children and adolescents with insomnia: a systematic review and meta-analysis. Braz J Med Biol Res. 2018;51(6):e7070.
56. Alimoradi Z, Jafari E, Broström A, Ohayon MM, Lin CY, Griffiths MD, et al. Effects of cognitive behavioral therapy for insomnia (CBT-I) on quality of life: a systematic review and meta-analysis. Sleep Med Rev. 2022;64:101646.
57. Gold MA, Dahl RE. Using motivational interviewing to facilitate healthier sleep-related behaviors in adolescents. In: Behavioral treatments for sleep disorders. Elsevier Inc.; 2011. p. 367–81.

Index

R. W. Apple et al. (eds.), *Using Integrated Behavioral Health in Pediatric Practice*, https://doi.org/10.1007/978-3-031-85784-3

MIX
Papier aus verantwortungsvollen Quellen
Paper from responsible sources
FSC® C105338

If you have any concerns about our products,
you can contact us on
ProductSafety@springernature.com

In case Publisher is established outside the EU,
the EU authorized representative is:
Springer Nature Customer Service Center GmbH
Europaplatz 3, 69115 Heidelberg, Germany

Printed by Libri Plureos GmbH
in Hamburg, Germany